D1621139

Coping with
Methuselah

Coping with Methuselah

The Impact of Molecular Biology on Medicine and Society

Henry J. Aaron
William B. Schwartz

Editors

BROOKINGS INSTITUTION PRESS
Washington, D.C.

Library of Congress Cataloging-in-Publication data

Coping with Methuselah : the impact of molecular biology on medicine and
society / Henry J. Aaron, William B. Schwartz, editors.
      p.   cm.
Includes bibliographical references and index.
  ISBN 0-8157-0040-7 (cloth : alk. paper)
  ISBN 0-8157-0039-3 (paper : alk. paper)
  1. Longevity—Social aspects. 2. Life expectancy—Social aspects. 3.
Old age—Social aspects. 4. Medical technology—Social aspects. I.
Aaron, Henry J. II. Schwartz, William B., 1922–

  HQ1061.C654 2003
  304.6'45—dc22   2003019908

9 8 7 6 5 4 3 2 1

The paper used in this publication meets minimum requirements of the
American National Standard for Information Sciences—Permanence of Paper for
Printed Library Materials: ANSI Z39.48-1992.

Typeset in Adobe Garamond

Composition by Circle Graphics
Columbia, Maryland

Printed by R. R. Donnelley
Harrisonburg, Virginia

Contents

Foreword

Here's a Brookings book that truly relates to all of us. It's natural, indeed healthy, to be in favor of long lives. On birthdays, we wish one another many more years. But along with those hopes for ourselves, our loved ones, and our friends as individuals, we need, as a society, hard-headed thinking about the implications of collective longevity for our economy and the quality of the services provided by our government, our other public institutions, our insurance, pharmaceutical, and health care industries. That's exactly what *Coping with Methuselah* provides: research, analysis, and recommendations about a hitherto largely underexamined area of public policy.

From the time of the ancient Greeks, the prospect of eternal life has been viewed as a divine attribute denied to humans. Methuselah made it into the Book of Genesis largely because he was, at 969 years, rather an exception to the three-score-and-ten span that was considered about the maximum in those days. In recent decades, the examination of the charms and pitfalls of perpetual life was the province of authors of science fiction and undergraduate participants in philosophy seminars. Recent developments in molecular medicine have moved this topic into prestigious journals of science. What was once a fantasy has become a prospect.

What has been missing, however, is much serious consideration of the questions like the following: Is there a reasonable prospect that life expectancy, now in the high seventies or low eighties in the most advanced nations, will reach 100 during the first half of the twenty-first century? Yes, say the authors of the first chapter. If that should happen, what will be the impacts on the demography of the United States and on the health and pension programs that businesses and governments now sponsor for American workers? Are American workers likely to extend their working lives or to devote substantially all of their extended lives to retirement leisure? Will a dearth or a glut of saving ensue as workers prepare for their retirement years? How will the changes in financial flows affect U.S. foreign trade? While a definitive answer to none of these questions is now possible, it is time to begin to think about them and to identify likely pressure points. In short, it is time to take seriously the prospect that people will routinely live to ages of which human beings have heretofore been able only to dream.

The two editors of this book—my Brookings colleague Henry Aaron and University of Southern California physician William B. Schwartz, both noted experts on national health policy—have put their heads together to tackle challenging issues like this one before. About twenty years ago, they examined the controversial issue of rationing health care in a major book, *The Painful Prescription,* one of the most influential books Brookings has published and one of the first to articulate the difficult choices and sacrifices Americans would need to make to control health care costs.

In the present case, with the generous support of the Robert Wood Johnson Foundation, they gathered together a distinguished group of economists, physicians, attorneys, and journalists, first for a planning meeting at Stanford University in August 2001, and then for a follow-up conference at which draft papers were presented and discussed. This is the result of their efforts, and it merits careful attention—and given the subject, I suspect it will get it.

STROBE TALBOTT
President

November 2003
Washington, D.C.

Acknowledgments

T HE CHAPTERS IN this volume emerged from a planning conference held at Stanford University in August 2001 and were presented at a conference held at the Brookings Institution in April 2002. In addition to the authors and discussants, whose contributions appear in this volume, other attendees included Jodi Allen, *U.S. News and World Report;* Jordan Cohen, American Association of Medical Colleges; David Colby, Robert Wood Johnson Foundation; Samuel Hellman, University of Chicago; Janet Miller, Massachusetts General Hospital and Harvard University; Alicia Munnell, Boston College; John Palmer, Maxwell School at Syracuse University; Robert Reischauer, Urban Institute; Stanford Ross, Arnold and Porter law firm; David Schlessinger, National Institutes of Health; and Charles Schultze, Brookings Institution.

Support for the conferences, authors, and publication comes from the Robert Wood Johnson Foundation. At Brookings, Kathleen Elliot Yinug was instrumental in organizing the meeting; Emily Y. Tang and Ben Harris provided research assistance; Diane Hammond edited the papers emanating from that meeting and appearing here. Gloria Paniagua and Emilia Richichi checked the papers for factual accuracy, while Inge Lockwood proofread the typeset pages and Julia Petrakis provided an index.

Coping with
Methuselah

HENRY J. AARON
WILLIAM B. SCHWARTZ

Introduction

THE CAPACITY TO manipulate the genetic templates that shape all living beings was long the plaything of science fiction. That humans could mold the biological determinants of their own character was eerie and unreal. But then, in the final decades of the twentieth century, intellectual alchemy transmuted genetic tinkering from dream into reality. In 1953 two young scientists identified the double helix, composed of four nucleotides, containing the code of all life. In so doing they opened the first chapter in the saga of molecular biology. In 2001 two scientific teams, competing to read the components of the human genome, wrote another chapter. But these events are the barest beginnings of the gradually emerging understanding of the forces that shape humans, that cause them to sicken, and that eventually cause them to die.

Commentators still remain free to imagine futures as they will, much as observers of the first steps of industrialization saw quite different worlds emerging from the new machines. Some looked at machines and saw dehumanization and the demise of skills. Others looked and saw abundance and leisure. What none could fully apprehend was that the vision of people who lived with the new technology would be fundamentally and irreversibly different from that of people who only imagined what the future might hold.

1

Those alive after the advent of electricity, mass production, modern telecommunications, air travel, and computer science have been shaped by those technologies in ways that those born in earlier times could not imagine. Not even the cleverest person in 1800 could fathom the effects of these future technologies, not least because they could not even imagine what all of those technologies would be. Nor, perforce, could they see the future through eyes of those who would be alive to experience the as-yet-undiscovered technologies.

The molecular biology century, as the twenty-first century may well be called, will almost certainly change how humans see the world and themselves. Even if an eighteenth-century artisan who had cried jeremiads against the dehumanization of machine production was somehow teleported into the present and said, See, I told you so, we would not take such testimony seriously. Such criticism would be pointless—quaint and irrelevant commentary from inhabitants of a world now as imaginary to us as ours was to them. For these reasons, those who pass moral judgment on the new world to which revolutionary advances in molecular biology will give birth are engaging in a kind of romantic irrelevance—attempting to apply early-twenty-first-century standards to a future world as different from our own as ours is from the artisanal life of the eighteenth century.

We present the following essays in that spirit. We are persuaded that molecular biology will alter human lives and consciousness at least as profoundly as did the industrial revolution, modern telecommunications, mechanized travel, and the information revolution. Side by side with these developments came improvements in public health, nutrition, and medical treatment. Birth rates plummeted. Life expectancies soared. And the content of lives changed.

No one can predict the precise extent or timing of advances in molecular biology. No one can foresee when particular diseases will be prevented or cured. No one can know exactly when or even if human aging will be slowed or stopped. No one yet knows for sure whether the genetic makeup of humans limits life span or, if it does, what those limits might be. Some families include more nonagenerians and centenarians than any roll of nature's dice can explain. This fact suggests that genetic inheritance powerfully influences longevity. Average human life spans longer than any nation's current average may be achievable without genetic tinkering. Even if life span now has limits, molecular biology may reveal that these limits are variables, not constants, and provide ways to slow aging and to prevent or cure illnesses that cause physical decline and death.

The Frontiers of Molecular Medicine

John T. Potts and William B. Schwartz open this volume by describing the channels through which such advances could occur. Humans have been trying to cure their own diseases for millennia. Potts and Schwartz make clear that scientific advance has revolutionized the assault on human illness. Current methods flow directly from the emergence of a detailed understanding of the functioning of human cells and an emerging understanding of the structure and function of human genes and their protein products.

Physicians have long understood, in some sense, the basis of successful medical treatments. Still, the underlying processes by which these interventions worked their magic remained hidden. The first antibiotics, for example, were more or less serendipitous discoveries. The death of bacteria led an astute observer to recognize the potential value of a mold as a source of penicillin for the treatment of infection. Later antibiotics resulted from systematic searches. But the fundamental reasons why antibiotics killed pathogens for decades remained as mysterious to the discoverers and to the physicians who used the drugs as they were to the patients whose lives they saved.

Safe correction of genetic defects through insertion of normal genes into the patient's DNA (dioxyribonucleic acid) seems to be an ever-retreating target. The more promising near-term approach is likely to be through identifying the pathologic proteins specified by an abnormal gene and synthesizing a drug that can offset its effects. Whether progress will be fast or slow cannot be forecast because this new field—structural genomics—must surmount major obstacles before it yields effective therapeutic agents. But expectations are high that intense research—by government-supported scientists and by drug companies with dollar signs dancing before their eyes—will lead to a wide range of breakthrough agents. Portents for the discovery of cures for major diseases within the first half of the twenty-first century are extremely encouraging. If each disease resulted from a single genetic defect, progress could be extremely rapid. Unfortunately, only a few illnesses are directly traceable to a single genetic flaw. Most illnesses result from multiple genetic mutations and the expression of a vast number of proteins. This painful reality guarantees that major resources over many decades will be required to produce the promised cornucopia of new drugs.

Potts and Schwartz provide a *tour d'horizon* of the multiple frontiers of biomedical advance. No brief chapter can encompass the enormous range of current biomedical research. Nonetheless, their chapter identifies a variety of fields in which progress is particularly encouraging. For example, molecular biology has created a whole new field of therapy: regenerative medicine. Skin, tissue, and whole organs may be grown in the laboratory and implanted in living humans to repair injuries and replace worn-out body components. Organs may soon be grown in animals that have been biologically modified so that human recipients will not reject the organs. Stem cells may be harvested and reimplanted to enable humans to regenerate their own organs—or so cutting-edge researchers believe.

Cancer presents the largest target and what may be the greatest challenges for molecular biology. Cancer results directly from the breakdown of genetic instructions for cell replication. The result is unlimited and uncontrolled cell growth. Understanding the multiple mechanisms by which genes instruct cells on when to divide and to self-destruct and the many ways error creeps into these instructions is the first objective. Techniques designed to check abnormal cell growth include antibodies and enzymes that inactivate the receptors that tell the cell to divide and factors to inhibit growth of the blood vessels that nourish the rapidly growing cancer tissues. Other interventions will facilitate the normal processes of cell death, which are suppressed in cancer cells, or will reverse mutations that block natural body defenses against cancers. In an interesting twist on the virus problem, viruses will be used to infect or poison cancer cells.

Molecular biology also carries hope of preventing or curing cardiovascular illness, the number-one killer disease in the United States. Some people have a genetic predisposition to high levels of the form of cholesterol associated with cardiovascular disease. Interventions to correct this defect or to block it from boosting cholesterol would reduce the likelihood of heart disease. Effective measures to encourage the growth of blood vessels could spare victims of coronary thrombosis from the damage to the heart that results from blocked coronary arteries. Recent work also indicates that inflammation of the coronary arteries may be responsible for as many as half of heart attacks.

Perhaps the greatest medical advance of the twentieth century is the development of antibiotics. Unfortunately, strains of bacteria have emerged that resist all known antibiotics. Now that the genomes of many pathogens have been identified and the genes responsible for the harmful effects have been brought into view, molecular biology represents the best hope of forestalling this threat. With that understanding, scientists will be able to design therapeutic agents that circumvent these bacterial defenses. Prospects are also improving for the development of agents that successfully combat viral infections, which with few exceptions have resisted treatment.

As the twenty-first century begins, the hit-or-miss search for new drugs and for other ways to cure or prevent many illnesses is ending. A new era is emerging in which scientists work from a fundamental understanding of cells, proteins, and genes to design interventions that reverse, block, or otherwise forestall illnesses. In the words of the Nobel prizewinner Alfred Gilman, scientists are now "able to complete [their] understanding of the wiring diagram of the signaling switchboard in each type of cell." With that knowledge in hand, they now—or soon will—have the means to design drugs or to directly change how cells operate to correct the genetic defects that each person inherits or acquires during life from mutations or other sources.

Molecular biology also provides weapons for combating a few illnesses that have become increasingly frequent as incomes have risen—obesity and senile dementia. Increasing incomes and decreasing activity are leading to a veritable epidemic of diabetes and other illnesses of the indolent overfed. An emerging understanding of cell metabolism and the brain chemistry that leads to overeating is helping scientists to find other ways to prevent or lessen the harmful consequences of excessive caloric intake.

While cancer has historically been the paradigmatic dread disease, senile dementia—Alzheimer's disease in particular—has become the new terror of those who can expect to live into old age. With improved understanding of the process by which this disease corrodes cognitive capacity and then destroys personality and physical functioning is coming the realistic prospect of interventions to prevent the disease or forestall its harmful consequences. Whether increased longevity will be a blessing or a curse, for the elderly themselves and for society, hinges in part on the success of this endeavor.

Our Uncertain Demographic Future

Even without accelerated medical advance, demographers project that longevity will increase and that the elderly will comprise a growing proportion of the U.S. population. Biomedical advance could intensify these trends. The reduction in mortality from heart disease by more than 50 percent since 1960 demonstrates the feasibility of such improvements.

Henry J. Aaron and Benjamin H. Harris explore the demographic implications of accelerated reductions in mortality rates and review various demographic models for human mortality. One such model suggests that reductions in mortality rates could average 2 percent a year, approximately the rate of decline in Japan during the 1970s and 1980s. According to another view, mammalian life span has a natural limit. After reproduction, it is argued, survival serves no useful evolutionary purpose, and early demise after reproduction may aid evolutionary success by reducing pressure on resources. The finding by the nineteenth-century scientist August Weismann that cells stop reproducing after a certain number of divisions seems consistent with this hypothesis.[1]

Even if a natural limit exists, however, the practical questions are whether that limit is near or much above current average life span and what can be done to modify those processes. Aaron and Harris conclude that the most helpful theory of the aging process is an analogy of humans to a machine that consists of many components, each essential for the machine's operation. Each component remains functional until too many of its constituent parts fail. Engineers have shown that machines fail over time in patterns that closely resemble human mortality rates. The machine model suggests that medical progress comes through interventions that prevent or postpone the failure of the constituent parts of each of the biological systems essential for life.

Rapid reductions in mortality rates quickly affect longevity but alter the population profile only with considerable delay. Social Security Administration projections, which assume no acceleration in reductions in mortality rates, posit that people born in 2030 will have a life expectancy at birth of just over 84 years; for those born in 2075, the average is 86 years. But if mortality rates decline 2 percent a year, babies born in 2030 could expect to live 104 years, and those born in 2075, more than 115 years. Even this rapid rate of improvement would not have much effect on the population distribution until the second half of the century. During the first half, the dominant event will be the aging and retirement of the baby-boom generation.

Whether reduced mortality increases or reduces disability depends on whether mortality is measured as years since birth or as years until death. If disability rates depend on years since birth, the number of disabled would skyrocket as the aged population rises. If it depends on years until death, disability would probably change little. The same holds for the cost and burden of supporting the elderly and the disabled. If delayed aging or public policy encourage later retirement, the ratio of retirees to active workers might increase only slightly. If current retirement age patterns persist, however, the cost of increased longevity would rise sharply as people spend ever more years outside of the labor force.

Work

If the proportion of each age group that works is unchanged, declining mortality cannot much affect the labor force. The reason is that few of the

1. See Gavrilov and Gavrilova (1991).

elderly work. Even if their numbers greatly increased, the impact on the labor force would be tiny. Only if people change the timing of retirement could increased longevity have large labor market effects. Gary Burtless poses the question of whether such changes are likely.

Economic theory by itself does not suggest that increased longevity will cause people to change their retirement plans—unless public policy is changed. If increased longevity does not affect wage rates, workers could rationally choose to allocate their increased life expectancy entirely to work, entirely to leisure, or partly to both. Each choice is consistent with the precepts of economic theory. Historically, longevity and incomes have risen and men have retired at progressively earlier ages. Increasing longevity could encourage later retirement if it changed the lifetime earnings profile. Because most workers earn less when old than when middle aged, the cost of retiring, measured by loss of potential lifetime consumption, declines as workers age. If increasing longevity keeps workers' productivity and earnings high until later ages, increased longevity would boost lifetime consumption possibilities. On the other hand, if the added years are ones of very low productivity, average lifetime consumption would necessarily fall.

Many private pension plans encourage retirement because annual benefits do not increase enough when workers defer retirement to ensure them the same total lifetime pension benefit they would receive if they retired earlier. Changes in pension policy that maintain the value of lifetime benefits if workers defer retirement would remove this disincentive to work.

Burtless finds little in economic theory or empirical evidence to suggest that sharply increased longevity will have a major direct effect on retirement behavior. But increased longevity would boost pension costs, which in turn would probably force changes in public policy to encourage workers to extend their working lives. Higher pension costs would necessitate sharply higher charges on workers to support public pensions, greatly increased contributions by workers or their employers to support private pensions, higher taxes to support public pensions, benefit cuts, or increases in the age at which pensions are first paid. All of these changes would likely cause workers to stay in the paid labor force longer than they now do.

Government Finance

Increased longevity is certain to have a large effect on government revenues and spending. It will increase revenues if it leads to extended working lives. A larger labor force would earn and produce more. The resulting increase in taxes could largely or fully offset increased spending to support an increased elderly population. But estimating the impact on revenue of an enlarged work force is subject to enormous error and uncertainty.

To sense the magnitude of effects flowing from increased longevity, one can consider the consequences of a 10 percent increase in average working lives, which would add about 7 percent to output if the added years of work were of unchanged quality—that is, if the education, experience, and other worker characteristics were unaffected. Such an increase in output would boost government revenue by $150 billion to $200 billion in 2004. While the actual increase could be considerably larger or smaller, it clearly would offset many of the added costs of a growing elderly population.

Increased longevity would also boost government spending. John B. Shoven provides estimates of this impact on the three largest domestic government programs serving the elderly: Social Security, Medicare, and Medicaid (programs that also, incidentally, serve the nonelderly). Outlays for all three programs are projected to grow rapidly as the baby-boom generation becomes eligible for benefits. The question that Shoven considers is whether a major reduction in mortality rates would significantly increase spending above these steeply rising trends.

Social Security costs, measured as a share of taxable earnings, are officially projected to nearly double between now and 2080. The payroll tax necessary to just cover outlays for Old-Age, Survivors, and Disability Insurance is projected to increase from just under 11 percent to just over 20 percent. This projection assumes that mortality rates will decline by about 0.6 percent annually. If mortality rates were to fall 2 percent annually but the duration of working lives were to stay at the official projection, the cost of Social Security would rise to more than 25 percent of payroll. A policy of raising the age at which full Social Security benefits are paid by one month a year starting in 2018 would eliminate most of the additional longevity-related cost. Shoven's message is simple and clear: As longevity increases, so too do Social Security costs.

Projecting the effects of longevity on Medicare and Medicaid costs is much trickier because program outlays depend not only on the number of beneficiaries but also on trends in the per capita costs of medical care. Medical spending is projected to rise over time as new technologies become available. But medical spending also rises with age because people's bodies gradually wear out or become subject to disease. Shoven considers whether increasing longevity would change the age profile of health care spending. According to one view, decline is an immutable consequence of age since birth. Increased longevity means that more people will reach ages when per capita medical costs are high. According to another view, which Shoven regards as more plausible, medical spending depends not on years since birth but on years until death. In this view, if the eighty-year-olds of the future have the same remaining years until death as, say, today's sixty-five-year-olds, then the ratio of the cost of medical care for these eighty-year-olds to the health care spending for, say, forty-year-olds will be the same as today's ratio of health care spending for sixty-five-year-olds is to that of forty-year-olds. Various facts persuade Shoven that the second view is the more plausible, including the fact that disability rates have been falling as mortality rates have been improving.

The difference between projections based on these alternative assumptions depends directly on the speed with which mortality improves. Under all assumptions, projected Medicare and Medicaid costs will increase greatly because per capita medical costs for everyone will increase. If mortality declines at historical rates, as assumed by government actuaries, projections based on the years-since-birth assumption show 2070 Medicare costs as a portion of gross domestic product at about 2 percent more than costs projected using the years-until-death assumption. The difference jumps to roughly 5 percent of GDP if mortality rates fall 2 percent a year. In the case of Medicaid, the cost difference in 2070 between projections is a bit over 1 percent of GDP if mortality declines at officially assumed rates but is nearly 6 percent if mortality rates fall 2 percent a year.

The story that emerges is straightforward. Costs of Social Security, Medicare, and Medicaid will rise during the early part of the twenty-first century. The major reasons are the aging of the baby-boom generation and, in the case of the health programs, the assumed general increases in medical costs. Accelerated increases in longevity will make their effects felt primarily in the second half of the century and beyond. How much health costs rise depends on whether reduced mortality is associated with delayed physical decline. If it is, then the added effect of increased longevity on health costs will be modest. If working lives increase, the added revenues from increased output of an enlarged labor force will help defray these costs.

Alan M. Garber and Dana P. Goldman examine in more detail whether increased longevity will slow the age-related increase in health care spending. They conclude that such a delay is quite likely. Nonetheless, they calculate future health spending based on the alternative assumption—that relative health expenditures on various age-sex groups will remain unchanged. They begin by projecting how many people in various age-sex categories will be alive in the future and how much will be spent on health care if disease prevalence is unchanged. Medical advances may well reduce the prevalence of some diseases. Changes in behavior—the increase in obesity, for example—could boost the frequency of other diseases. They proceed by estimating how much the elimination of one disease—like heart disease, diabetes, or cancer—will change health care spending. The effect is a significant, but modest, decline. Reductions are largest in the case of heart disease and smallest in the case of cancer. The reason for the difference is that heart disease strikes middle-aged people more than does cancer, which occurs predominantly among the old, when other fatal illnesses also often strike.

Trends in health care spending are acutely sensitive to insurance coverage. Garber and Goldman point out that rapid increases in the cost of new medical interventions will have two offsetting effects. They will increase the need for health insurance, but they will also raise the price of insurance. As a result, insurance may become too costly for many, especially those with low incomes, to afford. If rising health costs swell the ranks of the uninsured, they could intensify ethically troubling inequalities in access to what is likely to be increasingly beneficial medical care.

The extent and nature of health insurance also influences the nature of medical innovation. Health insurance weakens the sensitivity of patients to the price of health care because third parties bear much of the cost at the point when it is used. Such price insensitivity encourages the development of high-quality, high-priced services rather than somewhat lower-quality but lower-priced services. If rapid growth in the cost of health care causes more people to be uninsured or to elect less complete coverage, Garber and Goldman hypothesize that the increased cost sensitivity of patients will cause the development of lower-cost innovations.

A Global Perspective

The effects of a sharp increase in longevity would not be confined to a single nation. The swelling ranks of the elderly threaten pension systems in many nations and may have important effects on international capital flows. Economists have studied the effects of demographic change on national saving, investment, and output. These studies provide some basis for anticipating the consequences of the dramatic increase in longevity examined in this book.

Barry P. Bosworth and Benjamin Keys present new estimates showing that such a development would render retirement systems in most developed nations unsustainable without significant changes. These trends could also prevent many developing nations from borrowing to finance growth because of declining saving rates in developed nations. (Changes in labor force participation and in immigration could modify these projections, but Bosworth and Keys do not consider these.)

Declining birth and mortality rates have occurred in nearly every nation at some time during the past 150 years. Whether birth or mortality rates fell first and by how much strongly influences a nation's population profile. From the standpoint of economic development, the ideal pattern is a drop in birth rate followed some years later by declining mortality. This pattern produces a period during which the ratio of the working-age population to the total population is high. Because the cost of the economically inactive is low during this period, domestic saving can support high rates of investment. Eventually, however, the aged population increases. If birth rates remain low, overall population, excluding immigration, will fall.

Bosworth and Keys point out that if major increases in longevity depend on costly medical interventions, they are likely to be confined to wealthy nations. Because mortality rates are already low among those under age fifty in developed nations, the principal effects of declining mortality rates are likely to show up as increases in the size of population groups over age fifty. The largest increases in the ratio of the elderly to the working-age population would therefore occur in wealthy nations. The effects in middle-income nations would be modest and in poor nations very small. The most extreme effects would show up in nations such as Japan, where the elderly population is already 71 percent as large as the working-age population. If mortality rates fall 2 percent a year, the elderly population could grow to 117 percent of the working-age population. The effect in the United States will be much smaller because above-average birth and immigration rates are projected to maintain some growth of the working-age population.

Bosworth and Keys find that currently foreseen population aging is likely to cause both saving and investment to decline in high-income countries. In both middle-income and poor nations, saving would increase. These shifts would push the foreign trade balances of rich nations into deficit and those of the rest of the world into surplus. Reductions in mortality rates of 2 percent annually, the central assumption of this volume, will intensify these effects. Saving would decline sharply, investment somewhat less. Because the impact of medically based increases in longevity are likely to be greatest in nations that can afford such innovations, these results suggest that increasing longevity will be associated with trade deficits in rich nations.

Bosworth and Keys emphasize the sensitivity of their results to a variety of factors that they do not examine. Among the most important are how increasing longevity affects labor force participation. If people work until older ages, the increased labor force will create a demand for additional investment, lower the cost of private and public pensions, and reduce the amount that individuals need to save on their own to sustain preretirement living standards. Technological change influences investment opportunities and the call on saving to finance that investment. But regardless of the strength of these influences, the core fact remains: Extending longevity is likely to be quite expensive, and rich nations are more likely than poor nations to incur those costs.

The Ethical Dilemmas of Increasing Longevity

The prospect of an engineered extension of human life has created a major stir among ethicists, some of whose theories Alexander M. Capron examines. Such interventions should be evaluated, he suggests, on three criteria. Is the goal legitimate? Are the means to achieve the goal acceptable? Are the consequences benign? Capron divides ethical questions into three categories: interpersonal, intergenerational, and fundamental (meaning questions regarding the basic legitimacy of efforts to extend the human life span).

To begin with, Capron points to the obvious fact that interventions that have extended human lives are not exactly new. Throughout the twentieth century public health advances, rising income, and medical discoveries combined to add decades to life expectancy at birth. The decline in infant mortality and the lives saved by antibiotics raised few moral questions. To be sure, life extension resulting from these sources has brought a variety of practical problems, such as how to pay for pension and health costs for the elderly. They have raised some ethical problems as well: whether it is ever right—and if so under what circumstances and after what steps—to curtail care for extremely ill patients or to allow severely damaged newborns to die. In the past anyone who ever questioned whether clean water, the reduction of poverty, or effective antibiotics were ethically desirable would have been regarded by most people as deranged, but the problem, Capron argues, is now different. Past life-extending developments simply extended to the many the opportunities previously available to the few. In contrast, he suggests, some interventions now in prospect would change the fundamental character of humans—by changing their genes or replacing their organs, for example.

The ethical issues raised by life extension depend in part on the consequences of life extension. To sharpen this point, Capron (adopting a suggestion of his discussant, Margaret P. Battin) presents several possible scenarios of life extension. The most benign scenario, he suggests, is if human decline mimics that of Oliver Wendell Holmes's wonderful one-hoss shay, which lasted a hundred years and a day and then instantly fell apart. The most problematic scenario is an increase in the average age at death without any decrease—and possibly with significant increase—in the amount and duration of physical and mental decline. If one knew in advance which of these outcomes would materialize, it would be possible to judge the desirability of the result. But as Capron points out, no one can foresee whether the myriad scientific advances contributing to the extension of life will add decades of mental and physical vigor or decades of senility and debility.

The ethical issues raised by life extension will also be shaped by the means used to achieve that end. Capron argues that irreversible interventions, such as alteration of human genes, raise more questions than do interventions that can be stopped, such as a hormone that a patient can stop taking. Other issues concern payment: When does a service become standard and normal and therefore one that private and public insurance are expected to cover, and when may it be regarded as experimental and be legitimately excluded from standard insurance? The larger point is that many of the innovations that hold the promise of extending life will require risky experimentation that itself requires stringent procedural safeguards.

Capron also addresses social questions that sharply increased longevity could raise. The first concerns the added costs for public pensions and health benefits that a larger aged population will generate. Capron argues that fairness dictates that some of these costs should be borne by the beneficiaries of these services through longer working lives and notes that the feasibility of this form of cost sharing depends sensitively on which pattern of physical decline eventuates. Another issue concerns the fairness of access to life-extending interventions. Capron dismisses the views of some ethicists that after the achievement of a "normal" life span equitable access to life-extending care is not ethically required. Both the duration of normal lives and the content of normal interventions is inescapably elastic. Both depend on expectations that are themselves influenced by technological possibilities. Finally, Capron points to suicide and passive euthanasia as questions that are likely to become increasingly prominent. Should the failure to use the capacity to extend life be regarded as euthanasia? Or is it suicide if patients actively reject such treatment?

Capron concludes his exploration of ethical issues by confronting the criticisms advanced by Leon Kass, Francis Fukuyama, and others that life extension is not a legitimate goal of science and that success in such an endeavor threatens to deprive people of essential attributes of their humanity. Finitude, it is argued, lends life savor, sweetness, and value. The quest for superhuman intelligence, looks, or longevity is quite literally inhuman. Gradually, step by step—like the person immersed in a bath gradually warming from comfortable to lethal—humans would surrender what it means to be human by a series of steps each seemingly reasonable but cumulatively dehumanizing. Capron holds that these concerns are far less likely to have substance than those arising from the possibility that successful life extension could easily produce a dystopia with ever-larger parts of life spent in dependence.

The title of this collection of essays invokes the name of the biblical figure alleged to have lived longer than anyone else: 969 years. Methuselah's life was relatively uneventful, if fathering a child at age 187 can fairly be described as uneventful. His grandson, Noah, lived nearly as long and, by some standards, went through a good deal more stress. This comparison highlights two important facts: that longevity seems to run in families and that lives of similar duration may be associated with both easy and troubled times.

A well-known Scottish economist, sensitive to the vagaries of prediction, advised forecasters, Give a number or a date; never both. We think that the scenario addressed in this book—a world in which living to a hundred or even beyond will one day be common if not typical—is a reasonable extrapolation of the revolution in molecular biology that is only now gaining momentum. That is the number. No one can forecast the date. The various threats to extended life—pandemics, terrorism, and the remarkable capacity of humans to behave self-destructively—may offset part or all of what biomedical science does. After all, the twentieth century witnessed remarkable advances in science, public health, and income, all of which contributed to longer life expectancy, but increases in life expectancy did not accelerate. Past rates of increase in longevity could continue or even slow. But we believe that a flowering of biomedical science is at hand and that it has created another possibility—still by no means a certainty—that declines in mortality rates will accelerate.

This book is dedicated to the proposition that it is worth thinking seriously about the implications of such a development. Writers always place utopias and dystopias in the imagined future. Qualification or complexity do not dilute these worlds, elysian or hellish, because they are imaginary. Readers may be repelled by the nightmares of the *Brave New World* or *1984,* chilled by the cold impersonality of *The Rise of the Meritocracy,* or swept by the romantic notions of *Looking Backward.* The authors of these imagined futures had a free hand to paint with their chosen palettes.

Historians and social scientists, in contrast, have no such license. The contributors to this volume have written with academic detachment about some of the problems we may face if living to ninety, a hundred, or beyond becomes common. What emerges are problems, challenges, and opportunities. Utopias do not adorn the pages of honest histories and analyses.

Reference

Gavrilov, L. A., and N. S. Gavrilova. 1991. *The Biology of Life Span: A Quantitative Approach.* New York: Harwood Academic Publishers.

JOHN T. POTTS
WILLIAM B. SCHWARTZ

1 The Impact of the Revolution in Biomedical Research on Life Expectancy by 2050

WITH THE CHARACTERIZATION of the structure of the human genome, the stage is set for a new era of genetic medicine. In the past physicians could treat only the consequences of disease. They can now begin to seek ways to interrupt the pathways leading from genes to illness. In his 1994 lecture Alfred Gilman, the Nobel laureate in medicine, envisioned the future this way. "Identification of all these components [of the cellular switchboard] seems certain in the next decade or so. With this information in hand, we will be able to complete our understanding of the wiring diagram of the signaling switchboard in each type of cell. Such knowledge, coupled with both increasing sophistication in rational drug design and increasingly clever approaches to screen huge chemical libraries, will revolutionize both pharmacology and therapeutics."[1]

The result could well be a dramatic increase in life expectancy, as outlined in the chapter by Henry Aaron and Benjamin Harris. The more optimistic projections suggest that life expectancy in 2050 could reach ninety years or more; others believe this estimate is overly positive in outlook.[2] Some emphasize the risk of worldwide pandemics of infectious diseases for which no effective treatments have been found and that could spread rapidly through

1. Gilman (1996).
2. Perls and others (2002); Olshansky, Carnes, and Désesquelles (2001); Hayflick (2000).

16

global travel, such as severe acute respiratory syndrome (SARS). These risks exist but so too does the potential for the emerging science of molecular medicine to respond effectively to such threats. Others fear that longer lives may not be healthier lives, a development that could put enormous stresses on social and economic institutions. Still others question the morality or wisdom of using science to tamper with the natural limits to the human life cycle.[3]

Later chapters in this book explore these issues. This chapter gives a selective and necessarily cursory sketch of some of the most promising research advances in molecular medicine. Success in all lines of research is unlikely, but we believe that success in many is highly probable. As a result, the problems and opportunities of greatly extended human longevity are worth thinking about now. The examples here highlight the therapeutic potential of medical science based on molecular biology and medical genomics. Many of the therapeutic techniques we describe have not yet moved beyond the laboratory. Some may never prove to be clinically practicable. Many, however, will reach the bedside during the lives of readers of this book.

Before turning to the potential for treating specific diseases, we review some of the basic strategies that underlie new molecular approaches to therapy. These include replacing missing or damaged genes; interfering with the process of gene expression; mitigating or neutralizing the effects of missing or abnormal proteins resulting from abnormal gene expression; designing probes and technologies that can detect disease-associated mechanisms; and when all else fails, providing "spare parts."

Genomics and Genetics

The sequencing of the human genome holds enormous promise for improvements in human health.[4] The impact of this advance on biology will likely resemble that occurring in chemistry at the end of the nineteenth century, when Mendeleyev developed the periodic table of elements. Chemistry, a science whose accomplishments have so transformed society, leaped forward when it was appreciated that the chemical elements could be grouped logically according to their capacity to combine with one another. The periodic table facilitated predictions about chemical reactions for which previously

3. Hayflick (2000); Cohen (2000); Dye and Gay (2003).
4. International Human Genome Sequencing Consortium (2001); Venter and others (2001); Hollon (2001); Davaluri, Grosse, and Zhang (2001); Shouse (2002); Claverie (2001). For a survey of genetic medicine, see Guttmacher and Collins (2002).

there had been no foundation. Biologists believe that the map of the human genome will foster a similar revolution in understanding and treating disease.

Human deoxyribonucleic acid (DNA) consists of sequences of approximately three billion nucleotide bases (see box 1-1). Upon initial inspection, DNA resembles an undecipherable encyclopedia written in an obscure language consisting of just four seemingly randomly repeating letters. Much of this encyclopedia appears to be meaningless. Sandwiched among this gibberish are the important parts, the genes, which compose only 1–1.5 percent of the entire sequence of nucleotides.[5] The genes are a blueprint for all the components of the body. They contain the information needed to make proteins, the functioning elements that determine the structure and function of each cell and organ.[6] A system of controls specifies which genes will be active and, therefore, which proteins are to be made at any given time, depending on the type of cell and the state of its activity or development.

At one point, scientists expected the human genome to contain as many as 100,000 genes.[7] To their surprise, they initially counted a comparatively modest 30,000–45,000, only twice the number found in the genome of such simple organisms as worms. Disputes about this estimate continue, but even 30,000 genes can dictate the great complexity of the human organism, because each gene can make multiple proteins by being spliced together to form other proteins or by modifications in the proteins after production.[8]

Human proteins are built with combinations of twenty amino acids arranged in linear sequence. The length of this chain, the characteristics of the component amino acids, the order in which the amino acids are arranged, and the way the chain is folded determine the property of the protein. Proteins are the assembly units of the body's organization. They drive the construction of the body's constituent parts and influence metabolic activity. Because every human illness has a strong genetic component, understanding genes and the proteins they encode can help in the diagnosis and treatment of virtually all diseases.

5. International Human Genome Sequencing Consortium (2001); Venter and others (2001); Hollon (2001); Davaluri, Grosse, and Zhang (2001); Shouse (2002); Claverie (2001); Wade (2001). For a survey of genetic medicine, see Guttmacher and Collins (2002).

6. Wade (2001).

7. Hollon (2001); Davaluri, Grosse, and Zhang (2001); Shouse (2002); Claverie (2001); International Human Genome Sequencing Consortium (2001); Venter and others (2001). For a survey of genetic medicine, see Guttmacher and Collins (2002)

8. Hollon (2001); Davaluri, Grosse, and Zhang (2001); Shouse (2002); Claverie (2001).

Box 1-1. *A Vocabulary of Molecular Biology*

Amino acids: Units that, when joined end to end, form proteins. All amino acids have identical complementary ends, but their center sections vary considerably in size, polarity, and other chemical characteristics.

DNA: Long molecular chains held together in pairs as a double helix by the nucleotide bases.

DNA code: The code by which genes can be translated to make a protein. Sequences of three nucleotide bases code for amino acids, the components of proteins. Since there are 4^3 (that is, 64) possible codes and only 20 amino acids, there is more than one code for many amino acids. There are also codes that designate the beginning and the end of a gene.

Gene: A sequence of DNA bases that codes for a protein. Many genes are active only within certain cells or at a particular stage of development. When a gene is active, the process of translating the code and protein synthesis is known as *gene expression.*

Genome: The blueprint of instructions to make all the components of a living being, in the form of DNA in all cell nuclei.

Nucleotide bases: Adenine, thymine, guanine, and cytosine, abbreviated as A, T, G, and C. A always links to T and G to C. These linkages make replication of DNA possible. When the DNA chains are separated, the pairing system ensures that copies are made in exactly the same sequence of bases as the original pair.

Proteins: Chains of amino acids, linked end to end and twisted and folded into specific three-dimensional shapes ranging from fibrous to globular and determined by their amino acid composition. Proteins play many roles in the body, including those of enzymes (catalysts for metabolic events), cell-surface receptors that transmit messages from outside the cell to the inside, hormones, growth factors and other signaling proteins, antibodies, and many structural entities.

RNA: A copy of the code that is formed when the gene is expressed. RNA, similar in structure to DNA, migrates out of the nucleus to the protein-making machinery of the cell.

SNP: A single nucleotide polymorphism, a substitution of one base for another in the DNA sequence. SNPs may be within a gene or between genes. Many SNPs result in little or no alteration in protein structure and function. They account for the normal variation within a species, and some may, in combination with others, convey disease susceptibility or result in variations in drug response. All can be useful markers for geneticists, who can study the co-inheritance of SNPs and disease susceptibility to hone in on and identify genes associated with disease susceptibility.

Single-Gene Mutations and Disease

Before the complete human genome sequence was mapped, scientists had already made considerable progress in identifying some single-gene (mono-genic) defects responsible for disease, such as in 1983 the gene responsible for Huntington's disease, a progressive degeneration of key brain function.[9] They have since identified many other genes responsible for monogenic disorders, including the genes responsible for pathologically high cholesterol levels, which cause early heart disease; for hemophilia, which causes excessive bleeding because of a deficiency of a critical clotting protein; and for a variety of rare syndromes associated with the early onset of certain cancers. More than 1,100 genes responsible for approximately 1,500 hereditary human diseases have now been identified. The number of diseases exceeds the number of genes, because more than one kind of error can occur in a gene and each error can produce a different protein abnormality. An understanding of a particular hereditary disease may be poor even if it is linked to a specific gene, because other genes, still unrecognized, may modify the severity of the disease. For this reason, families with the same mutant gene may show strikingly different severities of the resultant disease. Future treatment of such genetic disorders will, therefore, focus not only on reversing the effects of the defective gene but also on ascertaining the genes that modify the clinical expression of the illness.

Genetic Variation and Susceptibility to Disease

Common illnesses such as heart disease, cancer, and diabetes result from the combined effect of several variations in a person's genome that interact with environmental factors. The Pima Indians illustrate this interaction in a particularly dramatic way. These people rarely suffered from type 2 diabetes until they replaced their traditional diet with the standard U.S. diet, which is high in both fat and sugar. As the incidence of obesity among the Pima rose, the frequency of diabetes skyrocketed and now affects over half of adult Pimas. Scientists speculate that endemic genetic variations that allowed many of the Pimas to survive on the cusp of starvation in a harsh desert environment predispose them to disease when food is plentiful.[10]

To link genes to disease susceptibility, investigators need to be able to find the genes. Fortunately, the Human Genome Project has provided genetic

9. Peltonen and McKusick (2001).
10. Wilson and others (1999).

markers, or tags, to pinpoint genes linked with disease. More than 1.4 million variations in single nucleotides—so-called single-nucleotide polymorphisms (SNPs, pronounced "snips")—account for variations among individuals.[11] SNPs occur throughout the genome, both in genes and in nongene regions. They do not necessarily cause disease on their own, even when they change the composition of a gene and the protein product of that gene.[12] Together with the products of other variant genes, however, they may convey susceptibility to disease. Whether or not they are within a gene, SNPs are valuable as markers of correlations between the occurrence of a disease in certain members of a family and the inheritance of SNPs, whose position in the genome is known. These patterns provide clues to potentially responsible genes and have led to some intriguing early findings. For example, a variant of a hormone receptor involved in fat metabolism has been identified as a contributor to type 2 diabetes.[13] This hormone receptor is the target of a drug used to treat type 2 diabetes; the finding may serve to explain how this drug works. Future research will focus on identifying multigene causes of and susceptibility to disease and on effective treatments.

Genetics and Medical Practice in the Twenty-First Century

Genetics, heretofore an arcane specialty, will soon become part of routine clinical practice. For example, new technology in the form of DNA chips, or gene arrays, can be used to determine which genes are either overexpressed or suppressed in both normal and diseased tissues.[14] DNA chips have already been applied to the study of lymphoma and breast cancer. They have shown better diagnostic capacity than traditional methods used by pathologists. They have also been used to help determine the aggressiveness of a cancer and how rapidly it will spread, thereby guiding therapy.[15]

Progress being made in the ease, speed, and accuracy of genomic sequencing will make possible inexpensive analysis of an individual's genome.[16] The genetic profile will permit physicians to determine a person's risk of developing such diseases as cancer and cardiovascular disease and to predict how

11. International SNP Map Working Group (2001).
12. International SNP Map Working Group (2001); Sunyaev and others (1999).
13. Altshuler and others (2000).
14. Wade (2001); Shipp and others (2002); van't Veer and others (2002); Marx (2000a); Ramaswamy and others (2001); Lakhani, O'Hare, and Ashworth (2001).
15. Shipp and others (2002); van't Veer and others (2002); Marx (2000a); Ramaswamy and others (2001); Lakhani, O'Hare, and Ashworth (2001).
16. Ratain and Relling (2001).

a patient will respond to drugs so that drug selection and dosage can be individualized. The result will be increased efficacy and safety.[17] One such genetic variation of a liver enzyme has important implications for the dosing level of about 20 percent of commonly prescribed drugs. Another mutation—of an enzyme found in red blood cells—affects the metabolism of a family of drugs used for treating leukemia and rheumatic disease and for preventing the rejection of transplanted organs. Roughly 10 percent of the population with lower levels of this enzyme retain drugs in their bodies longer than normal. Such patients should receive much lower than normal doses to avoid toxic or even fatal reactions.[18]

As detailed knowledge of the genome and its protein products expands, possible interventions will grow in number. About 500 genes are currently targets for drug development, but this number is expected to increase tenfold.[19] Drugs will be developed not only to activate suppressed genes and to suppress overactive genes but also to replace missing proteins or to counter the harmful effects of abnormal proteins produced by mutant genes.

Gene Therapy

Gene replacement is one of the most dramatic strategies arising from the characterization of the human genome, and for over a decade much effort has gone into developing gene therapy. Gene therapy remains controversial, however, in part because progress has been slow and marked by serious setbacks.[20] Even a striking success, the apparent cure of eleven French children suffering from a severe immunodeficiency disease, has been set back seriously by the development of a form of leukemia in two of the treated children.[21] Many trials of gene therapy are in progress, especially in cancer, but other trials have been halted because of the complications in the case of the French children.

To successfully treat a disease resulting from a genetic deficiency, genes must be delivered efficiently into cells. Once there, the genes must work effectively for years to produce the proper amounts of the needed protein. In diabetes, for example, a gene that produces too little insulin would be ineffective. One that produces too much would be harmful. In certain other

17. McLeod (2001).
18. McLeod (2001); McLeod and others (2000).
19. Bumol and Watanabe (2001).
20. Pfeifer and Verma (2001).
21. Hacein-Bey-Abina and others (2002); Verma (2003); Bonetta (2002).

diseases, the exact level of activity of the introduced gene is not as critical. In hemophilia, for example, even a little of the missing anticlotting factor is helpful, and even moderately high levels are not predicted to be harmful.[22]

Viral-Based Gene Therapy

Most research on gene replacement has used viruses to deliver the genes because viruses can enter human cells efficiently. As noted, this method was used for the successful treatment of immunodeficient French children.[23] These children suffered from a mutation in a critical receptor that completely disrupts the development of all immune cells. In such cases, any infection can be lethal. A virus was used to deliver the missing receptor to stem cells that had been isolated from the children's bone marrow. The modified stem cells were then reinfused, and the defect in immunity was corrected. The approach used must be modified for safety, however, because leukemia appeared in two of the children. Despite the promise of the approach for treatment of other gene-deficiency diseases, many other barriers stand in the way of success (such as limited survival of the modified cells).

Interfering with RNA

Many of the virus-based gene-delivery trials resulted in the production of antibodies that destroyed both the viruses and their human gene cargo. Nonviral methods avoid the problems of rejection but have thus far failed to deliver genes efficiently.

Ribonucleic acid (RNA), the critical component linking the gene to protein synthesis, is a promising target for therapy. RNA takes instructions from the gene-forming messenger RNA, which travels to the ribosomes (key components of human cells), where the coded instructions direct protein synthesis. For some time, investigators tried to deliver into the cells strands of RNA that are mirror images of the messenger RNA. These strands—called antisense RNA—were used to bind to and thus inactivate the messenger RNA, effectively silencing the gene.

Initial studies of this technique were disappointing. A new approach, using double-stranded RNA, is far more efficient in silencing the gene. Dubbed RNAi (interfering RNA), this method can silence a target gene in every cell of an organism (experiments have been successfully conducted on

22. Miller and Stamatoyannopoulos (2001).
23. Somia and Verma (2000); Cavazzana-Calvo and others (2000).

worms).[24] Recent technical changes suggest it may be possible to use the approach in humans as treatment, based on success in blocking infection in human tissue culture cells.[25]

Gene Therapy and Cancer

Gene therapy holds its greatest immediate promise in the treatment of cancer when the long-term survival of modified cells needed in treatment of most deficiency diseases is not an issue. The genetic modification of cancer cells in preliminary studies has successfully goaded the previously dormant immune system into attacking the cancer. In another approach, viruses have been genetically modified to take advantage of mutations in cancers, allowing the viruses to selectively infect and kill tumor cells while leaving normal cells untouched.[26]

Proteomics

Proteomics is the study of the nature of the proteins produced by genes and of the way they interact with one another to build and regulate every cell in the body.[27] Cellular proteins vary according to cell type, cell cycle, and overall growth rate. Protein composition also changes in response to the cellular environment. By studying proteomics, scientists hope to catalog proteins in various kinds of cells to determine their roles in cell function and to explore how these proteins interact to form functional networks.

Proteomics promises to revolutionize the search for new drugs. Physiological changes in disease result from abnormal protein activity, caused by genetic mutation or in response to a disease-provoking agent. Determining the protein changes in disease will provide targets for intervention, since protein structure provides clues to the identity of the parent gene. When a given genetic abnormality is discovered, the changes in the associated protein can be tracked. The aberrant protein can then be made a target for a new drug, which will either substitute for or block the action of the disease-causing protein.

In principle, the discovery process is straightforward. In practice, it will be daunting. The problem is that there are far more proteins—200,000 to

24. Hammond, Caudy, and Hannon (2001).
25. Paddison, Caudy, and Hannon (2002).
26. Dranoff and others (1993); Dranoff and Mulligan (1995); Hodi and others (2002); Hermiston (2000); Kirn, Martuza, and Zwiebel (2001).
27. Ezzell (2002).

2 million—than genes.[28] Proteins can be cleaved and their activity modified or altered in a variety of ways after they are synthesized. Proteins also fold into a variety of three-dimensional structures in response to interactions with other molecules, which alter their functions. In addition, they form networks that themselves have unique functions. These variations create massive identification problems, yet the opportunities have attracted wide support from scientists, the National Institutes of Health, and from industry.[29]

Regenerative Medicine

Many of the most fruitful advances in therapy will take the form of new techniques for replacing failing components of the human body. These techniques will produce implantable body tissue, expand the range of transplants, and enable regeneration through the introduction of stem cells.

Tissue Engineering

Tissue engineering can be used to replace damaged tissues and organs, to repair congenital defects, and to replace tissue that has failed because of disease.[30] New emphasis on disease prevention could dramatically lower rates of organ or tissue failure. Nonetheless, population aging and the distressing ways many people abuse their bodies are still likely to cause an increase in the need for tissue engineering and regenerative medicine.

The first step in engineering replacement tissue and organs is to fashion a three-dimensional "scaffold" from biodegradable polymers that is shaped like the desired organ. The next step is to implant this form with cells taken from the patient or a donor. Though still at an early stage, this procedure has claimed some remarkable successes. Tissue-engineered skin has been used to promote the healing of venous and diabetic ulcers. It is also used for grafts in the treatment of third-degree burns. Cartilage cells are being used to regenerate the smooth cartilage that lines normal joints but that is lost in arthritic joints. Tissue-engineered corneas, blood vessels, heart valves, and urinary bladders are being produced.[31] Nutrients and oxygen can diffuse through a thin layer of tissue, but scaffolds for larger organs such as the liver

---

28. Service (2001).
29. Service (2001).
30. Nasseri, Ogawa, and Vacanti (2001); Griffith and Naughton (2002).
31. Griffith and others (1999).

must be designed to induce tissue-engineered blood vessels to grow and to provide the vital supplies.[32] Tissue engineers believe that they will eventually be able to produce whole organs, such as breasts, livers, and kidneys.[33]

Animals with severed spinal cords resulting in paralysis of their hind limbs have been treated in a novel and effective way to restore mobility. Undifferentiated spinal cord cells, laid onto a tissue-engineering scaffold, were used to bridge the gap in the cord. The development and growth of these cells effectively restored the ability of these animals to respond to sensory stimuli, allowed them to support themselves on all four legs, and partially restored their ability to walk.[34] Whether this technique can be extended to humans remains unclear.

Xenotransplantation

The transplantation of organs from one species to another—xenotransplantation—is a potential answer to persistent shortages of critical organs.[35] The organs of miniature swine, whose adult weight is comparable to that of humans, are anatomically and physiologically suitable for transplantation.[36] Unfortunately for this purpose, the human immune system rejects foreign organs by humoral (antibody) and cellular mechanisms. By removing the pig genes responsible for antibody reactions, it may be possible to overcome the antibody barriers, but difficult issues of cellular tissue rejection remain to be resolved.[37] Even if all rejection problems are overcome, xenotransplantation carries the risk that the animal organ may infect humans with an as-yet-unknown pathogen. Many feel that this threat is exaggerated; given the severe shortage of human organs, they argue that animal organs should be tried when the immunologic problems are solved.[38]

Stem-Cell Therapy

Stem-cell therapy is one of the most exciting advances in regenerative medicine. Stem cells can self-replicate endlessly. In response to signals, they can also differentiate into specialized cells. Bone marrow transplants from closely

32. Kaihara and others (2000).
33. Mooney and Mikos (1999).
34. Vacanti and others (2001a).
35. Organ Procurement and Transplantation Network, P.O. Box 13770, Richmond, VA 23225-8770 (www.optn.org).
36. Cooper, Gollackner, and Sachs (2002).
37. Cooper, Gollackner, and Sachs (2002); Lai and others (2002).
38. Cooper, Gollackner, and Sachs (2002); Lai and others (2002).

related donors—a form of stem-cell transplantation—has become an established treatment for certain cancers. In this procedure, radiation is used to kill the patient's cancerous blood-forming cells. Donated normal stem cells are then used to repopulate the patient's bone marrow. Experiments in animals and some early clinical trials indicate that stem cells could effectively treat such failing organs as the heart and the liver.[39]

Human embryonic stem cells were first isolated and grown in culture in 1998.[40] These cells, which can give rise to every type of cell, are a ball of cells found in the core of embryos about six days after fertilization and before the embryo normally becomes implanted in the uterus. Because extracting stem cells destroys the embryo, the use of these cells has provoked intense controversy.[41] Even when the embryo has been discarded—for example, in the course of fertility therapy—and will be destroyed, some critics still strenuously object to their use in research. For this reason, President George W. Bush in 2001 issued a regulation that fully satisfied neither the scientific community nor those opposed to stem-cell harvesting. Under this regulation, government funding is limited to research on embryonic stem cells from some sixty cell lines that already exist; these lines were derived from embryos produced for infertility treatments and no longer needed for this purpose.

Immune rejection is a potential limitation to the use of embryonic stem cells, since cells from any source other than an identical twin may be sensed by the body as foreign. An alternative approach—so-called therapeutic cloning—may forestall immunological rejection. Therapeutic cloning entails taking a cell from a patient, removing its nucleus, and placing the nucleus into a donated human ovum (egg cell) from which the nucleus has been removed. The resulting fused cell, with a nucleus from the patient and the cell body of a donated ovum, will act like a human ovum that has been normally fertilized by a sperm cell: It will begin to divide in tissue culture, just as do egg cells fertilized in vitro for infertile couples. When the ovum develops into an early embryo, the stem cells can be extracted.[42] These cells could be used as therapy for the donor of the nucleus. Because the cells are an exact genetic copy of the patient's cells, they will evade immunological rejection.[43]

39. Kaji and Leiden (2001); Quaini and others (2002); Orlic and others (2001); Ng, Alonso, and Bezerre (2000).
40. Thomson and others (1998).
41. Thomson and others (1998).
42. Committee on Science, Engineering, and Public Policy (2002).
43. We do not explore the issues regarding the use of this technique with implantation of the embryo into a woman's uterus to make an identical copy of an individual—so-called reproductive cloning—as support for this procedure is almost nonexistent. Unfortunately, therapeutic cloning is currently banned from federal funding.

Controversy regarding the use of embryonic stem cells derived from discarded embryos or from therapeutic cloning would likely wane if adult stem or stemlike cells retain the capacity to develop into any type of cell needed for organ replacement or cell therapy.[44] Research is under way to develop therapy using cells derived from adults for regenerative purposes, particularly for the failing heart.[45] Such cells, if isolated from each individual, would be free of rejection-related problems. The apparent complexity and expense of isolation, expansion, characterization, and directed differentiation of cells for each individual—whether from adult stem cells or via therapeutic cloning—are formidable. Thus efforts continue to determine whether stem cells from an unrelated donor may actually evade immunological rejection if their use is properly managed.

Whether embryonic stem cells from established cell lines, cells derived by therapeutic cloning, or adult stem cells prove most effective or practical, the ability to harness these cells to provide cells to regenerate failing organs promises a revolution in treatment for many of humanity's most serious diseases.

Disease Control and Life Expectancy

Projecting progress in controlling death from major diseases is subject to three factors that have been found to be true of studies in electronics, computer technology, and telecommunications.[46] First, predictions often overestimate change in the short term. As applied to longevity, this rule reminds us that projections that highly specific and effective therapies for various cancers will be available in just a few years may be overly optimistic. Because of the complexity of human biology and the difficulty in evaluating the safety and efficacy of treatments in human clinical trials, more time than is currently estimated may be required to achieve the enormous potential of recent advances in cancer biology. Second, forecasters tend to underestimate long-term change. For example, no early designer of mainframe computers foresaw that personal computers would replace mainframes for most uses. Fifty years hence, historians may marvel at the failure of most early twenty-first-century observers to anticipate the range or magnitude of improvements in medical care. Third, the more specific the prediction, the less likely it is to

44. Pittenger and others (1999); Toma (2002); Toma and others (2001); Vacanti and others (2001b); Palmer and others (2001); Zulewski and others (2001).
45. Taylor (2001); Hagège and others (2001); Anversa and Nadal-Ginard (2002).
46. Cringely (1998).

be correct. Some of the medical advances we describe as probable may not materialize. And as-yet-unimagined developments may emerge as the most important new treatments in the decades ahead.

At the beginning of the twentieth century, infectious disease was the major killer. Tuberculosis was rampant, and no specific therapy was available. Many common bacterial infections that are now cured with antibiotics were responsible for high death rates from infancy onward. A combination of improved diet, cleaner water and air, and advances in medical care combined to raise life expectancy from forty-nine years at the start of the twentieth century to seventy-seven years at its close.[47]

Heart disease and cancer now head the roster of mortality causes.[48] Heart disease and stroke will kill an estimated 13.6 percent of all men between the ages of sixty and seventy and 28.5 percent between the ages of seventy and eighty. They will kill 7.9 percent and 18.9 percent of women in the same age spans. Although shocking, these mortality rates have been falling recently and are projected to continue to fall.[49] In contrast, the frequency of cancer has been rising. The major cancers—lung, colon, and prostate—now kill 12.3 percent of men and 10 percent of women between the ages of sixty and seventy. Cancer deaths exceed those of heart disease and stroke after age seventy. Given these trends, cancer is likely to become the major cause of death.[50]

Eliminating either cancer or cardiovascular disease would obviously be a boon. But to have a major effect on life expectancy, progress on treatment for all major diseases must be achieved simultaneously. We explain below why advances in treatment—even cures and prevention—are likely also for such major causes of death as Alzheimer's disease and obesity. Control of resistant bacterial infections poses another major challenge to science and medicine; intensified efforts are needed to combat rising bacterial resistance. The expectation that progress will be made against major diseases simultaneously is what underlies the projections of sharply increased longevity presented by Henry Aaron and Benjamin Harris (this volume).

Cancer

An increased understanding of the genetic changes that cause cancer and, with it, the growing list of cancer therapies warrant the view that deaths from

47. Centers for Disease Control/National Center for Health Services (2002, pp. 1–2).
48. Anderson (2001); Woloshin, Schwartz, and Welch (2002).
49. Laura Meckler, "Fifty Years Saw Big Gains in Life Expectancy," Associated Press, September 13, 2002.
50. Woloshin, Schwartz, and Welch (2002).

this disease can be sharply reduced over the next few decades. A few spectacular successes have already been achieved.[51]

Genetic Mutations and Cancer

All cancers begin as abnormal growth in a single cell. Without effective treatment, the cell goes through initial rapid growth followed by states in which the cell no longer responds to the signals that normally control growth. Eventually, growth becomes aggressive, spreads to many sites in the body, and causes disabling symptoms and death.[52] Mutations in critical genes are responsible for initiating this malignant sequence of events.[53] Some gene mutation is inevitable in every individual, but the rate may be accelerated by exposure to harmful chemicals or damaging environmental factors.[54] Fortunately, most such mutations do not occur in genes that precipitate cancer.

Genetic changes that cause cancer are of two principal types. Tumor-suppressor genes limit the rate of growth and cell division, keeping cell growth down to a normal, healthy rate. Loss of both copies of such genes is analogous to the loss of brakes in a car. Other cells, protooncogenes, control the signals stimulating cell growth. Mutations of these cells also lead to cancer in a manner that is comparable to a permanently depressed accelerator pedal. The mutation of even one copy of a protooncogene is sufficient to cause cancer. An example is chronic myelogenous leukemia, a form of leukemia occurring in the elderly; it is driven by a single genetic change, increasing the activity of a regulatory enzyme called tyrosine kinase.[55] More than twenty tumor-suppressor genes and a similar number of protooncogenes are known to be involved in the development of human cancers.[56]

In hereditary cancers, one copy of a tumor-suppressor gene that controls cell growth is already disabled in every cell.[57] Because two copies of each gene are present in each body cell, the remaining normal gene compensates for the mutated one. A spontaneous mutation of the remaining normal gene in a single cell is, however, sufficient to initiate cancer. For cancers due to loss of growth-controlling genes in individuals who are not born with a disabled

---

51. D. Steinberg (2002a); Livingston and Shivdasani (2001); van Dyke and Jacks (2002); Johnstone, Ruefli, and Lowe (2002); Reed (2002).

52. Wilson and others (1999).

53. Haber and Fearon (1998).

54. Livingston and Shivdasani (2001); Druker and Lydon (2000).

55. Livingston and Shivdasani (2001); Druker and Lydon (2000).

56. Haber and Fearon (1998).

57. Haber and Fearon (1998).

copy of the gene, spontaneous mutations must occur in both copies of the gene. Fortunately, this is a rare event and explains why cancer incidence increases with age; hereditary cancers, which are uncommon, occur much earlier in life.[58]

Because cancer cells divide more rapidly than do normal cells, genetic mistakes accumulate over time, some involving additional cancer-promoting genes. These genetic changes interact to make the cancer more malignant.[59] In colon cancer, in which many genes are involved, years may elapse before a sufficient number of genetic mutations accumulate to cause the cancer to spread throughout the body.[60]

Selectivity and Synergy in Cancer Treatments

Several approaches have been designed to attack each of several critical points in cancer development. Cancer cells depend not only on increasingly hyperactive growth but also on the formation of blood vessels to supply these cells with nutrients and oxygen.[61] As cancer cells accumulate genetic mutations they become not only more aggressively malignant but also more vulnerable to sudden death—that is, cells with genetic defects are normally programmed to commit suicide (apoptosis). Cancer cells, however, evolve strategies to evade apoptosis. These features—rapid growth, elaborate supply lines (blood vessels), and other evasive tactics—provide opportunities for therapeutic attack.

Antibodies. Antibodies have been developed that bind to and block the activity of receptors critical to cancer cell growth. One antibody blocks the activity of a growth receptor overexpressed in about 25 percent of breast cancers. Another inactivates a growth receptor on the surface of colon cancers as well as on other solid tumors.[62] Still other antibodies block a signaling-recognition molecule on the surface of the malignant lymphocytes that cause lymphomas. The sudden loss of the growth signal that these antibodies induce leads to the death of the cancer cells. Clinical trials of these antibodies have produced dramatic benefits in many patients. Outcomes range from significant prolongation of life in patients with breast cancer to long periods of

---

58. Haber and Fearon (1998).
59. Vogelstein and Kinzler (2001).
60. Haber and Fearon (1998).
61. Livingston and Shivdasani (2001); Folkman (1996); Ferrara and Alitalo (1999).
62. D. Steinberg (2002a, b); Druker and Lydon (2000); Schnipper and Strom (2001).

improved health or even cure in some lymphoma patients. To increase the effectiveness of these therapies, the antibodies are now being armed with toxins or radioactive molecules so that the antibodies not only block tumor growth directly by interfering with their growth signaling but also poison the cancer cells or kill them with radiation.

Enzyme Inhibitors. Other treatments directly attack the critical enzymes called protein kinases, growth promoters that are hyperactive because of genetic changes within the cancer cells. Uncontrolled growth makes the cells not only malignant but also vulnerable to death if they are denied critical growth signals. The drug Gleevec™ takes advantage of this vulnerability by inhibiting the abnormal tyrosine kinase in patients with chronic myelogenous leukemia.[63] It is one of the first treatments that acts on a specific genetic fault in a cancer. Many patients with chronic myelogenous leukemia given this drug were alive and well two years and more after their treatment. With the best conventional therapy most patients would have died within months. A drug similar to vitamin A, called transretinoic acid, blocks another abnormally active growth-promoting protein and kills malignant cells in a different form of leukemia. These impressive results are stimulating efforts to identify more such critical targets in cancer cells.

Antiangiogenesis. The invading mass of malignant cells secrete, or induce normal cells around them to secrete, factors that stimulate the production of blood vessels for the tumor mass. Targeting these factors, one of which is called vascular endothelial growth factor (VEGF), prevents tumor growth. In preliminary patient trials and in animal models, drugs or antibodies have been used to block these angiogenic factors, sometimes with dramatic results.[64]

Promoting Apoptosis. Programmed cell death, or apoptosis, typically occurs when a cell recognizes that it has an internal error (genetic mutation).[65] Cancer cells should die because their genetic machinery is deranged, but they have evolved strategies to evade this mechanism. In normal cells, inhibitors at multiple points keep apoptosis in check. Some of these inhibitors are over-

63. Livingston and Shivdasani (2001); Druker and Lydon (2000).
64. Livingston and Shivdasani (2001); Folkman (1996); Ferrara and Alitalo (1999); Schnipper and Strom (2001).
65. Reed (2002).

expressed by cancer cells, thereby blocking cell death, but new drugs have been developed that block the action of such inhibitors. Cancer cells also prevent apoptosis by blocking signals to receptors on the cell surface by secreting decoy receptors. To counter this effect, excess quantities of apoptosis-inducing molecules are administered to patients. The cancer cells die, but normal cells remain unaffected.[66] Yet another approach is to directly stimulate the enzymes, called caspases, that trigger apoptosis.[67]

Activating Inhibited Tumor-Suppressor Genes. Mutations that inactivate the pathways of two tumor-suppressor genes, TP53 and RB, are present in more than half of cancers. When these genes are normally active, their protein products help regulate cell growth and division. When mutations disable these gene pathways, the cells they regulate grow rapidly; reversing this effect by causing the abnormal protein to fold normally helps it to regulate cell division.[68]

Gene Therapy and Cancer. One approach to cancer treatment by gene therapy takes advantage of the mutations that cause the loss of the product of the TP53 gene, p53, which plays a key regulatory function in cells. Normal cells protect themselves from infection in part by using signaling proteins such as p53 to resist viral invasion. Some viruses have evolved anti-p53 genes, which overcome this defensive strategy. If these viruses are selectively modified to remove their anti-p53 gene, they can still infect and kill tumor cells lacking p53 but leave normal cells unharmed.[69] These replication-selective, or oncolytic, viruses offer a promising direction in cancer therapy. They can be altered to deliver an enzyme not found in normal cells, which converts a drug administered in an inactive form into a toxic, active form. This conversion occurs only in cells that have the converting enzyme delivered by the virus. Thus chemotherapy is effectively delivered only to the cancer cells. Oncolytic viruses are being evaluated in animals; some are being tested in preliminary human clinical trials. Various problems must still be solved, however; for example, oncolytic viruses incompletely penetrate solid tumors. Furthermore, they are attacked by the body's natural immune response. Research is now exploring the capacity of further modifying oncolytic viruses to overcome these shortcomings.

66. Reed (2002).
67. Livingston and Shivdasani (2001); Johnstone, Ruefli, and Lowe (2002); Reed (2002).
68. Livingston and Shivdasani (2001); Johnstone, Ruefli, and Lowe (2002); Reed (2002).
69. Hermiston (2000); Kirn, Martuza, and Zwiebel (2001); Dranoff and others (1993).

Immunotherapy

Another use of gene therapy in cancer is to help stimulate the immune system to attack the malignancy. The immune system does not typically attack proteins made by healthy cells but recognizes and attacks foreign proteins, such as those from an infecting microbe. As the malignant transformation of cancer cells progresses, many of the proteins on their surfaces undergo mutations, which should make them seem foreign. Nevertheless, through unknown mechanisms these cancer cells evade attack by the immune system.[70]

One gene therapy approach uses cancer cells themselves to stimulate attack from the immune system.[71] A virus inserted into cancer cells that have been surgically removed from a patient delivers a protein known to stimulate an intense immune response. When these cells are reimplanted, the immune system responds by attacking them and, once aroused, goes on to attack the tumor that it had previously ignored. To prevent the modified, reimplanted cells from developing into cancer themselves, they are irradiated to make sure that they die within a few days. Results are striking in animal models and are encouraging in preliminary use in patients with melanoma, leukemia, and prostate, pancreatic, and lung cancer.

New Horizons in Cancer Treatment

The full promise of these treatments is being realized only slowly. All of them must be tested carefully and systematically in patients with different types of cancer before they can be evaluated. A variety of efforts is under way to determine if synergy in the killing of cancer cells can be successfully exploited. Genetically engineered mice, for example, that faithfully reproduce the exact steps in the initiation of human cancer provide a model that greatly facilitates this effort.

In contrast to standard radiological techniques, which are blind to fewer than hundreds of millions to a billion cancer cells, new molecular imaging techniques can detect a few thousand cancer cells in animals, enabling investigators to monitor the progress of cancer through its successive phases.[72] Current clinical trials follow many patients to determine the effectiveness of a given drug and its optimal dose, a process that takes many months. Using the new techniques investigators will be able to evaluate the effectiveness

70. Hermiston (2000); Kirn, Martuza, and Zwiebel (2001); Dranoff and others (1993).
71. Jaffee (1999); Jaffee and others (2001); Simons and others (1999); Soiffer and others (1998).
72. van Dyke and Jacks (2002); Weissleder (2001).

of treatment immediately, monitor cancer treatment in patients in real time, and observe the effects of increased doses, of adding a second agent, or of changing a drug.

Gene-array technology provides the capacity to quickly and fully characterize the range of genetic defects in cancer specimens. Knowledge of these defects helps physicians determine the aggressiveness of the cancer and therefore how vigorously to treat it. In just a few years this information will be used routinely to determine which of the growing range of possible treatments should be used.[73]

Cancer cells grow fast and undergo frequent genetic changes. These characteristics make cancer a formidable disease but also make cancer cells vulnerable to treatment. The number of therapeutic approaches is expanding at unprecedented speed: None of those described here was available just a few years ago. The virtual explosion of new insight into cancer's mechanisms and of new strategies for dealing with them suggests that many forms of cancer will be curable by 2040 or 2050. The conquest of this major disease would have enormous impact on life expectancy.[74]

Cardiovascular Disease

Heart attacks and strokes remain the leading causes of death in the United States, although mortality rates have diminished sharply in recent decades. Until recently, however, these advances have come not from an understanding of the basic mechanisms behind heart disease but from practical advances: improved diets, early and effective control of hypertension, and reduced smoking.[75]

Preventive measures focus on lowering cholesterol to block the formation of cholesterol plaques that can rupture and obstruct a coronary vessel. Furthermore, advances in acute medical treatments to support the damaged heart—drugs that strengthen heart performance and cardiac monitors and defibrillators to detect and reverse otherwise potentially fatal cardiac arrests—have boosted the chances that a heart attack patient will survive. Mortality rates from cardiovascular disease have declined significantly in the recent past and are likely to continue falling.[76]

73. Shipp and others (2002); van't Veer and others (2002); Marx (2000a); Ramaswamy and others (2001); Lakhani, O'Hare, and Ashworth (2001).
74. Woloshin, Schwartz, and Welch (2002).
75. Anderson (2001); Braunwald and others (2001).
76. Lefkowitz and Willerson (2001).

Management of Coronary Artery Disease

Even before a major heart attack, (chest) pain brought on by exercise—
so-called chronic stable angina, which indicates coronary disease—may be
present for months before being diagnosed.[77] Angioplasty, which widens
obstructed arteries, may reduce or eliminate the pain and may be lifesaving.
Because restenosis (a second narrowing of the vessel) often occurs just months
after surgery, mechanical props that keep the vessels open (stents) are commonly used.[78] If the obstruction cannot be dealt with through angioplasty,
a coronary bypass graft is the treatment of choice.

Cholesterol in Heart Disease

Cholesterol causes problems if low-density lipoprotein (LDL, or "bad" cholesterol) is too high or high-density-lipoprotein (HDL, or "good" cholesterol) is too low. At least part of the problem may be genetic. Members of a
family on Tangier Island located in the Chesapeake Bay suffer from a rare
condition characterized by vanishingly low levels of HDL.[79] Called Tangier's
disease, this hereditary disorder results from a defect in the mechanism that
normally moves cholesterol out of cells, where it is picked up by proteins for
transport to the liver and recycling back to the cells. Investigators have identified the genes responsible for this disturbance in HDL transport, opening
the way to the development of drugs to stimulate these transport mechanisms and thereby to elevate HDL levels.

A natural defense mechanism normally protects people against the harmful consequences of ingesting too much cholesterol, causing the intestinal
absorption of cholesterol and other dietary sterols to slow naturally. People
whose bodies fail to make this adjustment—and who then develop high
levels of LDL—often suffer from increased formation of coronary plaques.
Analysis of a rare metabolic defect called sitosterolemia has opened the way
to an understanding of excessive intestinal cholesterol absorption. Patients
with sitosterolemia accumulate abnormally high amounts of dietary sterols
(such as cholesterol) and have impaired elimination of sterols from the liver
into the bile. These people develop early heart disease and die young.

Studies of such patients have identified two genes whose products normally act to limit the intestinal absorption of sterols. In sitosterolemia, the

77. Braunwald and others (2001).
78. Cascieri (2002); Libby (2002), Braunwald and others (2001).
79. Bodzioch and others (1999); Brooks-Wilson and others (1999); Rust and others (1999).

mutant genes lead to massive cholesterol accumulation. If, as investigators now suspect, less severe defects in these genes and their protein products may lead to increased cholesterol in many otherwise normal individuals, drug treatments can counter this metabolic abnormality, possibly reducing the incidence of heart attacks. Recently, a drug that indirectly counteracts the defect in cholesterol accumulation in patients with sitosterolemia has been approved for use.[80]

Inflammation

Americans have higher cholesterol on average than residents of countries with a low incidence of heart disease.[81] However, cholesterol is not the only culprit in coronary artery disease. Even if cholesterol is in the normal range (in the United States), arterial inflammation has been shown to be responsible for heart attacks associated with unstable angina—defined as angina that has recently become more severe, that occurs even during bed rest, or that intensifies with a level of exercise that previously produced no symptoms. Inflammation, whether triggered by cholesterol deposits or other causes, seems to be another critical factor in the formation of plaque.

Evidence of inflammation has been identified by direct observation of the inflammatory cells in the coronary lesion and can now be predicted by measurements of key blood markers of immunologic activity.[82] One such marker is C-reactive protein (CRP). Elevated CRP indicates an increased likelihood of an impending heart attack even when cholesterol levels are normal, but the risk is much higher if both CRP and cholesterol are elevated.[83] New plaque fostered by inflammation probably explains why blockages recur in arteries soon after angioplasty. Coating stents with inflammation-fighting drugs discourages the recurrence of such blockages.

Some investigators speculate that bacterial infection may contribute to inflammation in coronary arteries just as Helicobacter pylori contributes to stomach ulcers. In fact a bacterium—Chlamydia pneumoniae—has been identified in many diseased coronary arteries, although a cause-effect relationship is still only speculative. Just as combining antibiotic therapy with standard antiulcer treatment greatly improves control of ulcers, so too some

---

80. Berge and others (2000); Allayee, Laffittee, and Lusis (2000); Earl and Kirkpatrick (2003).
81. Daniel Steinberg (2002).
82. Libby (2002); Buffon and others (2002); Keaney and Vita (2002); Daniel Steinberg (2002).
83. Libby (2002); Buffon and others (2002); Daniel Steinberg (2002).

patients with coronary artery disease may also respond to treatment of infection in future years. The observed reduction of heart attacks in patients treated with statins may be due to the combined effects of lowering cholesterol and reducing inflammation.[84] Better understanding of the role of inflammation as well as improving its management may help treat coronary artery disease.

Stimulating Blood Vessel Growth

As coronary arteries become blocked, the flow of oxygen to the heart muscle diminishes, and angina (pain) results. When an artery is entirely blocked, the part of the heart muscle served by the blocked artery receives no oxygen and dies. One way to treat coronary artery disease is to improve the blood supply to the oxygen-starved heart by stimulating the growth of new blood vessels. And one way to stimulate the growth of new blood vessels is by increasing the amounts of vascular endothelial growth factor (VEGF) in the heart tissue, either by injecting the DNA for VEGF directly into the heart tissue or through viral gene therapy.[85] Experiments with delivering VEGF into the cardiac muscle of heart patients and of experimental animals with induced coronary artery disease have indeed increased the growth of blood vessels. The results in the animal experiments are encouraging. Although only limited success is so far reported in the human trials, optimism that the approach will be useful remains high.

Cardiovascular Disease in the Future

Over the next several decades some or all of the new approaches for dealing with heart disease will likely have major beneficial effects. Progress is being made in discovering how stem cells—the early-stage, undifferentiated human cells capable of growing into various specialized forms—might be used to repair hearts damaged by coronary disease. Better control of blood levels of fat, ways to raise HDL cholesterol and lower absorption of total cholesterol, methods of reducing coronary artery inflammation, techniques for stimulating new growth of blood vessels in the heart, and ability to repair damaged hearts with stem cells are likely, in one combination or another, to further decrease mortality from heart attacks.

84. LaRosa, He, and Vupputuri (1999).
85. Freedman and Isner (2002).

Infectious Disease

Infectious disease once led all illnesses as a cause of death. Advances in medical care—the development of antibiotics and improvements in public health (notably clean water and vaccinations)—have sharply lowered death rates from infectious disease over the last century. Unfortunately, infectious disease remains a latent danger.

A major problem is that some bacteria are now resistant to all known antibiotics. A second issue is the ever-present possibility of widespread viral infections, against which antibiotics are largely ineffective. Until the last few decades, bacterial, not viral, infection was the principle cause of fatal infectious disease. However, viruses now pose a rising global health problem: the human immunodeficiency virus (HIV), the hepatitis B virus, and the hepatitis C virus are currently worldwide infections (although in the United States and other sociologically stable societies, the diseases spare most of the population). Although the influenza virus is checked in part by vaccination, it remains a threat. In the 1918 pandemic, one variant caused the deaths of 21 million people worldwide (500,000 of them in the United States).[86] Intense activity by international public health organizations has contained such contagious and lethal viruses as Ebola and Hanta, but future success with other viruses is not ensured (as emphasized by the 2003 SARS outbreak). A deadly contagion could devastate today's world, with its much larger population, increased urbanization, and global travel; a second pandemic such as in 1918 is only too possible. Finally, bioterrorists could deliberately create epidemics. All these threats are real, but so too is the possibility that medical and scientific advances could largely eliminate infectious disease as a cause of death and disability.

Why Antibiotic Resistance Arises

Antibiotics attack critical steps in bacterial life cycles, such as stopping formation of cell walls or blocking synthesis of critical proteins or bacterial DNA. However, bacteria divide very rapidly. A mutation in a single bacterium may produce a variant that is resistant to antibiotics and therefore can quickly become dominant.

The molecular mechanisms that create such resistance have been identified, and other new antibiotics have been found to kill the resistant bacteria by attacking at different steps in bacterial reproduction. Bacterial mutation,

86. Cohen (2000).

unfortunately, eventually overcomes the effectiveness of a second (and even a third) antibiotic. Although some infectious disease experts are concerned that we are losing the battle, rapid advances in the characterization of complete bacterial genomes offer many new targets for antibiotic development and therefore give promise that bacterial infection can be controlled.[87]

Overcoming Bacterial Resistance

Currently available antibiotics target only about twelve gene products of disease-causing bacteria, but scientists, using techniques developed in the Human Genome Project, have identified the complete genome of many pathogenic bacteria, including cholera and tuberculosis.[88] Efforts are now under way to determine which of the many genes discovered are critical for bacterial reproduction and which are potential targets for new antibiotics.[89]

The success in combating the rapidly mutating HIV virus with several independently acting antiviral agents used simultaneously suggests a new strategy for controlling bacterial infection. The various agents act at different critical loci in viral replication. One blocks an enzyme that translates the viral genome; another blocks the formation of the protein coat that the virus needs to spread to other cells; while a third blocks the point of entry of HIV into the cells.[90] Blocking the virus at several points makes it statistically unlikely that enough mutations will occur for the virus to escape all lines of attack. The multiyear survival of many HIV patients in the United States attests to the success of this strategy.[91]

Host Resistance Genes

Certain genes appear to confer heightened resistance to infection.[92] Because people of European ancestry apparently have a variant receptor on immune cells, they are in general more resistant to HIV infections than people from Africa, the Middle East, and Asia. Molecular detectives note that this recep-

---

87. Cassell and Mekalanos (2001).

88. International Human Genome Sequencing Consortium (2001); Cassell and Mekalanos (2001).

89. Dziejman and others (2002); Cassell and Mekalanos (2001).

90. Hammer (2002); Pomerantz and Horn (2003).

91. The treatment sometimes fails, perhaps because of drug side effects and the complex and demanding treatment schedules that make adherence to treatment protocols difficult.

92. Cassell and Mekalanos (2001).

tor confers resistance to the organism responsible for plague and hypothesize that the prevalence of this gene increased in the Middle Ages, when individuals with the variant receptors were those more likely to survive the plague.[93]

Other gene mutations contribute to resistance to malaria.[94] One mutation normally plays an important role in the function of red blood cells (the target of malaria) and renders them resistant to infection through processes that are not yet fully understood. This mutation arose in African and Mediterranean populations 2,000 or more years ago, when malaria first appeared with devastating effect. The improved survival of people with this mutation explains its persistence in these African and Mediterranean populations.

The identification of additional hereditary resistance factors and the mechanism by which they foster resistance to infection would offer a new way to combat infection. Simultaneous study of the genes of the microbe and the host should lead to better tools for control of infections through a two-pronged approach: the development of new antibiotics and antiviral agents and using them synergistically; and the development of drugs that strengthen human resistance.

Frontiers for Viral Therapy

As knowledge of entire viral genomes increases, specific antiviral therapies should follow. A few successes point the way, most notably the great strides in treatment of AIDS. New drugs inhibit influenza virus replication by inhibiting an enzyme—neuraminidase—that is critical to the release of newly formed influenza viruses from infected cells. Drugs that inhibit this enzyme reduce the severity of influenza if given immediately after infection. They also prevent infection when given to those who have been in close contact with infected people but have not yet developed the disease.[95]

Recent identification of a previously unknown role for RNA may lead to a new form of antiviral therapy based on the application of a newly discovered cellular system—termed RNA$_i$—that can destroy the specific messenger RNA molecules that direct protein synthesis. RNA molecules can thus be designed to recognize and inactivate unwanted viral RNA messages, thereby specifically blocking viral infection. Studies with human cells grown in tissue

93. Chakravarti (2001).
94. Volkman and others (2001); Tishkoff and others (2001); Luzzatto and Notaro (2001).
95. Elliott (2001).

culture indicate that the technology can protect against the polio virus and HIV; these results will now be tested in experimental animals.[96]

The Potential of Vaccines

Over the last century vaccines were successful in combating viral and, more recently, bacterial infection. A weakened strain of bacteria, virus, or inactivated toxin is administered to stimulate the immune system and to provide long-term protection without causing debilitating infection or toxicity. Smallpox has been entirely eliminated. Polio may be next. Childhood diseases such as tetanus, pertussis, diphtheria, measles, mumps, and rubella (German measles) have been greatly reduced.[97] Antibacterial vaccines have been effective against pneumococcal pneumonia, and a vaccine is under development against the toxin produced by anthrax. In general, vaccines can be the ideal method of counteracting disease: In the case of AIDS, for example, the cost and complexity of current antiviral treatment means that vaccination may be the only economically feasible method to stop the spread of HIV in poor nations. Vaccines may also be the only practical way to control malaria and tuberculosis. Perhaps the RNA$_i$ approach will develop into an entirely new concept in vaccination: an intracellular vaccination against HIV and other infectious agents.

Infectious Disease in the Twenty-First Century

The first goal of the struggle against infectious disease must be to sustain the progress already made. Historically, such bacterial infections as tuberculosis, bacterial pneumonia, meningitis, and septicemia (bloodstream infection) were deadly. In the last half of the twentieth century antibiotics arrested these scourges. Rapid increases in drug resistance threaten to undo these gains, but emerging strategies to counter the threat are encouraging. New classes of antibiotics will be developed and used in combination to prevent resistance.

---

96. Either of two approaches works well. One involves designing RNA molecules that are an exact copy of a critical piece of the viral RNA and delivering them into cells before infecting the cells with virus. The second involves genetically modifying the cells so that they themselves make the short fragment of viral RNA. When the virus enters these latter cells and attempts to reproduce, the blocking RNAi is produced, and the viral infection is stopped completely. Much further work on these approaches will be needed, including use of live animal models to test efficacy and safety before considering human testing. These methods, however, could be the antiviral treatments of the future. Carmichael (2002); Jacque, Triques, and Stevenson (2002).

97. Palese and Garcia-Sastre (2002a, 2002b).

Simultaneously using drugs that promote host resistance provides an entirely new approach, as do emerging antiviral therapies and vaccines.

Obesity

At an estimated 300,000 deaths a year, obesity is beginning to rival cancer and heart disease as a leading cause of death in the United States. If it goes unchecked, obesity may replace these diseases, particularly if progress continues in their prevention and treatment. Up to one-third of the U.S. population is now obese.[98] The rate is even higher in children, particularly in inner-city schools. Obesity increases the risk of hypertension, heart disease, stroke, cancer, diabetes, and early death.[99] Roughly half of obese individuals suffer from type 2 (insulin-resistant) diabetes, which increases the complications of other obesity-related illness. It aggravates heart disease; causes kidney, eye, and nerve degeneration; and increases susceptibility to infection.[100]

The Cause Lies in Our Genes

There is no satisfactory answer for this vast increase in obesity. Genetic factors determine body mass, leanness, and tendency to obesity. Human genes have not suddenly changed, but our environment has. Humans existed on the cusp of starvation for thousands of years. Genes promoting the ability to store fat when food is plentiful are important for survival during periods when nourishment is severely limited and starvation threatens. An obese human of 250 pounds has enough stored fat to serve as an energy source to survive a total absence of food for up to 150 days. Fat is the ideal way to store energy because it takes up the least space. When food is limited or periodically unavailable, fat storage may be lifesaving. However, most contemporary Americans face the opposite problem.

Strong evidence suggests that humans have genes that predispose them to obesity. In carefully controlled overfeeding experiments, it has been shown that although pairs of twins differ considerably from one another in the amount of fat they accumulate, the amount of fat accumulated by each twin within a pair is nearly identical. Obese twins have the genetic disposition to gain excess fat when food is plentiful.[101]

98. Spiegelman and Flier (2001).
99. Spiegelman and Flier (2001); Friedman (2000).
100. Shulman (2000).
101. Friedman (2000); Spiegelman and Flier (2001); Savage and O'Rahilly (2002).

The Brain and Appetite Control

We are increasingly aware that weight is physiologically controlled by certain genetic factors and that being overweight is not simply the result of bad behavior. A number of genetic mutations have been found in obese people, and even more are being found in inbred strains of mice.[102] Studies of naturally obese mice led to the discovery of the hormone leptin and its receptor. Mice that lack either leptin or the leptin receptor become massively obese. Their body weight returns to normal when leptin is administered. Manipulation of this and other complex genetic systems that determine body mass may provide the basis for new treatments of obesity. Only a small fraction of obese people are leptin-deficient, but those who are respond well to leptin infusions—appetite diminishes and body weight returns to normal.

Other hormones help balance energy intake and use. It is now known, for example, that special regions of the brain control appetite through the production of particular proteins that stimulate or suppress appetite. The production of these appetite-regulating proteins are, in turn, controlled by leptin. As body fat increases, leptin production rises, the brain output of appetite-stimulating proteins is reduced, and the production of appetite-suppressing proteins is increased. These proteins then cause the brain to produce yet other hormones that directly control appetite.

Specific mutations in a key brain area cause severe obesity in mice; 4–5 percent of humans with severe obesity have a mutation in the same receptor.[103] This genetic defect, like the failure to produce leptin or the leptin receptor, joins the small list of genetic defects recognized in human obesity. Although most cases of obesity are not linked to any known genetic defect, still-unrecognized genes undoubtedly influence appetite.

Energy Consumption

Small cell components, the mitochondria, are the fuel centers of the body. They determine whether sugars and fats are stored or used immediately to generate heat. This heat generation is referred to as adaptive thermogenesis, the rate at which absorbed nutrients generate calories of heat.

Proteins in the mitochondria apparently control this process. Mutations in these proteins in mice cause the animals to become either massively obese or extremely sensitive to cold.[104] Drugs that stimulate these proteins hold out

102. Friedman (2000); Spiegelman and Flier (2001); Savage and O'Rahilly (2002).
103. Friedman (2000); Spiegelman and Flier (2001); Savage and O'Rahilly (2002).
104. Friedman (2000); Spiegelman and Flier (2001); Savage and O'Rahilly (2002).

the prospect that the body might be fooled into burning, rather than storing, calories. Thyroid hormone promotes weight loss in just this way and has occasionally been used in weight reduction programs. Most physicians regard such therapy as too dangerous to use routinely, however, because excess thyroid can damage the heart and weaken muscles. Recent research on the newly recognized mitochondrial proteins that more selectively control adaptive thermogenesis is quite promising.[105]

The Stomach

While the leptin-brain regulatory system influences appetite over days or weeks, ghrelin, a hormone produced in the stomach, influences appetite immediately.[106] Infusing this hormone into animals causes a massive increase in food intake and weight gain. It also makes humans feel hungry. Strict diets have been shown to boost ghrelin levels, a response that helps explain why such diets often fail. Many massively obese and desperate individuals undergo gastric bypass surgery to reduce the physical size of their stomachs. The mechanism was thought to be that reduction of stomach volume makes overeating uncomfortable and thus often leads to major weight loss. The surprise is that ghrelin levels fall dramatically in such patients. Reduced ghrelin production, rather than reduced stomach volume, may explain why this extreme intervention succeeds. If so, finding ways to block ghrelin production by drugs may replace the need for surgery.

Diabetes

With increased obesity has come a striking growth of insulin-resistant (type 2) diabetes, which, according to current estimates, will affect one American in four by the age of sixty-five.[107] Insulin resistance can often be detected before diabetes (defined as loss of blood sugar control) develops. Recent work suggests that the high fatty acid levels in blood that occur in obesity trigger insulin resistance. Understanding the causes of insulin resistance will pave the way for its reversal by appropriate medication.

The successful treatment of a rare disease called lipodystrophy has yielded a dramatic and encouraging approach to the treatment of both type 2 diabetes and insulin resistance. In lipodystrophy an almost complete absence of

---

105. Friedman (2000); Spiegelman and Flier (2001); Savage and O'Rahilly (2002).
106. Flier and Maratos-Flier (2002).
107. Shulman (2000).

body fat is accompanied by severe insulin resistance and diabetes. Patients with the disease have practically no leptin, since they have no fat cells. Infusions of leptin dramatically reverse their insulin resistance.[108] Some obese individuals appear to have partial leptin deficiency. If administration of leptin in cases of lipodystrophy successfully treats diabetes, it might be possible that treating obese patients with inadequate leptin levels will also improve their diabetes.[109]

Obesity in the Future

Increased understanding of the fundamental control of fuel in the body and the causes of obesity offer some exciting possibilities for treatment. Effective new drugs to combat obesity and type 2 diabetes are likely to be discovered in the next two decades. In addition, improved diets (particularly for children) and exercise programs can avert what otherwise could become a major obstacle to increased longevity. It is known, for example, that weight reduction and exercise in patients with insulin resistance can prevent the development of full-blown diabetes.[110]

Neurodegenerative Disease

Few effective treatments for neurodegenerative diseases have been found.[111] Only modest and transient benefits come from interferon treatment for multiple sclerosis, drugs to increase dopamine levels for Parkinson's disease, and agents to block the enzyme that degrades the neurotransmitter acetylcholine in Alzheimer's disease.[112]

Alzheimer's disease is the leading cause of dementia or senility in the elderly. It affects one eighty-five-year-old in three but can occur as early as the thirties in families with hereditary predisposition.[113] Victims initially suffer difficulties in cognition, particularly in short-term memory, and later become disoriented, apathetic, and unable to perform the activities of daily living, such as dressing and eating. Eventually, intellectual function completely dete-

108. Friedman (2000); Spiegelman and Flier (2001); Savage and O'Rahilly (2002).
109. Friedman (2000); Spiegelman and Flier (2001); Savage and O'Rahilly (2002).
110. Kenneth Chang, "Diet and Exercise Are Found to Cut Diabetes by over Half." *New York Times,* August 9, 2001, p. 16.
111. Martin (1999).
112. Braunwald and others (2001).
113. Martin (1999); Hardy and Selkoe (2002).

riorates. Autopsies of patients who died with advanced Alzheimer's reveal widespread death of brain cells, neurofibrillary tangles, and deposits of beta-amyloid, an abnormal protein.[114] According to one hypothesis, initial errors in metabolism of a normal brain protein leads to accumulations of beta-amyloid, which in turn kills brain cells. A test now exists for early detection of abnormal beta-amyloid accumulation, offering an opportunity to monitor the effectiveness in humans of animal experiments designed to reverse beta-amyloid buildup.[115]

In families with early-onset Alzheimer's disease and in genetically engineered mice, certain mutations greatly increase the production of beta-amyloid. Certain enzymes normally cut a protein, the amyloid precursor protein (APP), into fragments, which the body then eliminates. As a result of the mutations, more sticky pieces of APP are formed; these clump into beta-amyloid deposits. Accumulation of the beta-amyloid in the brains of experimental mice is associated with impaired brain behavior. Recently developed drugs block the effect of the enzymes that produce beta-amyloid in animals, reverse the protein buildup, and improve brain function. These drugs have yet to be tested in humans to evaluate safety and efficacy.[116]

It is still not established conclusively, however, that the buildup of beta-amyloid deposits initiates brain cell death. The correlation between mouse brain function and amount of amyloid is imperfect. And tests of brain function in mice are crude at best for predicting human cognitive behavior. Some but not all forms of beta-amyloid may be toxic, which could explain the poor correlation between size of deposits and their effect on brain function. Nonetheless, the bulk of evidence suggests that excess beta-amyloid formation and accumulation are central to the development of Alzheimer's disease.[117]

A reliable test to show increased beta-amyloid in the brains of patients with early-onset Alzheimer's, and in suspected cases in the elderly, is critical to detection and treatment. A recently developed radiological test to detect amyloid has generated excitement. A radioactive substance that binds to amyloid plaque is injected into the patient, after which a PET (positron emission tomography) scan is used. Large deposits of plaque appear only in the brains of patients with the cognitive deficiencies characteristic of Alzheimer's

114. Martin (1999); Hardy and Selkoe (2002).
115. Helmuth (2002).
116. Martin (1999); Hardy and Selkoe (2002); Maher (2002); Gerlai (2001); Esler and others (2002); Hock and others (2002); Selkoe (2001); Schenk, Games, and Seubert (2001).
117. Martin (1999); Hardy and Selkoe (2002); Maher (2002); Gerlai (2001); Esler and others (2002); Hock and others (2002); Selkoe (2001); Schenk, Games, and Seubert (2001).

disease and only in characteristic sites. In addition to enabling early detection, this test can be used to evaluate the success of treatment.[118]

One treatment uses antibodies to remove the amyloid deposit; other treatments use immunization, both active (giving beta-amyloid to elicit antibodies) and passive (giving preformed antibodies directed against the amyloid).[119] Passive immunization has shown promising results in mice: Amyloid plaques have been cleared from the brain, improving brain function. Serious complications have occurred, however, in early clinical trials of active immunization. Whether the approach might be made safer remains to be determined; some benefit has been reported in certain treated patients.[120] If indeed amyloid deposition proves to be key to the development of Alzheimer's disease, a new possibility may be opening for the management of this grim and relentless disorder.

Limits to Life Expectancy

In addition to demographic evidence of increasing mortality with age, there is support for the inevitability of senescence from basic theories of biological evolution. Steps in this reasoning are as follows.

The forces of natural selection operate to preserve the species primarily by success in reproduction. Genetic mutations, many of which are silent, occur at a constant rate in all species. Mutations that confer a functional advantage, however, are preserved because reproduction of these individuals is favored. The favorable gene is passed on; harmful mutations tend to disappear, since weakened individuals are less likely to reproduce. Deleterious mutations that arise after successful reproduction, however, have no selection pressure operating against them; the accumulation of harmful mutations in an individual after reproductive age is of little consequence to the health of the species but make the aging of the individual inevitable.[121] Unrelated, independent,

118. Bacskai and others (2001); Helmuth (2002).

119. D. Steinberg (2002b); Hock and others (2002); Barinaga (1999).

120. Because some patients immunized against beta-amyloid developed a severe brain inflammation, the trial was halted. The patients improved after treatments to reduce inflammation. They are being carefully followed to determine whether brain function improves. Further studies of these immunized patients has already provided some encouraging information. Samples of blood and spinal fluid from the treated patients were obtained, and the nature of the antibodies was carefully examined. They were directed against the "bad" beta-amyloid only, not the normal proteins of the brain, such as the amyloid precursor. This result suggests that using antibody approaches may still be useful, but safety issues, careful patient selection (milder cases), and many related factors need to be properly addressed. Use of slowly increasing doses of preformed antibodies made against beta-amyloid might be safer.

121. Charlesworth and Partridge (1997).

but harmful genetic events happen in a random manner with time and have a cumulative deleterious effect, it is argued, so that aging and death are inevitable.

The Experimental Evidence

An impressive body of data gathered in recent decades counters this view, however.[122] Evidence that certain genes can determine longevity comes from experiments involving selective breeding only of long-lived members of a group of fruit flies; mating cycles repeated many times produced a cohort of uniformly longer-lived fruit flies, with an average life span double that of the starting population.[123] These experiments are a form of directed evolution under controlled conditions in a laboratory setting, where the effort is to favor life span increase (mere survival is not the issue, as it is in natural evolution). The success of such experiments in part counters the evolutionary argument that aging is genetically inevitable due to an accumulation of errors. Genes for longevity (even capable of overriding or correcting harmful genetic mutations) existed in humans but were not apparent since they had little impact on survival under the harsh environmental circumstances that caused early death of humans for millennia. The existence of such genes would only become apparent in recent human history.

That prolongation of life may involve only a few genes is supported by other studies in fruit flies, worms, and yeast; it has been demonstrated that even single gene mutations can remarkably increase life span.[124] Gene mutations associated with longer life span were similar in each species. Some genetic changes increase resistance to injury from agents that tend to oxidize and kill cells. Others involve reduction in the activity of insulinlike genes.[125]

The life spans of mammals have also been greatly increased experimentally. Caloric restriction increases life span significantly in rodents. Caloric restriction seems to operate through insulin sensitivity, one of the genetic changes important in the prolongation of life span in fruit flies and worms. Another spontaneously arising gene mutation in mice has been shown to extend life span by about 30 percent; the mutation helps cells resist death from harmful

122. Helfand and Inouye (2002).
123. Strauss (2001); Melov and others (2000); Wolkow and others (2000); Lee and others (1999); Alfred (2001); Migliaccio and others (1999); Fabrizio and others (2001); Guarente and Kenyan (2000).
124. Strauss (2001); Melov and others (2000); Wolkow and others (2000); Lee and others (1999); Alfred (2001); Migliaccio and others (1999); Fabrizio and others (2001); Guarente and Kenyan (2000).
125. Parkes and others (1998).

agents that cause oxidative damage, the other genetic mechanism that operates in fruit flies.[126]

The Evidence in Humans

Laboratory evidence that division of human cells grown in the laboratory stops after fifty to sixty divisions (replicative senescence) was used to argue the inevitability of aging in humans.[127] It is now clear, however, that cell division does not stop because random mutations destroy the viability of the cell. Rather, each cell has a remarkable mechanism that keeps track of the number of its divisions and stops dividing after the preset number is reached. Sections of DNA called telomeres lie at the end of each chromosome.[128] With each cell division the telomeres shorten unless the enzyme telomerase is present in amounts sufficient to relengthen them. When telomeres become quite short, the cell stops dividing. When telomerase is introduced artificially, the cell becomes essentially immortal and continues to divide indefinitely.[129]

Other evidence reveals that normal human aging results from coordinated, rather than random, genetic changes and that this process may be subject to genetic control. A systematic study of gene activity reveals that, in all individuals studied, 1 percent of some 6,000 genes have consistent patterns of change with aging. Children suffering from progeria, a rare but well recognized disease of premature aging, display the same pattern of changes in gene activity but decades earlier than in normally aging individuals.[130] Because only one or at most a few genetic mutations explain progeria, perhaps just a few genes control the several hundred that regulate normal aging.

A growing body of demographic evidence in humans suggests that aging is influenced by genetic factors.[131] For example, a surprising number of centenarians have been verified among a rather closed population in Sardinia. In France, a study of some five generations of the family of a woman who died at the age of 122 (the longest documented life span) reveals a much higher proportion of long-lived individuals than in a control group. In the United States, the life spans of approximately 2,000 siblings of centenarians were

---

126. Strauss (2001); Melov and others (2000); Wolkow and others (2000); Lee and others (1999); Alfred (2001); Migliaccio and others (1999); Fabrizio and others (2001); Guarente and Kenyan (2000).
127. Hayflick (2000).
128. Stewart and Weinberg (2002).
129. Stewart and Weinberg (2002).
130. Marx (2000b).
131. Perls and others (2002); Puca and others (2001); Koenig (2001); Robine and Allard (1998).

compared with life spans of siblings of noncentenarians.[132] Siblings of the centenarians lived sixteen to seventeen years longer than those in the control population, strongly suggesting a genetic basis of longevity. One group believes they have identified a gene locus for longevity in American centenarians.[133]

Therapeutic and Ethical Considerations

Longevity may not be synonymous with health and vigor. Are some centenarians vigorous because their genes resist disease, or do they have genes that slow the onset of coordinated genetic changes that cause aging (identified in children with progeria and in normally aging individuals)? The evidence leads to the cautious prediction that there may indeed be the latter type of gene, one that slows coordinated change. If this is true, it may be possible to increase the human life span without senescence. If and when genes associated with longevity are identified, pressure will be overwhelming to test the effects of the products of such genes to prolong life in humans. Obviously, great caution will be needed. Interfering with telomere shortening, for example, may increase the risk of cancer, since telomeres operate on the same checkpoint controls where mutations induce cancer.

The biology of senescence is complex, and current knowledge is fragmentary. Fortunately, model systems such as that of the mouse, which has been used to study the functions of human genes in cancer, could be used to study the activity and safety of genes or gene products identified as candidates for healthy longevity. Numerous ethical questions will arise if it ultimately develops that it is possible to significantly prolong health and vigor along with life span. For example, can studies in longevity be justified given the gap in health care between advanced and developing nations and given that so many people die young from lack of simple public health care measures?

On the other hand, with growing success in reducing death from disease comes the need to ensure that the elderly maintain their vigor and independence. Otherwise, what we anticipate as progress would become a disaster if the result is a large population of weak and dispirited elderly. As with other, sometimes startling, challenges arising from the current revolution in biology, a responsible ethical pathway will need to be found.

The following chapters present analyses by economists, ethicists, and other social scientists who consider the problems as well as the opportunities that will arise from an accelerated pace in present-day biomedical progress.

132. Perls and others (2002); Puca and others (2001); Koenig (2001); Robine and Allard (1998).
133. Puca and others (2001).

COMMENT
Nicholas Wade

The chapter by John Potts and William Schwartz provides an authoritative description of the present ferment in biomedical research and the high hopes that this very interesting brew will prove to be a significant tonic for human health. Here, I assess the ways in which this research might effect human longevity; I then consider some of the practical difficulties that could hinder its implementation.

The New Interest in Longevity

It is certainly remarkable that the possibility of a major increase in life expectancy has now become the subject of serious discussion. The search for the fountain of youth has long been regarded as an archetypal human delusion. Rejuvenation treatments have been in distinct disfavor since the 1930s, when patients paid large sums to be injected with extracts of goat or monkey glands. Until recently, research on aging was something of a scientific backwater, and there were powerful reasons for thinking that no dramatic change in human longevity would ever be possible.

The change in outlook has been prompted by the recent undermining of three tenets that seemed to place ineluctable constraints on human longevity. These are the Gompertz rule, the theory of evolutionary biology, and the Hayflick limit. The first, laid down in the nineteenth century by the mathematician Benjamin Gompertz, holds that after puberty the human death rate doubles every eight years. These are hard odds to beat. Evolutionary biologists meanwhile formulated the theory that evolution favors any gene that helps an animal survive to the age of reproduction but not beyond. Moreover, so many genes must be involved in determining senescence that there is no practical way of altering all of them. The Hayflick limit is the observation by Leonard Hayflick that human cells grown in culture will grow and divide a finite number of times, usually about fifty or so, depending on the cell type. This limit seemed firmly to constrain human life, since it was easy to imagine the body's cells eventually losing their regenerative powers after they had used up their allotted number of divisions.

These constraints have not been overthrown, but each now seems far less ironclad than before. Human populations live longer than they did in Gompertz's day, and we can see that the Gompertz curve tends to flatten out. Past a certain age, the increase in the death rate decelerates, as if once you make it to a certain age, around seventy-five to eighty-nine, your chances of dying worsen much more slowly.

The gloomy expectations of the evolutionary biologists have also been contradicted, it would seem, by experimental biologists who, by manipulating single genes in worms or fruit flies, have made these animals live significantly longer. The strong implication here is that the genetic manipulation of life span may be less daunting than the evolutionary biologists have made it appear. And the Hayflick limit has now been broken; biologists have acquired a detailed understanding of the cells' system for counting cell divisions; they know, too, how to override the division-counting mechanism and "immortalize" the cells, which, in biologists' parlance, means enabling cells in a petri dish to grow and divide indefinitely.

There is therefore the beginning of a surprising new optimism among cell biologists that something can be done to extend human longevity, just as soon as they can understand the genes that control it.

The advances described by Potts and Schwartz lead in many directions, but I think it is useful to distinguish between the steady upward drift in human life spans and a sharp increase that some dramatic advance might bring about. We can assume that medical research will continue in a general way to contribute to the steady upward drift in human longevity. Our social and financial systems have already learned how to accommodate the gentle age inflation that has now been under way for at least a century in most developed countries. But the focus of this volume is a major increase in longevity, which I assume implies some advance or set of advances that causes a sharp departure from the background trend. There are at present three sources from which such an advance might come: regenerative medicine, caloric restriction, and life-span manipulation.

Regenerative Medicine

Regenerative medicine is a therapy that at present exists almost entirely on paper but that seems to have a strong future. Its basic idea is that the body knows better how to heal itself than we do. It does so with stem cells and the signaling factors that control and cue them. The surgeon's knife and the pharmacist's potent chemicals are crude tools compared with the body's own cells, if only we knew how to direct them.

A major premise of regenerative medicine is that the body is a self-assembling system. With the mouse, at least, you can take an embryonic stem cell and drive it down the lineage toward becoming a pancreatic islet cell. In test tube experiments, the cell will differentiate into the four cell types of the islet, one of which produces insulin, and the cells will assemble themselves into structures that resemble those seen in natural islets.[1] This leads one to hope that we can grow new organs without fully understanding what we are doing; just get the right stem cells and let *them* figure out what is needed.

One of the most elegant ideas for deploying stem cells concerns repair of the heart. People have been looking for years for the heart's stem cells, without success. It now seems they were looking in the wrong place. The heart's stem cells apparently reside in the bone marrow, not the heart. And the bone marrow's stem cells can be mobilized by special hormones that make them rush out into the bloodstream and look for damaged tissue. So it could be that this mobilizing hormone, already used widely as a substitute for bone marrow transplants, could also treat heart attacks, a possibility now being addressed in rats.[2]

Stem cells are the basic clay from which the body is sculpted. The embryonic cells form the body in the womb, then disappear, bequeathing to the adult stem cells the duty of maintaining the body's tissues throughout life. It remains to be seen how far we can shape this living clay to our purposes. But suppose that we learn how to take a patient's own stem cells and use them to repair or replace damaged organs. We would have fashioned an extraordinary technique for overcoming many of the degenerative diseases of old age. Such an advance could well lead to a quantum leap in life expectancy.

Caloric Restriction

A second line of research that might provide a sharp increase in longevity is that of caloric restriction. A calorically restricted diet includes all necessary vitamins and minerals; it differs from a normal diet simply in having 30 percent fewer calories. This is the one easy intervention that we know increases the longevity of rats and mice. (Castration, too, prolongs life.) The increase is dramatic: up to 40 percent if the diet is started in infancy. There is still a benefit, though smaller, if the diet is started in later life. This is an important fact; if caloric restriction should work for people, too, it means the diet could be started later, perhaps after the childbearing years. We do not yet know

1. Lumelsky and others (2001).
2. Orlic and others (2001).

if caloric restriction will work in humans; monkey experiments have been under way for some years, but since the normal life span of rhesus monkeys in captivity is forty years, it takes a long time to show results.[3]

It seems quite probable, however, that the life extension caused by caloric restriction is shared by all animals. What is happening is that a calorically restricted diet triggers an ancient reflex, that of postponing reproduction when food is scarce. The body's resources are switched from breeding to body maintenance, in the hope that the organism can ride out a famine and produce its progeny when good times return. Some of the genes that extend life span in experimental roundworms or fruit flies probably work by triggering this mechanism.

Assuming that the caloric restriction mechanism exists in people too, would it help increase life span? By itself, probably not. We do not possess the will power to reduce our calories by 30 percent, not even if an extra twenty years of life might depend on it. Half of Americans are overweight, and 20 percent are obese.[4] Biologists therefore hope that they will be able to identify the genes that mediate the caloric restriction response and then to devise drugs to switch on this genetic circuit. Such a drug could have a major impact on populationwide longevity because, unless it were very expensive, large numbers of people might start taking it immediately. Calorically restricted animals enjoy good health; with luck, everyone would live longer and be a lot thinner.

The caloric restriction pill is likely to have important side effect, however. Evolutionary biologists like to point out the frequent trade-off between longevity and fertility. Live quickly and breed prolifically, like the rabbit, or live long and gestate slowly, like the elephant. Mice on a calorically restricted diet switch their resources from breeding to bodily maintenance. They do not reproduce at all. Their Darwinian fitness has been reduced to zero. So the caloric restriction pill, it might seem, would do double duty as a birth control pill.

Life-Span Manipulation

A third possible source of a major increase in longevity would be the discovery of genes that control life span itself. The caloric restriction mechanism

3. Wade (2001).

4. Humphrey Taylor, "The Obesity Epidemic Is Getting Even Worse," March 6, 2002 (www.harrisinteractive.com/harris_poll/printerfriend/index.asp?pid=288).

does not itself determine life span; it simply modulates some deeper program. Though biologists understand little about this deeper program, it is clearly tunable by evolution.

Mice in the wild live about four months. Suppose you design a mouse that could live a hundred months. It would never get to enjoy 96 percent of them. So nature has designed mice to live in the fast lane, breeding prolifically before the barn owl strikes. Elephants, on the other hand, with no natural predators except people, have evolved a life span of seventy years. Many shellfish, like the common mussel, live more than a hundred years. Redwoods can live beyond a thousand years. The bristlecone pine lives five thousand years.[5] It is evident, therefore, that living cells can support a wide range of life spans. This is a provocative fact because if life spans are tunable they are under genetic control, and once we discover those genes and how they work we will in principle be able to manipulate them.

Some biologists believe life span is controlled as directly as puberty and menopause, by hormones released from the brain. Gary Ruvkun, a cell biologist at the Massachusetts General Hospital, has found indirect evidence for a youthfulness hormone at work in roundworms.[6] The hormone, in his view, works to keep the worm young and vigorous until it has reproduced. After reproduction, the hormone is switched off, and the worm's whole body falls apart. Such a mechanism might explain why in people sometimes everything seems to give out at about the same time. Many other biologists, however, remain to be persuaded that any such process is at work in people.

Suppose we do learn to manipulate life span, whether through a putative youthfulness hormone or other means. How far might we extend it? We are only just beginning to understand the rules for the construction and maintenance of multicellular organisms, but it is clear that our bodies, despite their eventual fragility, are extraordinarily robust. Many of our organs are constantly renewed. Red blood cells get replaced every 120 days. The intestinal lining is continually sloughed off and replenished. Our skin regularly turns over, though we shed it cell by cell, not whole like a snake. Even the skeleton is replaced every seven years. No one knows why the renewal does not continue indefinitely, unless perhaps the stem cells that govern the repair of each tissue themselves fail to renew.

Not only are many organs continually renewed, but also the cells of which they are composed are robust. For long-lived animals, the problem is how

5. Finch (1990, p. 208).
6. See Wolkow and others (2000).

to constrain and limit the cells' vigor. That is probably the reason for the Hayflick limit, whose constraint on the number of permissible divisions serves as a last-ditch defense against cancer. A special class of our cells is in fact so vigorous that they are immortal, at least in the sense that biological time stands still for them. These of course are the egg and sperm cells. These germ line cells do not age. The proof is the fact that babies are born equally young, whatever the age of their parents.

Given the underlying robustness of cells and organs, it seems quite possible that human lifetimes of great length could in principle be supported once we understand how to manipulate the genes that influence longevity.

Longer Life and Its Opponents

When can we expect to enjoy these major increases in longevity? Potts and Schwartz give no timetable for the implementation of the advances they describe, and I follow their prudent example. But I would note a curious fact of trying to forecast biotechnology (which others have remarked on): that small advances often seem to take much longer than expected and big ones much less. The remarkable new drug Gleevec, which secures remissions in most early cases of chronic myelogenous leukemia, stems directly from discoveries made in the early 1980s; it is hard in retrospect to understand why it took twenty years to develop this drug. On the other hand, probably few people expected the human genome to be sequenced, at least in draft form, as soon as it was. Longevity increases might be one of those big steps that arrive much sooner than expected. However, genomics, expected to be a major driver of pharmaceutical innovation, has so far produced only indigestion. Research and development costs have soared, but the number of new drugs approved has slumped.[7] Gene therapy, as Potts and Schwartz point out, has been consistently disappointing.

Even if a technical means of increasing longevity is developed, one cannot assume that it will be free of political and ethical controversy. This may seem surprising, since extra life with good health seems so obviously desirable. But some people object on various grounds to extending life span. Many fear it would lead to an unwelcome and unmanageable increase in population. Others feel that extreme longevity is a somehow sacrilegious interference in the natural human cycle of birth, procreation, and death.

7. Pollack (2002).

What single property would more profoundly change human nature than immortality?

At a conference on immortality, several ethicists and theologians pronounced themselves seriously opposed to specific attempts to increase human life span.[8] The Reverend Richard J. Neuhaus, of the Institute on Religion and Public Life, calls the search for immortality "a pagan and sub-Christian quest" driven by the "essentially amoral and mindless dynamic of the technological imperative joined to an ignoble fear of death."

The ethicist Leon Kass, then of the University of Chicago and now the chairman of the President's Council on Bioethics, says that "to argue that human life is better without death is to argue that human life would be better without being human." The finitude of human life, in his view, "is a blessing for every individual whether he knows it or not." Kass's belief is that death gives meaning to life and that without a clear end point we would accomplish nothing—a point familiar enough to journalists, whose productivity depends on firm deadlines. Kass also notes that the new immortals "would not be like us at all." Even a doubling, say, of human life span would create a class of people with such different horizons that they might differ profoundly in nature from their fellow citizens.

Though I do not think Kass would win an election on this prodeath platform, his reservations cannot be airily dismissed. The gift of many extra years of life and health, however desirable, is not one to be accepted lightly.

8. Wade (2001).

References

Alfred, Jane. 2001. "The Fly That Won't Die." *Nature Reviews Genetics* 2 (2): 83.

Allayee, Hooman, Bryan A. Laffittee, and Aldons Lusis. 2000. "An Absorbing Study of Cholesterol." *Science* 290 (5497): 1709–11.

Altshuler, David, and others. 2000. "The Common PPARgamma Pro12Ala Polymorphism Is Associated with Decreased Risk of Type 2 Diabetes." *Nature Genetics* 26 (1): 76–80.

Anderson, Robert N. 2001. "Deaths: Leading Causes for 1999." *National Vital Statistics Reports* 49 (11): 1–8.

Anversa, Piero, and Bernardo Nadal-Ginard. 2002. "Mycocyte Renewal and Ventricular Remodeling." *Nature* 415 (6868): 240–43.

Bacskai, Brian J., and others. 2001. "Imaging of Amyloid-Beta Deposits in Brains of Living Mice Permits Direct Observation of Clearance of Plaques with Immunotherapy." *Nature Medicine* 7 (3): 369–72.

Barinaga, Marcia. 1999. "An Immunization against Alzheimer's?" *Science* 285 (5425): 175–77.

Berge, Kjetil, and others. 2000. "Accumulation of Dietary Cholesterol in Sitosterolemia Caused by Mutations in Adjacent ABC Transporters." *Science* 290 (5497): 1771–75.

Bodzioch, Marek, and others. 1999. "The Gene-Encoding ATP-Binding Cassette Transporter 1 Is Mutated in Tangier Disease." *Nature Genetics* 22 (4): 347–51.

Bonetta, Laura. 2002. "Leukemia Case Triggers Gene-Therapy Controls." *Nature Medicine* 8 (11): 1189.

Braunwald, E., and others, eds. 2001. *Harrison's Principles of Internal Medicine.* 15th ed. McGraw-Hill.

Brooks-Wilson, Angela, and others. 1999. "Mutations in ABC1 in Tangier Disease and Familial High-Density Lipoprotein Deficiency." *Nature Genetics* 22 (4): 336–45.

Buffon, Antonio, and others. 2002. "Widespread Coronary Inflammation in Unstable Angina." *New England Journal of Medicine* 347 (1): 5–12.

Bumol, Thomas F., and August M. Watanabe. 2001. "Genetic Information, Genomic Technologies, and the Future of Drug Discovery." *Journal of the American Medical Association* 285 (5): 551–55.

Carmichael, Gordon G. 2002. "Silencing Viruses with RNA." *Nature* 418 (6896): 379–80.

Cascieri, M. A. 2002. "The Potential for Novel Antiinflammatory Therapies for Coronary Artery Disease." *Nature Reviews Drug Discovery* 1 (2): 122–30.

Cassell, Gail H., and John Mekalanos. 2001. "Development of Antimicrobial Agents in the Era of New and Reemerging Infectious Diseases and Increasing Antibiotic Resistance." *Journal of the American Medical Association* 285 (5): 601–05.

Cavazzana-Calvo, Marina, and others. 2000. "Gene Therapy of Human Severe Combined Immunodeficiency (SCID)-X1 Disease." *Science* 288 (5466): 669–72.

Centers for Disease Control/National Center for Health Services. 2002. "HHS Issues Report Showing Dramatic Improvements in Americans' Health over Past 50 years: Infant Mortality at Record Low, Life Expectancy at Record High." U.S. Department of Health and Human Services.

Chakravarti, Aravinda. 2001. "To a Future of Genetic Medicine." *Nature* 409 (6822): 822–23.

Charlesworth, Brian, and Linda Partridge 1997. "Aging: Leveling the Grim Reaper." *Current Biology* 7 (7): R440–R442.

Claverie, Jean-Michel. 2001. "What If There Are Only 30,000 Human Genes?" *Science* 291 (5507): 1255–57.

Cohen, Mitchell L. 2000. "Changing Patterns of Infectious Disease." *Nature Insight* 406 (6797): 762–67.

Committee on Science, Engineering, and Public Policy. 2002. *Scientific and Medical Aspects of Human Reproductive Cloning.* Washington: Board on Life Sciences, National Academy of Sciences.

Cooper, David K., B. Gollackner, and David H. Sachs 2002. "Will the Pig Solve the Transplantation Backlog?" *Annual Review of Medicine* 53: 133–47.

Cringely, Robert. 1998. "The Five Rules of Prognostication." *Forbes ASAP* 162 (November 30): 36.

Davaluri, Ramana V., Ivo Grosse, and Michael Q. Zhang. 2001. "Computational Identification of Promoters and First Exons in the Human Genome." *Nature Genetics* 29 (4): 412–17.

Dranoff, Glenn, and Richard Mulligan. 1995. "Gene Transfer as Cancer Therapy." *Advances in Immunology* 58: 417–54.

Dranoff, Glenn, and others. 1993. "Vaccination with Irradiated Tumor Cells Engineered to Secrete Murine Granulocyte-Macrophage Colony-Stimulating Factor Stimulates Potent, Specific, and Long-Lasting Antitumor Immunity." *Proceedings of the National Academy of Sciences USA* 90 (April): 3539–43.

Druker, Brian J., and Nicholas B. Lydon. 2000. "Lessons Learned from the Development of an Abl Tyrosine Kinase Inhibitor for Chronic Myelogenous Leukemia." *Journal of Clinical Investigation* 105 (1): 3–7.

Dye, Chris, and Nigel Gay. 2003. "Modeling the SARS Epidemic." *Science* 300 (5627): 1884–85.

Dziejman, Michelle, and others. 2002. "Comparative Genomic Analysis of *Vibrio Cholerae*: Genes That Correlate with Cholera Endemic and Pandemic Disease." *Proceedings of the National Academy of Sciences USA* 99 (3): 1556–61.

Earl, John, and Peter Kirkpatrick. 2003. "Fresh from the Pipeline: Ezetimibe." *Nature Reviews Drug Discoveries* 2 (2): 97–98.

Elliott, M. 2001. "Zanamivir: From Drug Design to the Clinic." *Philosophical Transactions of the Royal Society: Biological Sciences B* 356 (1416): 1885–93.

Esler, William P., and others. 2002. "Activity-Dependent Isolation of the Presenilin-Gamma-Secretase Complex Reveals Nicastrin and a Gamma Substrate." *Proceedings of the National Academy of Sciences USA* 99 (5): 2720–25.

Ezzell, Cora E. 2002. "Proteins Rule." *Scientific American* 286 (4): 40–47.

Fabrizio, Paola, and others. 2001. "Regulation of Longevity and Stress Resistance by Sch9 in Yeast." *Science* 292 (5515): 288–90.

Ferrara, Napoleone, and Kari Alitalo. 1999. "Clinical Applications of Angiogenic Growth Factors and Their Inhibitors." *Nature Medicine* 5 (12): 1359–64.

Finch, Caleb E. 1990. *Longevity, Senescence, and the Genome.* University of Chicago Press.

Flier, Jeffrey S., and Eleftheria Maratos-Flier. 2002. "The Stomach Speaks: Ghrelin and Weight Reduction." *New England Journal of Medicine* 346 (21): 1662–63.

Folkman, Judah, 1996. "Fighting Cancer by Attacking Its Blood Supply." *Scientific American* 275 (3): 150–54.

Freedman, Saul Benedict, and Jeffrey M. Isner. 2002. "Therapeutic Angiogenesis for Coronary Artery Disease." *Annals of Internal Medicine* 136 (1): 54–71.

Friedman, J. M. 2000. "Obesity in the New Millennium." *Nature* 404 (6778): 632–34.

Gerlai, Robert. 2001. "Alzheimer's Disease: Beta-Amyloid Hypothesis Strengthened!" *Trends in Neuroscience* 24 (4): 199.

Gilman, Alfred. 1996. "1994 Nobel Lecture: G Proteins and Regulation of Adenylyl Cyclase." In *Nobel Lectures: Physiology or Medicine, 1991–1995.* Singapore: World Scientific Publishing.

Griffith, Linda G., and Gail Naughton. 2002. "Tissue Engineering: Current Challenges and Expanding Opportunities." *Science* 295 (5557): 1009–14.

Griffith, May, and others. 1999. "Functional Human Corneal Equivalents Constructed from Cell Lines." *Science* 286 (5447): 2169–72.

Guarente, Leonard, and Cynthia Kenyan. 2000. "Genetic Pathways That Regulate Aging in Model Organisms." *Nature* 408 (6809): 255–62.

Guttmacher, Alan E., and Francis S. Collins. 2002. "Genomic Medicine: A Primer." *New England Journal of Medicine* 347 (19): 1512–20.

Haber, Daniel A., and Eric R. Fearon. 1998. "The Promise of Cancer Genetics." *Lancet* 351 (supp. 2): 1–8.

Hacein-Bey-Abina, Salima, and others. 2002. "Sustained Correction of X-Linked Severe Combined Immunodeficiency by Ex-Vivo Gene Therapy." *New England Journal of Medicine* 346 (16): 1185–93.

Hagège, Albert A., and others. 2001. "Regeneration of the Myocardium: A New Role in the Treatment of Ischemic Heart Disease?" *Hypertension* 38 (6): 1413–15.

Hammer, S. M. 2002. "Increasing Choices for HIV Therapy." *New England Journal of Medicine* 346 (26): 2022–23.

Hammond, Scott M., Amy A. Caudy, and Gregory J. Hannon. 2001. "Post-Transcriptional Gene Silencing by Double-Stranded RNA." *Nature Reviews Genetics* 2 (2): 110–19.

Hardy, John, and Dennis J. Selkoe. 2002. "The Amyloid Hypothesis of Alzheimer's Disease: Progress and Problems on the Road to Therapeutics." *Science* 297 (5580): 353–56.

Hayflick, Leonard. 2000. "The Illusion of Cell Immortality." *British Journal of Cancer* 83 (7): 841–46.

Helfand, Stephen L., and Sharon K. Inouye. 2002. "Rejuvenating Views of the Ageing Process." *Nature Reviews Genetics* 3 (2): 149–53.

Helmuth, Laura. 2002. "Long-Awaited Technique Spots Alzheimer's Toxin." *Science* 297 (5582): 752–53.

Hermiston, Terry. 2000. "Gene Delivery from Replication-Selective Viruses: Arming Guided Missiles in the War against Cancer." *Journal of Clinical Investigation* 105 (9): 1169–72.

Hock, Cristoph, and others. 2002. "Generation of Antibodies Specific for Beta-Amyloid by Vaccination of Patients with Alzheimer Disease." *Nature Medicine* 8 (11): 1270–75.

Hodi, F. Stephen, and others. 2002. "ATP6S1 Elicits Potent Humoral Responses Associated with Immune-Mediated Tumor Destruction." *Proceedings of the National Academy of Sciences USA* 99 (10): 6919–24.

Hollon, Tom. 2001. "Human Genes: How Many?" *Scientist* 1 (20): 14–15.

International Human Genome Sequencing Consortium. 2001. "Initial Sequencing and Analysis of the Human Genome." *Nature* 409 (6822): 860–921.

International SNP Map Working Group. 2001. "A Map of Human Genome Sequence Variation Containing 1.42 Million Single Nucleotide Polymorphisms." *Nature* 409 (6822): 928–33.

Jacque, Jean-Mari, Karine Triques, and Mario Stevenson. 2002. "Modulation of HIV-1 Replication by RNA Interference." *Nature* 418 (6896): 435–38.

Jaffee, Elizabeth M. 1999. "Immunotherapy of Cancer." *Annals of the New York Academy of Sciences* 886: 67–72.

Jaffee, Elizabeth M., and others. 2001. "Novel Allogeneic GM-CSF-Secreting Tumor Vaccine for Pancreatic Cancer: A Phase I Trial of Safety and Immune Activation." *Journal of Clinical Oncology* 19 (1): 145–56.

Johnstone, Ricky W., Astrid A. Ruefli, and Scott W. Lowe. 2002. "Apoptosis: A Link between Cancer Genetics and Chemotherapy." *Cell* 108 (2): 153–64.

Kaihara, S., and others. 2000. "Silicon Micromachining to Tissue Engineer Branched Vascular Channels for Liver Fabrication." *Tissue Engineering* 6 (2): 105–17.

Kaji, Eugene H., and Jeffrey M. Leiden. 2001. "Gene and Stem Cell Therapies." *Journal of the American Medical Association* 285 (5): 545–50.

Keaney, J. F., Jr., and J. Vita. 2002. "The Value of Inflammation for Predicting Unstable Angina." *New England Journal of Medicine* 347 (1): 55–57.

Kirn, David, Robert L. Martuza, and James Zwiebel. 2001. "Replication-Selective Virotherapy for Cancer: Biological Principles, Risk Management, and Future Directions." *Nature Medicine* 7 (7): 781–87.

Koenig, Robert. 2001. "Sardinia's Male Methuselahs." *Science* 291 (5511): 2074–76.

Lai, Liangxue, and others. 2002. "Production of alpha-1,3-Galactosyltransferase Knockout Pigs by Nuclear Transfer Cloning." *Science* 295 (5557): 1089–92.

Lakhani, Sunil R., Michael J. O'Hare, and Alan Ashworth. 2001. "Profiling Familial Breast Cancer." *Nature Medicine* 7 (4): 408–10.

LaRosa, John C., Jiang He, and Suma Vupputuri. 1999. "Effect of Statins on Risk of Coronary Disease: A Meta-Analysis of Randomized Controlled Trials." *Journal of the American Medical Association* 282 (24): 2340–46.

Lee, Cheol-Koo, and others. 1999. "Gene Expression Profile of Aging and Its Retardation by Caloric Restriction." *Science* 285 (5432): 1390–93.

Lefkowitz, Robert J., and James T. Willerson. 2001. "Prospects for Cardiovascular Research." *Journal of the American Medical Association* 285 (5): 581–87.

Libby, Peter. 2002. "Atherosclerosis: The New View." *Scientific American* 286 (5): 46–55.

Livingston, David M., and Ramesh Shivdasani. 2001. "Toward Mechanism-Based Cancer Care." *Journal of the American Medical Association* 285 (5): 588–93.

Lumelsky, Nadia, and others. 2001. "Differentiation of Embryonic Stem Cells to Insulin-Secreting Structures Similar to Pancreatic Islets." *Science* 292 (5520): 1389–94.

Luzzatto, Lusio, and Rosario Notaro. 2001. "Malaria: Protecting against Bad Air." *Science* 293 (5529): 442–43.

Maher, Brion. 2002. "Attacking Beta-Amyloid at Its Source." *Scientist* 16 (2): 25–26.

Martin, Joseph B. 1999. "Molecular Basis of the Neurodegenerative Disorders." *New England Journal of Medicine* 340 (25): 1970–80.

Marx, Jean. 2000a. "DNA Arrays Reveal Cancer in Its Many Forms." *Science* 289 (5485): 1670–72.

———. 2000b. "Chipping away at the Causes of Aging." *Science* 287 (5462): 2390.

McLeod, Howard L. 2001. "Pharmacogenetics: More than Skin Deep." *Nature Genetics* 29 (3): 247–48.

McLeod, H. L., and others. 2000. "Genetic Polymorphism of Thiopurine Methyltransferase and Its Clinical Relevance for Childhood Acute Lymphoblastic Leukemia." *Leukemia* 14 (4): 567–72.

Melov, Simon, and others. 2000. "Extension of Life Span with Superoxide Dismutase/ Catalase Mimetics." *Science* 289 (5484): 1567–69.

Migliaccio, Enrica, and others. 1999. "The P66shc Adaptor Protein Controls Oxidative Stress Response and Life Span in Mammals." *Nature* 402 (6759): 309–13.

Miller, D. G., and G. Stamatoyannopoulos. 2001. "Gene Therapy for Hemophilia." *New England Journal of Medicine* 344 (23): 1782–84.

Mooney, D. J., and A. G. Mikos. 1999. "Growing New Organs." *Scientific American* 280 (4): 60–65.

Nasseri, Boris A., Kohei Ogawa, and Joseph P. Vacanti. 2001. "Tissue Engineering: An Evolving 21st-Century Science to Provide Biologic Replacement for Reconstruction and Transplantation." *Surgery* 130 (5): 781–84.

Ng, V., M. Alonso, and J. A. Bezerre. 2000. "Hepatocyte Transplantation: Advancing Biology and Treating Children." *Clinical Liver Disease* 4 (4): 929–45.

Olshansky, S. Jay, Bruce A. Carnes, and Aline Désesquelles 2001. "Prospects for Human Longevity." *Science* 291 (5508): 1491–92.

Orlic, Donald, and others. 2001. "Mobilized Bone Marrow Cells Repair the Infarcted Heart, Improving Function and Survival." *Proceedings of the National Academy of Sciences USA* 98 (18): 10344–49.

Paddison, Patrick J., Amy A. Caudy, and Gregory J. Hannon. 2002. "Stable Suppression of Gene Expression by RNAi in Mammalian Cells." *Proceedings of the National Academy of Sciences USA* 99 (3): 1443–48.

Palese, Peter, and Adolfo Garcia-Sastre. 2002a. "New Directions in Vaccine Research." *Journal of Clinical Investigation* 109 (12): 1517–18.

———. 2002b. "Influenza Vaccines: Present and Future." *Journal of Clinical Investigation* 110 (1): 9–13.

Palmer, Theo D., and others. 2001. "Progenitor Cells from Human Brain after Death." *Nature* 411 (6833): 42–43.

Parkes, Tony L., and others. 1998. "Extension of Drosophila Life Span by Overexpression of Human SOD1 in Motorneurons." *Nature Genetics* 19 (2): 171–74.

Peltonen, Leena, and Victor A. McKusick. 2001. "Genomics and Medicine: Dissecting Human Disease in the Postgenomic Era." *Science* 291 (5507): 1224–29.

Perls, Thomas J., and others. 2002. "Lifelong Sustained Mortality Advantage of Siblings of Centenarians." *Proceedings of the National Academy of Sciences USA* 99 (12): 8442–47.

Pfeifer, Alexander, and Inder M. Verma. 2001. "Gene Therapy: Promises and Problems." *Annual Review of Genomics and Human Genetics* 2: 177–211.

Pollack, Andrew. 2002. "Despite Billions for Discoveries, Pipeline of Drugs Is far from Full." *New York Times,* April 19, p. C1.

Pomerantz, Roger J., and David L. Horn. 2003. "Twenty Years of Therapy for HIV-1 Infection." *Nature Medicine* 9 (7): 867–73.

Pittenger, Mark F., and others. 1999. "Multilineage Potential of Adult Human Mesenchymal Stem Cells." *Science* 284 (5411): 143–47.

Puca, Annibale A., and others. 2001. "A Genome-Wide Scan for Linkage to Human Exceptional Longevity Identifies Locus on Chromosome 4." *Proceedings of the National Academy of Sciences USA* 98 (18): 10505–08.

Quaini, Federico, and others. 2002. "Chimerism of the Transplanted Heart." *New England Journal of Medicine* 346 (1): 5–15.

Ramaswamy, Sridhar, and others. 2001. "Multiclass Cancer Diagnosis Using Tumor Gene Expression Signatures." *Proceedings of the National Academy of Sciences USA* 98 (26): 15149–54.

Ratain, Mark J., and Mary V. Relling. 2001. "Gazing into a Crystal Ball—Cancer Therapy in the Post-Genomic Era." *Nature Medicine* 7 (3): 283–85.

Reed, J. C. 2002. "Apoptosis-Based Therapy." *Nature Reviews Drug Discovery* 1 (2): 111–21.

Robine, Jean-Marie, and Michel Allard. 1998. "The Oldest Human." *Science* 279 (5358): 1831.

Rust, Stephan, and others. 1999. "Tangier Disease Is Caused by Mutations in the Gene-Encoding ATP-Binding Cassette Transporter 1." *Nature Genetics* 22 (4): 352–55.

Savage, D. B., and S. O'Rahilly. 2002. "Leptin: A Novel Therapeutic Role in Lipodystrophy." *Journal of Clinical Investigation* 109 (10): 1285–86.

Schenk, Dale, Dora Games, and Peter Seubert. 2001. "Potential Treatment Opportunities for Alzheimer's Disease through Inhibition of Secretases and A-Beta Immunization." *Journal of Molecular Neuroscience* 17 (2): 259–68.

Schnipper, Lowell E., and Terry B. Strom. 2001. "A Magic Bullet for Cancer—How Near and How Far?" *New England Journal of Medicine* 345 (4): 283–84.

Selkoe, Dennis J. 2001. "Alzheimer's Disease: Genes, Proteins, and Therapy." *Physiological Reviews* 81 (2): 741–66.

Service, Robert F. 2001. "High-Speed Biologists Search for Gold in Proteins." *Science* 294 (5549): 2074–77.

Shipp, Margaret A., and others. 2002. "Diffuse Large B-Cell Lymphoma Outcome Prediction by Gene-Expression Profiling and Supervised Machine Learning." *Nature Medicine* 8 (1): 68–74.

Shouse, Ben. 2002. "American Association for the Advancement of Science: Human Gene Count on the Rise." *Science* 295 (5559): 1457.

Shulman, Gerald I. 2000. "Cellular Mechanisms of Insulin Resistance." *Journal of Clinical Investigation* 106 (2): 171–76.

Simons, Jonathan, and others. 1999. "Induction of Immunity to Prostate Cancer Antigens: Results of a Clinical Trial of Vaccination with Irradiated Autologous Prostate Tumor Cells Engineered to Secrete Granulocyte-Macrophage Colony-Stimulating Factor Using Ex Vivo Gene Transfer." *Cancer Research* 59 (20): 5160–68.

Soiffer, Robert, and others. 1998. "Vaccination with Irradiated Autologous Melanoma Cells Engineered to Secrete Human Granulocyte-Macrophage Colony-Stimulating Factor Generates Potent Antitumor Immunity in Patients with Metastatic Melanoma." *Proceedings of the National Academy of Sciences USA* 95 (22): 13141–46.

Somia, Nikunj, and Inder M. Verma. 2000. "Gene Therapy: Trials and Tribulations." *Nature Reviews Genetics* 1 (2): 91–99.

Spiegelman, Bruce M., and Jeffrey S. Flier. 2001. "Obesity and the Regulation of Energy Balance." *Cell* 104 (4): 531–43.

Steinberg, D. 2002a. "Closing in on Multiple Cancer Targets." *Scientist* 16 (7): 29.

———. 2002b. "Testing Potential Alzheimer Vaccines." *Scientist* 16 (2): 23–24.

Steinberg, Daniel. 2002. "Atherogenesis in Perspective: Hypercholesterolemia and Inflammation as Partners in Crime." *Nature Medicine* 8 (11): 1211–17.

Stewart, Sheila A., and Robert A. Weinberg 2002. "Senescence: Does It All Happen at the End?" *Oncogene* 21 (4): 627–30.

Strauss, Evelyn. 2001. "Growing Old Together." *Science* 292 (5514): 41–43.

Sunyaev, Shamil, and others. 1999. "Prediction of Nonsynonymous Single Nucleotide Polymorphisms in Human Disease-Associated Genes." *Journal of Molecular Medicine* 77 (11): 754–60.

Taylor, Doris A. 2001. "Cellular Cardiomyoplasty with Autologous Skeletal Myoblasts for Ischemic Heart Disease and Heart Failure." *Current Control Trials in Cardiovascular Medicine* 2 (5): 208–10.

Thomson, James A., and others. 1998. "Embryonic Stem Cell Lines Derived from Human Blastocysts." *Science* 282 (5391): 1145–57.

Tishkoff, Sarah A., and others. 2001. "Haplotype Diversity and Linkage Disequilibrium at Human G6PD: Recent Origin of Alleles That Confer Malarial Resistance." *Science* 293 (5529): 455–62.

Toma, Catalin. 2002. "Human Mesenchymal Stem Cells Differentiate to a Cardiomyocyte Phenotype in the Adult Murine Heart." *Circulation* 105 (1): 93–98.

Toma, Jean G., and others. 2001. "Isolation of Multipotent Adult Stem Cells from the Dermis of Mammalian Skin." *Nature Cell Biology* 3 (9): 778–84.

Vacanti, M. P., and others. 2001a. "Tissue-Engineered Spinal Cord." *Transplant Proceedings* 33 (1–2): 592–98.

———. 2001b. "Identification and Initial Characterization of Spore-like Cells in Adult Mammals." *Journal of Cell Biochemistry* 80 (3): 455–60.

van Dyke, Terry, and Tyler Jacks. 2002. "Cancer Modeling in the Modern Era: Progress and Challenges." *Cell* 108 (2): 135–44.

van't Veer, Laura J., and others. 2002. "Gene Expression Profiling Predicts Clinical Outcome of Breast Cancer." *Nature* 415 (6871): 530–06.

Venter, J. Craig, and others. 2001. "The Sequence of the Human Genome." *Science* 291 (5507): 1304–51.

Verma, Inder M. 2003. "A Voluntary Moratorium?" *Molecular Therapy* 7 (2): 141.

Vogelstein, Bert, and Kenneth W. Kinzler. 2001. "Achilles' Heel of Cancer?" *Nature* 412 (6850): 865–66.

Volkman, Sarah K., and others. 2001. "Recent Origin of *Plasmodium Falciparum* from a Single Progenitor." *Science* 293 (5529): 482–84.

Wade, Nicholas. 2001. *Life Script.* Simon and Schuster.

Weissleder, Ralph. 2001. "A Clearer Vision for In-Vivo Imaging." *Nature Biotechnology* 19 (April): 316–17.

Wilson, Jean D., and others, eds. 1999. *Harrison's Principles of Internal Medicine.* 12th ed. McGraw-Hill.

Wolkow, Catherine A., and others. 2000. "Regulation of C. Elegans Life Span by Insulinlike Signaling in the Nervous System." *Science* 290 (5489): 147–50.

Woloshin, Steven, Lisa M. Schwartz, and H. Gilbert Welch. 2002. "Risk Charts: Putting Cancer in Context." *Journal of the National Cancer Institute* 94 (11): 799–804.

Zulewski, Henryk, and others. 2001. "Multipotential Nestin-Positive Stem Cells Isolated from Adult Pancreatic Islets Differentiate Ex Vivo into Pancreatic Endocrine, Exocrine, and Hepatic Phenotypes." *Diabetes* 50 (3): 521–33.

HENRY J. AARON
BENJAMIN H. HARRIS

2 *Our Uncertain*
Demographic Future

THE BIOMEDICAL REVOLUTION has created a historically
unprecedented prospect—that advances in medical
treatments for the major causes of disease may slash human mortality
rates and increase life expectancy. The same advances could also retard
aging and debility, thereby increasing the duration of active, productive
lives. Even without such advances, the aged will be a rapidly growing
proportion of the population in the United States and other developed
nations. Based on extrapolation of past declines in mortality rates, the
proportion of the population over age sixty-five is projected to approach
30 percent by the middle of the twenty-first century in several developed
nations. Further reductions in mortality rates would accentuate these
trends.

John Potts and William Schwartz, in their chapter in this volume, explain
how rapid achievement of the potential of molecular biology holds out the
possibility of truly revolutionary increases in longevity. Resulting medical
advances could lead to dramatic increases in life expectancy. Scientists will
identify genes that predispose people to longevity. Manipulation of such
genes to extend life could become commonplace. Conceivably, biologists
and physicians could learn how to stop the aging process entirely. One study,
for example, identifies genes that are infrequent in the general population
but are common to centenarians who also have extremely long-lived sib-

lings.[1] Control over portions of genes that govern cell replication could dramatically extend life.

In this chapter we explore the demographic implications of such medical advances. We present alternative population projections based on sharply lower mortality rates. These projections are based on improvements in mortality rates that are both extremely rapid and sustained but not so high as some rates that have been achieved for periods of one or two decades in some nations. We compare these projections to our baseline, the intermediate projections of the Social Security Administration (SSA) for the year 2001.[2] We show the implications of shifts in immigration rates and of extended working lives for the growth of the labor force. We present alternative projections of the impact of an increase of life expectancy on the number of people with disabilities and on the relative duration of years of healthy adulthood.

The projections should not be construed as forecasts but as an effort to explore the consequences should improvements in life expectancy, which are possible but by no means guaranteed, occur. Indeed, although the prospects for major medical advances are promising, there is some risk that life expectancy will fall. Some biologists and demographers fear that catastrophic worldwide pandemics could become common. The AIDS epidemic in some sub-Saharan African countries—which has slashed life expectancy by ten to twenty years in less than a decade—is illustrative. The globalization of trade and increased labor mobility heighten risks that horrific diseases—such as Ebola and hemorrhagic fever, for which no known cures or even treatments exist—could quickly spread worldwide.

Such cataclysms are conceivable, but they are not the subject of this volume. Nor do we consider the debilitating consequences of harmful behaviors, such as bad dietary habits. The sharp recent rise in obesity in the United States, for example, has fostered an epidemic of diabetes. We ignore the possibility that such developments could offset the effects of improved diagnosis, prevention, and treatment of disease.

To anticipate, we find that the U.S. population will age rapidly over the next three decades, whether mortality rates fall gradually or rapidly. Reduction in mortality rates will affect the U.S. population profile but will cause only small changes from baseline projections between 2000 and 2030. Rapid

1. Puca and others (2001). This study provides persuasive evidence that those who live very long lives possess certain genetic characteristics that differ from those of the general population.

2. The SSA 2002 trustees' report, which somewhat increases the rate at which mortality rates are projected to fall, appeared after we completed our projections. Had we used these later estimates, the difference between the Social Security actuary's projections and those presented here would have been somewhat reduced. Board of Trustees (2002)

reductions in mortality rates will eventually lead to quite impressive increases in the share of the population that is elderly. But even large drops in mortality rates would not produce major effects on the portion of the population over age sixty or age eighty until the second half of this century. The reason is that mortality rates among the young and prime-age adults are already so low that further reductions produce few detectable effects. In contrast, mortality rates among the very old are currently so high that drops over many years are necessary before life expectancy increases significantly at advanced ages. Increased immigration temporarily retards population aging because most immigrants are relatively young. But the effect is temporary, as immigrants age at the same rate as the indigenous population.

If people retire at the same ages as they do today, the ratio of dependent elderly to active workers will rise sharply. Should the historical trend toward ever-earlier retirement by men reverse, the increase in the ratio of the inactive elderly to the general population would be quite moderate. The implications of such a reversal depend on its cause. Extended working lives could result from reduced disability and delayed aging, with profound implications for human well-being. On the other hand, people might remain active not because of increased vigor but because changed economic incentives make continued work a necessity.

Models of Aging

Well-regarded scientists disagree profoundly on whether there is currently a limit to the human life span (and what that limit might be).[3] They also hold divergent views on the rate at which mortality rates will improve. Although these questions appear to be related, their answers are not. A maximum human life span might constrain growth or it might be far above current realized life expectancies, leaving room for rapid—even accelerating—declines in mortality rates. Similarly, prospects for near-term reductions in mortality rates could be rosy or bleak, even if no biological limit to longevity exists.

A summary measure of the rate of increase in life expectancy is the difference between period life expectancy and cohort life expectancy. Period life expectancy is based on mortality rates for all age cohorts at a given point in time. Thus the mortality of people born in, say, 2005 would be assumed to occur at rates applicable to people of all ages in the year 2005. For example, people age fifty in year 2055 are assumed to die at the same rate as did actual

---

3. This section borrows from Aaron and Harris (2002).

Figure 2-1. *Gap between Period and Cohort Mortality, Male and Female Life Expectancy, 2000*[a]

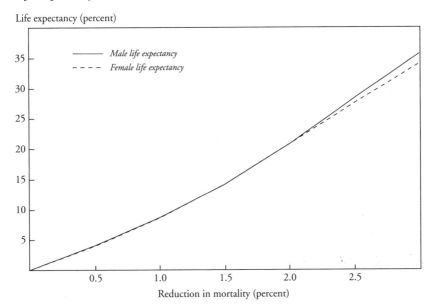

Life expectancy (percent)

Reduction in mortality (percent)

a. In the base case, mortality at 120 is assumed to be 100 percent for both men and women. The mortality rate is reduced by the assumed percentage reduction for age 120 in the first year, age 120 and 121 in the second year, and so on. The mortality rate is assumed to remain at 1.0 at age 130. Projections differ marginally from those of the SSA. We apply SSA methods but not its detailed model. Because of omitted details, the total differs marginally from published SSA estimates.

fifty-year-olds in 2005. To project cohort life expectancy, one computes average life expectancy for a cohort of newborns based on the assumption that as they age they will be subject to changing (and probably falling) mortality rates through time. For example, people age fifty in 2055 are assumed to die at rates based on projected mortality rates for fifty-year-olds assuming some annual rate of change in mortality rates from 2005. In brief, period life expectancy excludes anticipated changes in mortality rates, while cohort life expectancy includes them. If age-specific mortality rates were unchanging, cohort and period life expectancies would be identical. The difference between them is a measure of the anticipated reduction in mortality rates. Figure 2-1 graphs the two measures for varying assumed rates of decline in mortality rates for the U.S. population in the year 2000.

The Natural Limit Hypothesis

Several population analysts hold both that there is a limit to human longevity and that mortality rates will fall little. According to this view, biological organisms in general, and human beings in particular, are genetically programmed to have a limited life. Beyond a certain age, internal biological processes cause annual mortality rates to rise rapidly and to approach one.

Natural Selection. The evolutionary rationale for this view is that natural selection has no incentive to eliminate harmful mutations that diminish viability after reproductive age.[4] Evolution might even favor mutations that hasten death after reproduction. Death of the old would reduce competition for food or other resources. Other theorists speculate that natural selection might favor survival if the elderly aid the species in some way—such as by caring for children or by preserving information that is valuable to survival.

Cell Division. In the late nineteenth century August Weismann theorized that animals die because cells lose the capacity to divide after a certain number of divisions.[5] This theory enjoyed considerable popularity early in the twentieth century but then lost favor for a time. It has enjoyed a resurgence since 1961, when Leonard Hayflick and Paul Moorhead claimed experimental support for the proposition that normal human cells can divide only a finite number of times in vitro and inferred that similar limits applied in vivo. Hayflick later modified this proposition to hold that cell division slows with age but does not entirely stop. Those holding this view maintain either that cessation of cell division leads to the death of the organism or that the slowing down of cell division contributes to senescence and a greatly heightened vulnerability to disease.

Is the Limit Near? Without two additional assumptions, however, a natural limit to human life would impose few restraints on prospects for future increases in human life expectancy.

The first assumption is that the natural limit is not materially greater than current life expectancy in populations with the highest observed life expectancy. Some who believe that human life has a biological maximum

---

4. Olshansky, Carnes, and Désesquelles (2001).
5. For citations in this paragraph, see Gavrilov and Gavrilova (1991).

place that maximum so high that it constitutes no effective barrier to large and continuing declines in human mortality rates. A life-span limit of, say, 120 years would not materially impede rapid and prolonged reductions in human mortality rates.[6] In contrast, James Fries suggests that the limit to human life expectancy is approximately 85 years.[7] That age is close to the current period life expectancy of women in Japan, the country with the highest combined life expectancy for men and women in the world. Were mortality rates in Japan to fall 2 percent a year, Japanese women born in 2075 would have a cohort life expectancy of 180 years and a period life expectancy of 120 years.

The second assumption necessary for natural limits to constrain extension of life expectancy is that prospects for modifying that limit are poor. Such a view may have been quite plausible in the past. The newfound possibility of altering genetic composition, along the lines set forth by Potts and Schwartz, makes any such view hard to defend.

Historical Extrapolation

Statistical evidence has led many demographers to project continuing reductions in mortality rates and corresponding increases in life expectancy, persisting throughout this century and beyond.

—If a limit in life-expectancy were near, then one might expect rates of improvement to be lowest in countries with the highest life expectancies. Such is not the case. Japanese life expectancies, currently the highest in the world, have been rising at about 2 percent annually for two decades.

—Mortality rates in most developed nations have been falling for decades. They show no signs of stopping.

—If life expectancies in countries with the highest life expectancies were near a biological limit, one might expect male and female life expectancies to converge. In fact, such convergence is not commonly observed. In Japan, they have diverged for roughly a century. Stephen Goss, in his comment on this chapter, points out that convergence may be occurring in the United States, although the period over which it is observed is brief.

Extrapolation of past rates of decline is an art, not a science. The fall in mortality rates fluctuates widely from year to year and decade to decade. Demographers do not agree on what past period is appropriate or even on the

6. The highest documented age of death is approximately 120 years. Wilmoth (2000).
7. Fries (1980).

relative probative value of recent and past improvements. Consequently, one can find in past trends "evidence" to support a wide range of projections (see tables 2-5 through 2-10, part of Goss's comments on this chapter).

The fastest, sustained drop in mortality rates over the past half century has been in Japan. Following World War II, Japanese life expectancy soared at rates seldom seen before or since. For two decades or more, mortality rates fell at an annual rate of more than 5 percent a year. Life expectancy rose by five years a decade. The pace of advance has slackened somewhat in recent years. Even in the 1990s, however, mortality rates fell more than 2 percent a year and life expectancy rose two years.[8]

Since 1965 life expectancy in the United States has been lower than in Japan and has been rising more slowly. Nonetheless, official government agencies and many private demographers project improvements in life expectancy at approximately the same rate as that foreseen for Japan. The SSA and Bureau of the Census project an increase in U.S. life expectancy at birth from 76.7 years in 2000 to 81.7 years (SSA) and 84.0 years (Census Bureau) in 2050.[9] The Census Bureau projection is similar to that of Ronald Lee and Lawrence Carter, who in 1992 extrapolated improvements in U.S. mortality rates to project life expectancy at birth in 2050 at 84.3 years.[10] Dennis Ahlburg and James Vaupel suggest that 2 percent a year is a reasonable upper limit for sustained reductions in U.S. mortality rates.[11] They project period life expectancy at birth in 2080 of 100 years for females and 96 years for males.

Population Prometheans

Some demographers and a growing number of biological scientists project massive increases in life expectancy. It is important to distinguish between projections of very high life expectancy and estimates of high life-span limits. Some life expectancy pessimists put maximum life span at well above a hundred years.[12] Even genetically identical populations exhibit consider-

    8. Wilmoth (1996).

    9. Lee and Edwards (2001, p. 9).

    10. Lee and Carter (1992). The procedure was to fit the logarithm of the actual mortality rates for people of age x in year t, $\ln m_{x,t}$, to a function $a_x + b_x k_t$, where k is an index of the natural logarithm of mortality rates that decreases linearly at b per year, where the bs sum to 1 and the ks sum to zero. As a result, a_x are simply the average mortality rates at time t.

    11. Ahlburg and Vaupel (1990).

    12. Fries (1980) cites the *Guinness Book of World Records* for the longest documented life *span* of 114 years but puts maximum achievable life *expectancy* at not much more than 90 years. See also Gavrilov and Gavrilova (1991).

able dispersion in life span. Environmental conditions or inescapable causes of mortality powerfully influence mean life span. But even if conditions are optimal, deaths are widely dispersed over time. Genetic inheritance and environmental conditions can powerfully influence life expectancy. However, neither can much lower the variance of the date of death. The pattern of mortality bears a considerable resemblance to radioactive decay, a random process.

For this reason, the difference between the longest observed life span and life expectancy is bound to be a considerable. Advances in medical technology can increase the maximum life span. Environmental changes and human behavior can either raise or lower it. But changes in life span under ideal conditions provide only limited information about trends in life expectancy under average conditions.

The emergent optimism on life expectancy rests on the prospect that science will decode the basic genetic mechanisms behind diseases responsible for most deaths. After scientists understand what causes diseases, it is held, they will then find ways either to prevent or to cure them.

British philosopher John Harris captures this Promethean vision. "New research now allows a glimpse into a world in which aging—and even death—may no longer be inevitable. Cloned human embryonic stem cells, appropriately reprogrammed, might be used for constant regeneration of organs and tissue. Injections of growth factors might put the body into a state of constant renewal. We may be able to switch off the genes in the early embryo that trigger aging, rendering it 'immortal' (but not invulnerable)."[13] Harris injects a note of caution when he adds "We do not know when, or even if, such techniques could be developed and made safe, but some scientists believe it is possible." Others project that living to 130 or more by the middle of this century could become routine.[14]

Despite the vision sketched by Potts and Schwartz, caution regarding the vision of population Private is in order. Major advances in medical science and public health occurred during the twentieth century. The discovery and introduction of antibiotics dramatically lowered deaths from infectious diseases. Organ transplants and prostheses restored or replaced damaged, defective, or injured body parts. A veritable supermarket of

13. Harris (2000, p. 59).
14. Schwartz (1998) writes, "Although Census Bureau calculations project an increase in average life span of only 8 years by the year 2050, some experts believe that the human life span should not begin to encounter any theoretical natural limits before 120 years. With continuing advances in molecular medicine and a growing understanding of the aging process, that limit could rise to 130 years or more" (p. 150).

advanced diagnostic equipment facilitated diagnosis and treatment. These and other advances reduced mortality rates over the course of the twentieth century by a bit more than 1 percent annually. There are good reasons to believe that the new capacities of molecular biology may generate larger effects than did past advances, which were confined to single treatment modalities. But until there is strong evidence of discontinuous increases in life expectancy—evidence that is not yet apparent in mortality data—claims of the population Prometheans should be viewed as hopes, not description.[15]

What Is the Underlying Process?

Expectations regarding mortality rates should depend, in part, on one's model of why and how humans age and die. No model of aging is now generally accepted. Without such a model, one has no basis for deciding whether the discovery of a cure for a particular illness will have a large or a small effect on overall mortality rates. To illustrate the problem, we lay out three models of mortality.

The Independent Causes Model. Most countries collect information on causes of death. With these data, one can attribute each death to a particular illness or cause. In other words, each cause of death is assumed to operate independently. This approach is valid only if the ex ante probability of death from, say, respiratory disease is no higher or lower for those who, ex post, die from, say, heart disease than it is for any random person of the same age. To put matters another way, the assumption of independence is equivalent to saying that learning that a person died from a particular disease conveys no information about the prior likelihood that this person was vulnerable to other diseases. It is also equivalent to saying that a development that reduces mortality from one disease has no secondary effect on deaths from other diseases.

These assumptions are hard to defend.[16] Suppose that a medical advance dramatically reduces the likelihood of death from, say, cardiovascular disease. As a result, some of those who otherwise would have died from cardiovascular disease survive. Call this group "the spared." As explained in the next section, the prior health characteristics of the spared may differ from those of the general population. Furthermore, a new treatment that works by producing

---

15. Wilmoth (2000).
16. For a defense of using cause-specific methods, see Caselli and Lopez (1996).

some general improvement in health may lower mortality rates of the spared from other causes below those of the general population. In that case, the "cure" for cardiovascular disease would also lower mortality rates from, say, respiratory disease. Conversely, if the spared are particularly sickly, their mortality rate from many illnesses other than cardiovascular disease might well have been higher than that of the general population. In this case, a reduction in deaths from cardiovascular disease could increase average mortality from other causes. In general, one would expect to see different interactions with different treatments. What one would not expect is independence—although it is conceivable that the increases and decreases from causes of death other than the one for which improved treatment is found could just offset one another.

The Frailty Model. The independence assumption fails if people differ from one another systematically in their inherent susceptibility to illness.[17] Suppose that people differ in characteristic z and that each person's probability of dying from all causes is proportional to his or her endowment of z. People who are particularly frail—that is, they have high values of z—will be more likely to die in any given year than those who are less frail. Similarly, new cures are assumed to keep alive those with the lowest endowments of z who otherwise would have died. This assumption is equivalent to saying that the spared are frailer than average. Such variations in frailty could be genetically based, environmentally caused, or both. Over time, the surviving members of the cohort will have progressively lower values of z. That is, they will be progressively less frail than those who died previously.

One inference from the model leads to the conclusion that estimates of life expectancy, based on age-specific mortality rates, are lower than they would be if they were based on the frailty characteristics of the entire age cohort at birth. The frailty model also suggests that summing projected reductions in mortality rates from individual causes is likely to overstate reductions in total mortality rates. Those spared death by a medical advance will tend to be frailer than members of their population cohort who would have survived without the advance.[18]

17. Vaupel (1988); Manton, Stallard, and Vaupel (1981).

18. Those who die at any given time are not likely to be uniformly frail. As a result, the possibility exists that those spared death by some medical advance could be less frail than the average survivor. In that event, reductions in mortality from one cause would be associated with reductions, not increases, in age-specific mortality from other causes.

The Limited Reliability Model. Human death may be analogized to machine failure, which engineers have analyzed extensively.[19] Although the mechanics of machines differ from the biology of living organisms, they bear certain similarities. Each contains systems that must all operate, at least up to a minimal standard, if the entity is to remain functional. Each such system has more or less redundancy. That is, some elements of a system may fail before the system entirely ceases to work.

The time profile of human aging has three distinctive ranges. During early childhood, death rates are relatively high but quickly fall to very low levels. This stage is analogous to the burn-in period with some new machines, especially electronic equipment. Next comes a lengthy period during which human death rates are low but climb steadily and exponentially, following the repeatedly validated Gompertz-Makeham function:

$$\mu_x = A + Re^{ax},$$

where μ_x is the mortality hazard at age x and A, R, and a are positive parameters. That period may be regarded as analogous to the useful life of most machines. During this phase, machine failure also is initially low but climbs exponentially. In a third and final stage death rates are high and continue to rise, but the rate of increase is slower than it is during the second phase. Machines exhibit a similar phase, after the end of their useful lives. During this phase failure rates increase by less-than-exponential rates.

One way to develop a model of human mortality is to identify a type of machine for which the pattern of failure matches that of mortality rates observed in humans. One such machine consists of many component systems, each essential to the operation of the machine. A system consists of many elements. The system continues to work as long as any one element functions. That is, the systems are built with redundancy. Many of the elements are faulty at the outset of the period of useful life (or, in humans, the adult phase). The remaining elements fail at a constant rate. The machine fails when any system fails. The pattern of failure rates of such a machine resembles the mortality rates of adult humans (excluding the very elderly, whose mortality rates follow a different pattern). A second type of machine whose failure rates resemble mortality rates of humans consists of one or a small number of essential systems, obeys the other assumptions described above, and exhibits diversity with respect to the number of flawed elements in the component systems.

---

19. This section based on Gavrilov and Gavrilova (1991).

Table 2-1. *Life Expectancy at Birth, 2030, 2050, 2075*

	Period life expectancy		Cohort life expectancy	
Year and assumption	*Male*	*Female*	*Male*	*Female*
2030				
SSA	77.1	81.6	81.9	86.0
2 percent improvement	80.8	85.9	101.4	106.3
2050				
SSA	78.8	83.0	83.1	87.1
2 percent improvement	85.7	90.4	107.2	111.5
2075				
SSA	80.6	84.6	84.5	88.3
2 percent improvement	91.7	95.9	114.0	117.3

In either case, the pattern of machine failure rates mimics the pattern of human mortality rates.[20] If one assumes, in addition, that failure of a critical portion of elements degrades performance of that component and increases the failure rates of other components, one ends up with a model of senescence in which mortality rates from distinct causes are clearly interdependent.

Alternative Projections

The effects on life expectancy at birth of sharply lower mortality rates are large, even in the near term. In contrast, the effects on population size and the age distribution emerge only gradually.

Life Expectancy

Table 2-1 shows how life expectancy at birth will change if mortality rates decline at two alternative rates for people born in three future years, 2030, 2050, and 2075. The base case incorporates assumptions used by the SSA in its intermediate projections for 2001 (see box 2-1). Under these projections, mortality rates fall at an average annual rate of 0.68 percent. In addition to the SSA base case, we include an alternative projection, based on the assumption that mortality rates fall at approximately 2 percent a year.

---

20. The mathematical form is the Gompertz-Makeham function, $A + Re^{ax}$, where A, R, and ax are parameters and x is age.

Box 2-1. *How Social Security Projects Mortality Rates*

The U.S. Social Security Administration (SSA) groups all causes of death listed in the International Classification of Diseases (ICD) into eleven groups (heart disease, cancer, vascular disease, violence, respiratory disease, infancy, digestive diseases, diabetes, liver cirrhosis, AIDS, and all others). It reports mortality rates from each of these eleven grouped causes. That is, each age and sex group has a specific annual probability of dying from each of the eleven causes. SSA projects trends in overall mortality rates by projecting rates of change in age-sex-specific death rates from each of the eleven groups. SSA's projections of the rates at which mortality from each cause of death are changed over time are based on expert judgment and past trends. The change in aggregate mortality rates for each age-sex group is the weighted sum of the change in each of the eleven age-sex-specific mortality rates. Although SSA projects mortality from separate diseases, it does not subscribe to the view that causes of death are independent. Reductions in particular causes of death may be associated with increases or decreases in death rates from other causes.

Specifically, we assume that mortality rates fall annually at 2.8 percent among cohorts zero to fourteen years of age, 2.2 percent among those fifteen to sixty-four years of age, and 1.9 percent among those age sixty-five or older. In the year 2000 these fractions average out to a drop in mortality rates of 2 percent. In later years the improvement drifts toward 1.9 percent because nearly all deaths occur among those aged sixty-five or above.

The SSA projections come close to being extrapolations of recent historical experience. The 2 percent assumption produces life expectancies that fall well within the zone of the population Prometheans. The resulting cohort life expectancy exceeds 100 years by 2030, is just under 110 years by 2050, and reaches 115 years by 2075. Improvement in mortality at 2 percent a year is well outside U.S. experience for any extended period, although mortality improvement of as much as 2 percent has occurred for periods of a few years.

Population

The aging of the baby-boom generation has become a familiar theme—of government budget projections, the popular press, and scholarly research. A sharp increase in the fraction of the population over age sixty, a common threshold for senior discounts, will begin in 2005. The 70 million surviving boomers, born between 1946 and 1964, will become eligible for Social Security pensions starting in 2008 and for Medicare starting in 2011.[21]

Figures 2-2, 2-3, and 2-4 show the population distribution in four years for three age groups. The percentage of the population over age sixty, seventy, and eighty in 2000 is, respectively, 15.7, 8.6, and 3.0. The fraction of the population over age sixty rises quickly as the baby-boom generation reaches retirement age; it then levels off as the boomers age and are succeeded by younger, and only slightly larger, cohorts. As the boomers continue to age, older age groups expand because of increased survival rates among younger cohorts. Figures 2-5, 2-6, and 2-7 show the differences in the projected population shares over time for each projection. The second projection assumes a 2 percent annual improvement in mortality rates. It carries over all assumptions embodied in the SSA projections other than mortality rates. The third projection assumes that immigration doubles.

The figures make it clear that, even if mortality rates fall no more than SSA projections assume, the population will age significantly. Without increased immigration, the proportion of the population over age eighty is projected in the base case to increase 183 percent by 2050 and 251 percent by 2075. Under the assumption of continuous 2 percent drops in mortality rates, the fraction of people age ninety or older increases twelvefold by 2075. Increased immigration would substantially increase the nonaged population and modestly increase the number of elderly, thereby slowing the growth in the fraction of the population that is elderly.

Disability

The projections in figures 2-2 through 2-7 present population projections under various assumptions about future mortality rates, but they contain no information about morbidity. The social, economic, and legal challenges and opportunities posed by an increased population depend critically on whether a longer-lived population is fit or feeble.

Under one scenario, suggested by some models of aging, medical science could succeed in defeating one killer disease after another but fail to delay the onset of debility. Such a development would be consistent with the frailty model and the limited reliability model. The relatively frail would be kept alive at higher rates. Age-specific disability rates could actually increase even as life expectancy rose—indeed, precisely because life expectancy was rising. The failure of the last element of essential body systems would be delayed. The elderly population would continue to exhibit debilitating but not fatal

21. Aaron and Reischauer (1998, p. 1).

Figure 2-2. *Proportion of Population Age Sixty and Older, 2000, 2030, 2050, 2075*

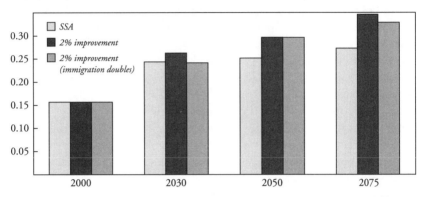

Figure 2-3. *Proportion of Population Age Seventy and Older, 2000, 2030, 2050, 2075*

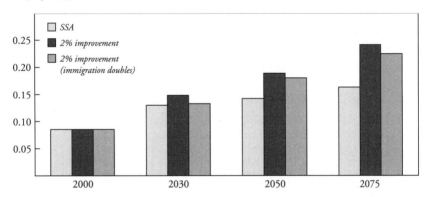

Figure 2-4. *Proportion of Population Age Eighty and Older, 2000, 2030, 2050, 2075*

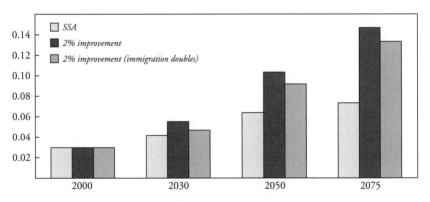

Figure 2-5. *Proportion of Population Over Time, Age Sixty and Older, Three Projections*

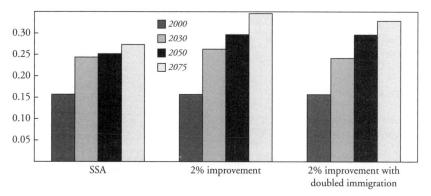

Figure 2-6. *Proportion of Population Over Time, Age Seventy and Older, Three Projections*

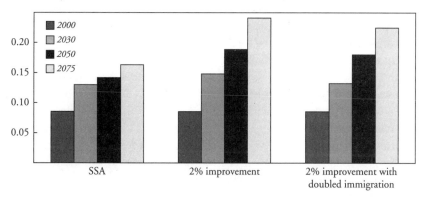

Figure 2-7. *Proportion of Population Over Time, Age Eighty and Older, Three Projections*

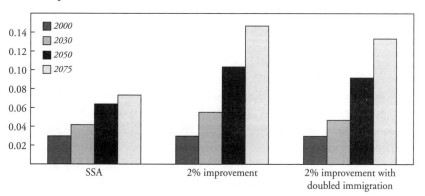

Table 2-2. *Percent of Adult Population with Severe Disability by Mortality Assumption and Method of Computing Disability Rates*

Assumption	Method of computing	2000	2050	2075
SSA population projections	SSA disability rates	15.5	19.1	19.9
SSA population projections	Disability rates based on remaining years of life	15.5	15.3	17.5
Population projections based on 2 percent annual reduction	SSA disability rates	15.5	21.7	24.4
Population projections based on 2 percent annual reduction	Disability rates based on remaining years of life	15.5	17.1	21.4

conditions at high, and possibly increasing, rates. Because the elderly population would greatly increase, the number of mentally and physically frail and disabled people would be vastly larger than it is today.

Under an alternative scenario medical advance not only would forestall death but also would delay or prevent chronic and debilitating conditions. The scientific skills that promise to defeat cancer and coronaries would simultaneously prevent such stigmata of aging as arthritis, Alzheimer's disease, and age-related loss of hearing, vision, and bone mass. The elderly would live healthier, as well as longer, lives. Age-related mental decline poses additional challenges. It is not clear how much of the age-related loss of memory and diminished capacity to learn new tasks is physiological and how much is social. Whether the medical advances that may spawn cures for life-ending illnesses will extend to the aging brain is unclear, as is the possibility that behavioral interventions could offset biological decline.

We project the growth of the disabled population with severe disabilities (see box 2-2 for definition and table 2-2 for projections). The first projection is based on the assumption that age-specific rates of severe disability remain as they were in 1996. If population grows at rates assumed in the SSA intermediate projections, the number of disabled people will grow from 15.5 percent of the population over age sixteen (34 million) in 2000 to 19.1 percent (58 million) in 2050, and 19.9 percent (65 million) in 2075. If mortality rates fall 2 percent annually and age-specific disability rates are unchanged, the proportion of the population with severe disability would increase to nearly one-fourth by 2075 (line 3, table 2-2). If disability rates were related to remaining years of expected life, the age of onset of disabil-

Box 2-2. *Severe Disability*

Disability takes many forms and comes in varying severity.[1] Furthermore, the term is often confused with impairment. Many people with impairments, even severe ones, function normally in most respects. A blind man sits on the U.S. Court of Appeals. A triple amputee was a U.S. senator. For statistical purposes, however, it is necessary to adopt a definition of *disability,* even if one recognizes that any given impairment is imperfectly correlated with capacity to function well in economic and social life.

The U.S. Census Bureau defines as severely disabled any person fifteen years old or older who falls in either of two categories. The first category includes all people who have any one of the following five characteristics:

—They use a wheelchair, cane, crutches, or a walker.

—They have a mental or emotional condition (frequent depression or anxiety, trouble getting along with others, trouble concentrating, trouble coping with day-to-day stress) that seriously interferes with everyday activities.

—They receive benefits based on inability to work.

—They have Alzheimer's disease.

—They are mentally retarded or have another developmental disability.

The second category includes people who are unable to perform or need help in performing one or more of the following activities:

—seeing, hearing, speaking, lifting and carrying, using stairs, walking, or grasping small objects

—getting around inside the home, getting out of bed or a chair, bathing, dressing, eating, and toileting

—getting around outside the home, keeping track of money and bills, preparing meals, doing light housework, taking prescription medicines in the right amount and at the right time, and using the telephone

—working around the house

—if ages sixteen to sixty-seven, have a condition that makes it difficult to work at a job or business.

1. Following information based on McNeil (2001).

ity would increase commensurately. Disability rates would still increase, but the effects would be somewhat attenuated (compare lines 2 and 4 with lines 1 and 3, table 2-2). However, unless disability rates fall, the burden of disability is bound to increase substantially as the population ages.

Recent trends strongly suggest that age-specific rates of disability are falling. Whether these trends will continue is less clear. Increasing prevalence of obesity and associated increases in diabetes, as well as the spread of asthma, pose identifiable threats. New illnesses, such as AIDS, could emerge.

But it seems unlikely that the medical advances that are expected to result in declining mortality rates will have no corresponding payoffs in cures or treatment for debilitating conditions. Furthermore, the trend to obesity could easily be reversed, much as rising death rates from cardiovascular disease were reversed starting in the 1960s, probably as a result of decreases in smoking and changes in diet.[22]

The Nonworking and the Working

To shed some light on the economic difference between the two scenarios, we compute the ratio of the population that is age sixteen or older that is in the labor force to the population in this age range that is not in the labor force under each of the population projections. Those not in the labor force include not only the retired but also nonaged adults who are not in the labor force for other reasons. This group includes students, parents who stay home with children, and all other adults who do not work in the paid labor force. This ratio gives some indication of the portion of current economic production that must be transferred from active to inactive adults.

Those who are currently economically inactive do not necessarily impose any economic burden on the active population. One cannot tell from the fact that people are currently economically inactive whether their lifetime earnings are sufficient to pay for their lifetime consumption—that is, whether they have saved enough or paid sufficient taxes to support their current and future consumption. If they have done so, these savings increased the stock of capital, domestic or foreign. This increased capital stock, in turn, generates higher incomes for its owners, individually and in the aggregate. Domestically located capital boosts domestic income. Foreign-located capital increases net transfers from abroad. Either way, the added income pays for the consumption of the economically inactive. As a result, they impose no burden on the rest of the population.[23] In human terms, retirees who have saved enough to support their consumption do not economically burden their children or anyone else.

The fundamental question is whether lifetime earnings of a person or age cohort equals or exceeds their lifetime consumption. If it does, they impose

---

22. Cutler and Meara (2001).
23. Increased saving that is invested domestically raises the earnings of labor and lowers average returns to recipients of capital income in addition to generating income for the saver. Under conditions in which payments to various factors of production just equal total production, the added production generated by that saving just equals income to savers plus added income to labor, less reduced

no burden on others, regardless of their numbers or how much of their lives they spend in retirement. For this reason, it is a mistake to infer from an increase in the numbers of elderly that workers must bear increased burdens. On the other hand, if the inactive consume more than they earned, they do impose a burden on the economically active population, whether they are many or few. The ratios shown in table 2-3 contain all people projected to be economically inactive, whether or not they consume more over their life-times than they earned. Not only do the numbers in the table exclude people younger than age sixteen, they also exclude any difference between the relative consumption of the economically active and inactive members of the population.

The SSA projections of the ratio of the dependent adult population to the labor force will increase 37 percent by 2050 and 47 percent by 2075. The increase occurs for two reasons: an anticipated drop in age-specific labor force participation rates and an increase in the proportion of the population in age cohorts (the elderly) with low labor force participation rates. Even a radical increase in immigration would slow this increase relatively little, if all other conditions are unchanged. Increased immigration does cause a major jump in population growth (436 million in 2050 and 500 million in 2075 with increased immigration, versus 373 million and 403 million, respectively, under baseline assumptions).

The projection based on the assumption that people somehow index their retirement to longevity is admittedly extreme. It entails a reversal of a long-term trend toward earlier retirement ages. Some increase in labor force participation may have occurred since the mid- to late-1980s, but analysts disagree on whether the uptick in labor force participation rates reflects a trend reversal or cyclical factors.[24] Many economists hold that people tend to spend some of their rising incomes on increased leisure time and, in particular, that leisure is a superior good, meaning that people spend an increasing proportion of their earning power to buy leisure as incomes rise. The trend toward later entry into the labor force and lower male age-specific labor force participation rates is consistent with that assumption. Increasing female labor force participation rates seems to contradict it. However, many regard this trend as a response to quite separate forces, which have expanded women's choices to pursue careers outside the home.

For people to hold constant the proportion of their adult lives spent in the labor force requires reversal of two of these trends. Any increase in college attendance rates or in time spent during adulthood on education would

24. Quinn (1999); Costa (1999).

Table 2-3. *Ratio of Nonworking Adults to Working Adults, 2000, 2050, 2075*[a]

Assumption	Baseline immigration			Double immigration		
	2000	2050	2075	2000	2050	2075
SSA mortality and labor force participation rates	.482	.662 *37*	.710 *47*	.482	.637 *32*	.687 *42*
SSA mortality, labor force spends unchanging fractions of adult life in retirement[b]	.482	.618 *28*	.617 *28*	.482	.594 *23*	.597 *24*
2 percent mortality improvement, SSA labor force participation rates	.482	.766 *59*	.900 *87*	.482	.708 *47*	.854
2 percent mortality improvement labor force spends unchanging fractions of adult life in retirement[b]	.482	.574 *19*	.586 *22*	.482	.527 *9*	.554 *15*

a. Numbers in italics signify the percentage increase from the year 2000 in the ratio of nonworking to working adults.

b. Labor force participation rates in 2050 and 2075 are computed so that labor force participation rates for each age cohort equals the labor force participation rate of an age cohort that in 2000 has the same ratio of remaining years of expected life to total adult years. We use Social Security Administration labor force participation rates for the year 2000, which come in five-year intervals. We assign that labor force participation rate to the annual age group in the center of the five-year cohort and interpolate. We derived a labor force participation rate for 70–74 year olds in 2000 by assuming that 90 percent of the workers in SSA's 70+ age bracket were workers in the 70–74 age group.

tend to reduce time in the labor force and raise the ratio of adults outside the labor force to adults in the labor force. Nonetheless, such a trend might arise if public policy shifted to discourage early retirement and if medical advances reduced physical and mental disabilities. In any event, the assumption that labor force participation is a function of remaining life expectancy is not a forecast. Rather, it is included to give some indication of the potential ramifications on public costs and labor force growth should age-specific labor force participation rates increase based on remaining life expectancy. Once again, increased immigration has relatively little impact on these adult ratios.

Labor Force

If labor force participation rates are based on remaining years of life, the labor force will become increasingly elderly (see table 2-4). With major increases

Table 2-4. *Age at Which Three-Fourths and Four-Fifths of Retirees Have Left the Labor Force, 2000, 2050, 2075*[a]

Assumption	Baseline immigration			Double immigration		
	2000	2050	2075	2000	2050	2075
SSA mortality and labor force participation rates	65/70	65/70	65/70	65/70	65/70	65/70
SSA mortality, labor force spends unchanging fractions of adult life in retirement	65/70	68/71	69/73	65/70	68/71	69/73
2 percent mortality improvement, labor force spends unchanging fractions of adult life in retirement	65/70	74/79	77/81	65/70	74/79	77/81
2 percent mortality improvement, labor force spends unchanging fractions of adult life in retirement	65/70	74/79	77/81	65/70	74/79	77/81

a. First number in each cell refers to the age at which three-fourths of the labor force has retired; the second number refers to the age at which four-fifths has retired.

in life expectancy, these assumptions imply a huge reversal of the historical lowering of retirement age. Such an increase would occur despite rising incomes, which historically have been associated with increased demand for leisure, part of which has taken the form of progressively earlier ages of retirement. Increases in labor force participation rates are unlikely to occur unless medical advances that extend life also reduce morbidity. It is not clear that both trends will materialize. On the frailty model, life-extending medical advances could raise, not lower, the incidence of debilitating conditions, as those spared death would disproportionately include the relatively frail.

On the other hand, recent trends indicate some reduction in disability rates, and the discovery of effective treatments for arthritis and Alzheimer's disease could dramatically extend mental and physical vigor. Further, increases in labor force participation would reduce the projected growth in the cost of retirement benefits by half or more. Some increase would occur because an increasing proportion of the population would have only a few years of expected life remaining.

The implications for growth of the labor force is also potentially important. With declining fertility rates, U.S. labor force growth is projected to

Table 2-5. *Labor Force in 2000, 2050, and 2075*[a]

	Baseline immigration			Double immigration		
Assumption	*2000*	*2050*	*2075*	*2000*	*2050*	*2075*
SSA mortality and labor force participation rates	**146.0**	**181.2** *0.43*	**191.1** *0.21*	**146.0**	**213.8** *0.77*	**239.8** *0.46*
SSA mortality, labor force spends unchanging fractions of adult life in retirement	**146.0**	**186.1** *0.49*	**202.1** *0.33*	**146.0**	**219.6** *0.82*	**253.7** *0.58*
2 percent mortality improvement, SSA labor force participation rates	**146.0**	**184.4** *0.47*	**196.8**	**146.0**	**216.1** *0.78*	**245.9** *0.52*
2 percent mortality improvement, labor force spends unchanging fractions of adult life in retirement	**146.0**	**206.9** *0.70*	**235.9** *0.53*	**146.0**	**241.8** *1.01*	**293.4** *0.78*

a. Labor force in millions in bold; annual percentage growth in italics.

slow dramatically and remain well under one-half of one percent a year throughout the twenty-first century (see table 2-5). Even with increased immigration, delayed retirement, and a rapidly aging labor force, growth rates will be well below rates common in the twentieth century. But the power of compound interest means that the total labor force will be sensitive to these assumptions.

Summary

The U.S. population, like that of most other developed countries, is aging. Changes in mortality rates from current levels are unlikely to materially change these trends for several decades. Eventually, however, a sharp reduction in mortality rates will result in a large increase in both life expectancy and the population profile. The effects will be relatively small among the young-elderly—those ages sixty to seventy—because mortality rates in these age cohorts will become low even without reductions in mortality rates beyond those in baseline projections. But the effect of sharply reduced mortality rates on the population over age seventy and, especially, over age eighty will be dramatic. By 2075 the number of people over age eighty will be as large as the population over age sixty-eight was in the year 2000.

The implications of these trends depend acutely on whether the medical advances that reduce death also increase mental and physical vigor. If aging and debility are delayed—that is, if tomorrow's eighty-year olds and ninety-year-olds resemble today's fifty-year-olds and sixty-year-olds—the capacity of people to work more years will increase and people will be able to choose between spending their extended lives at work or in retirement. If they choose work, the share of the adult population that is economically inactive would increase negligibly. Such a development would require major changes in the life cycle of work and in labor markets (see the chapter by Gary Burtless). In that event the problems confronting Social Security and Medicare could actually diminish. If despite improved health the healthy elderly choose retirement, it will become necessary for them to have saved more during their working lives or for the economically active to pay much steeper taxes than are customary today. In either case, these would be the choices of a physically vigorous population.

The more daunting prospect would be a world in which the population of the very old increases but the prevalence of disability and frailty does not diminish. In that event, the real burdens imposed by the economically inactive would multiply, with far-reaching implications for public budgets and the family and difficult ethical choices for us all.

Appendix 2A: Methods

The following section describes our methods for modeling future trends in mortality, life expectancy, population, and labor force participation rates.

Mortality

We projected death rates under two scenarios: the SSA baseline and the 2 percent annual mortality reduction.

The SSA mortality rates are those used in the 2001 Old-Age Survivors and Disability Insurance (OASDI) program. SSA forecasts age-specific mortality rates by sex in each year from 1999 to 2201, with a composite mortality rate for individuals age 100 and above. The composite is a blend of separate mortality rates for eleven mutually exclusive and totally exhaustive causes of death.[25] For these mortality rates, we assumed the given SSA rates for ages 0 to 99 and extended the composite 100+ rate for 100-year-olds through the maximum age of 130. SSA projects annual rates of decline in mortality rates for subsequent years.

For the 2 percent annual mortality reduction scenario, we assumed the annual rates of reduction for all primary causes of death to be 2.8 percent for ages 0–14, 2.2 percent for ages 15–64, and 1.9 percent for ages 65 and above. These percentage reductions, when applied to the 1999 population, yield an aggregate decrease in mortality rates of almost exactly 2 percent in the first year.

We then applied the annual rates of reduction to the 1997 calendar-year death rates from the Social Security Administration's 2000 trustees' report. The death rates are expressed as deaths per 100,000 by sex at age zero and subsequently in five-year age groups in addition to a 95+ group. In our simulation we summed the total deaths per 100,000 at each age and calculated the total death rate per 100,000. Due to the uniformity of the age 95+ total death rate, we realized that we would need to adjust the death rates from that age category in order to avoid unrealistic death patterns among the very old. In addition, we elected to insert a maximum-age assumption into the simulation. To create a mortality pattern among the very old, where chance of death increases greatly with age, we replaced the year 2000 age-95-and-older death rate category with age-specific death rates from SSA Actuarial Study 107.[26] We then calculated the annual rate of reduction in age-specific death rates for the age-95-and-above category for each year and applied it to the graduated age-specific death rate from the previous year, beginning in 2000. To illustrate, the age-95 male death rate from the actuarial study was 25.67 percent. In the 2 percent annual reduction scenario, this death rate was reduced by 1.9 percent. Therefore, the 2001 death rate for a 95-year-old was approximately equal to $.2567 \times (1 - .019) = .2518$. Following the identical procedure for the following year, we adjusted the age-95 male death rate to equal approximately .2470 in 2006, or $.2518 \times (1 - .019)$.

The maximum age assumption was straightforward. We assumed in the 2 percent annual reduction that the maximum age was 107 for males and 109 for females in 2000. We increased the maximum age by one year every two calendar years until the maximum age reached 130, the ultimate maximum age. After applying these procedures to obtain the various mortality rates, we then transformed the mortality rates into survival rates (one minus the mortality rate) for each age, sex, and year.

25. The primary causes of death are heart disease, cancer, vascular disease, violence, respiratory disease, infancy, digestive disease, diabetes mellitus, liver cirrhosis, AIDS, and all others.
26. Bell, Wade, and Goss (1992).

Life Expectancy

We calculated life expectancy using both the period and cohort methods. To determine cohort life expectancy at birth, we applied the survival rates from a particular scenario to a 100,000-person cohort. Survival rates were applied to the cohort as though it were aging, so the cohort would experience the survivor rate at age x in year y, and age $x + 1$ in year $y + 1$. From this procedure we derived the survivors from the original 100,000-person cohort at each age 0 to 130 (for life expectancy at birth), then calculated the number of deaths occurring at each age and, subsequently, the number of total years lived by individuals in the cohort dying at each age. We determined life expectancy at age x to be the sum of years lived between age x and age 130 and divided by the number of survivors in the cohort at age x. The result is the average number of years remaining in life, or life expectancy. To illustrate, under SSA mortality rates the male cohort born in 2000 had 86,368 survivors in year 2065. To calculate life expectancy of that cohort at age x, we applied the death rate for age 65 in year 2065 to the remaining cohort, then applied the death rate for age 66 in year 2066, 67 in year 2067, and so forth. We then calculated total years lived by those dying between 2065 and 2130 and divided the sum by 86,368 to determine life expectancy.

When using the method for period life expectancy, an identical procedure was used, except age-specific survival rates remained constant across years. The original 100,000-person cohort was still "aged" through the death rates, except the age-specific death rate would not change across years. The result was, predictably, a significantly lower life expectancy dependent on the degree of mortality improvement.

Population

Our method of simulating population growth incorporated four factors: mortality, immigration, fertility, and sex ratio at birth. We began with the January 1, 1999, population provided by the SSA, applied the 1999 SSA death rates, and added immigration to obtain the year 2000 starting population.

To the age- and sex-specific population at the beginning of a year we added immigration. We used the net immigration estimates (including illegal immigration) provided by the Social Security Administration (2001 trustees' report), where net immigration reaches an ultimate level of 900,000 in 2008.[27] We infused the net immigration numbers at the 'beginning' of the

27. In the double immigration scenarios, we assume an identical age distribution of net immigrants as in the standard immigration scenarios.

year, so that immigrants in a given year were immediately subject to the mortality rates in that year.

As with net immigration, we used the fertility rates provided by the SSA from the 2001 trustees' report. Fertility reached an ultimate level in 2025. We applied the fertility rates in a given year to the starting female population of that year to obtain total newborns. We then applied the sex ratio at birth employed by the SSA: 105 male newborns for every 100 female newborns. Newborns were inserted into the population at the beginning of the year so that the age-0 mortality rate could be applied. Our population estimates refer to the year-end population, including the mortality, fertility, and immigration implications for any given year.

Labor Force Participation Rates

Our forecast of future labor force participation rates (LFPRs) is based on the premise that individuals choose to participate in the labor force based on their expected remaining proportion of life. We first adjusted the SSA LFPRs in the 2001 trustees' report, which are expressed in terms of five-year age groups and an age 70+ category, by linearly interpolating between the midpoint of each interval (for example, for the 65–69-year age group we assumed the LFPR to be the actual value for age 67 and linearly interpolated between ages 67 and 62, the midpoint of the previous age group, to determine the LFPRs for ages 63–66). In addition, we modified the 70+ age category by assuming that 90 percent of the 70+ workers in 2000 were in the 70–74 age group and assigning that value to the midpoint of the 70–74 age group. We then linearly interpolated the other values as we did with younger age groups. Once we modified the year-2000 LFPRs, we calculated the remaining years of adult life (ages 16 and above) under each of the mortality scenarios using the period method of determining life expectancy. From these calculations we derived the expected proportion of adult life remaining.

Once we calculated remaining proportion of life by age, gender, and mortality assumption, we compared the remaining proportion of adult life in a future year to the expected remaining years of adult life in 2000 and assigned the LFPR in 2000 to the age with a corresponding remaining years of adult life in a future year. We linearly interpolated the difference in LFPR as a proportion as the difference in expected proportion of remaining years of adult life between ages. The value of the age-65 LFPR in 2050 is therefore equal to the proportion of difference between the proportion of expected remain-

ing years of adult life at ages 58 and 59, multiplied by the difference in
LFPRs, plus the lower LFPR. In mathematical terms:

$$LFPR_x = \frac{(PERYAL - F_x - PERYAL - P_y)}{(PERYAL - F_{y-1} - PERYAL - F_y)}$$
$$\times (LFPR - P_{y-1} - LFPR - P_y) + LFPR - P_y$$

where x = age in future, y = upper bound of corresponding ages in 2000,
$PERYAL$ = proportion of expected remaining years of adult life, P = value
in 2000, and F = value in future. The result is a gradual curve for LFPRs in
the future that approximately resembles the LFPR curve in 2000, shifted
outward to a degree dependent on improvements in life expectancy.

COMMENT
Stephen Goss

The chapter by Henry Aaron and Benjamin Harris explores one of the most challenging economic questions we will face in this century: How much longer will we be living and how will we afford it? The authors begin with a thorough but succinct description of the competing models of aging and the mortality process. Next, they present two alternative projections of mortality and the resulting patterns of life expectancy and population age distributions. These reflect the intermediate projection of the Social Security Administration plus an alternative mortality pattern with much more rapid decline in death rates, averaging about 2 percent a year. Finally, they explore two ways in which the nation might address the economic strains that would be caused by very rapid increases in life expectancy, involving increased immigration and increased labor force participation.

The material in each of these areas is enlightening and thought provoking. My discussion suggests some further considerations, following on from their work.

Models of Aging

The natural limit hypothesis has appeal in that a limit of around 110 years appears to have been fairly robust in the face of extraordinary progress in reducing mortality throughout the last century. This reduction has been predominantly at lower ages, at which the resulting gains in life expectancy at birth can be large. While a "hard" natural limit is out of favor, a "soft" limit seems reasonable. A soft limit might conceivably increase another ten or twenty years in the next century or so, at least for outliers in a population with optimal environmental and behavioral experience. As the authors point out, however, such a limit on the effective maximum life span places little constraint on possible improvement in mortality at all younger ages for the foreseeable future.

Extrapolation from historic trends is the nearly universal approach to projecting mortality. The authors suggest three reasons for taking this approach over the natural limit hypothesis. The reasons are, more specifically, arguments for the plausibility of continued extrapolation of rapid mortality improvement. However, two of these arguments are not well supported, at least for the United States. One of their arguments is that mortality decline has con-

Table 2-6. *Reduction in Mortality, Average Historic and Projected Rates,*
1900–2076[a]

| | Historic rate | | 1999–2076 rates | | |
| | | | SSA 2002 trustees report | | |
Population	1900–99	1982–99	Intermediate	Low mortality	2 percent improvement
Male, all ages	0.96	0.94	0.78	1.35	1.95
Female, all ages	1.26	0.40	0.72	1.29	1.94
Average, all ages	1.11	0.67	0.75	1.32	1.95
Male, 65 and older	0.59	0.79	0.73	1.29	1.89
Female, 65 and older	0.88	0.22	0.69	1.24	1.89
Average, 65 and older	0.74	0.51	0.71	1.27	1.89

Source: Office of the Chief Actuary, Social Security Administration, April 4, 2003.

a. Rates are age adjusted to the distribution of the population as of 1990; average is computed using the average of male and female annual rates of reduction in age-adjusted death rates.

tinued for decades and shows no sign of stopping. While this is true for at least the most prosperous nations, the pace of decline has been slowing in the United States (see table 2-6). Between 1997 and 1999 death rates for the aged declined at only 0.47 percent a year for men and actually increased by 1.2 percent a year for women. Experience varies greatly among the developed countries (see tables 2-7 and 2-8).

Another argument states that male and female life expectancies are not converging, and experience for Japan is cited. In the United States, however, since 1982 mortality has been improving considerably more rapidly for men than for women. As a result, the difference between female and male period life expectancy at age sixty-five has declined from 4.4 years for 1980 to only 3.2 years for 1999.[1]

The authors suggest caution in accepting the position of population Prometheans. Certainly major advances in our ability to postpone, avert, or reverse many diseases are on the horizon. How effective and affordable these will be is a major question. A very costly procedure may have little effect on overall population mortality if only the richest can afford it.

1. Board of Trustees (2002, p. 83).

Table 2-7. *Life Expectancy at Age Sixty-Five, Seventeen Countries, 1960–96*

Country	1960–66		1990–96		Per decade, 1960–90, over recent three decades	
	Male	Female	Male	Female	Male	Female
Australia	12.2	15.7	15.8	19.6	1.2	1.3
Austria	12.2	14.8	14.7	18.1	0.8	1.1
Canada	13.5	16.1	15.7	19.9	0.7	1.3
Denmark	13.8	15.1	14.1	17.9	0.1	0.9
Finland	11.3	14.1	14.6	18.7	1.1	1.5
France	12.7	16.1	16.1	20.6	1.1	1.5
Ireland	12.6	14.4	13.4	17.1	0.3	0.9
Italy	13.1	15.5	15.4	19.2	0.7	1.2
Japan	12.4	15.1	16.9	21.5	1.5	2.1
Netherlands	14.0	16.0	14.6	18.9	0.2	1.0
New Zealand	12.8	15.5	15.0	18.8	0.8	1.1
Norway	13.9	16.6	15.5	19.5	0.5	1.0
Spain	12.8	14.8	15.5	19.2	0.9	1.5
Sweden	14.0	16.5	16.1	19.7	0.7	1.1
Switzerland	13.0	15.6	16.3	20.3	1.1	1.6
United Kingdom	12.0	15.6	14.8	18.3	0.9	0.9
United States	12.9	16.2	15.6	18.9	0.9	0.9
Average	12.9	15.5	15.3	19.2	0.8	1.2

Source: United Nations.

This leads to the question, What is the underlying process? The authors effectively describe the complexity of interactions among death rates by cause and argue against the notion of independence of separate causes. The SSA's mortality projections incorporate separate assumptions for future rates of improvement by age, sex, and cause of death. However, the authors note that this approach is not intended to suggest that cause-of-death groups are independent of each other. In fact, there is strong interdependence among them, as suggested by the frailty model. Those who are "spared" from dying of one cause are likely to be more susceptible to other causes than is the rest of the population at that age. This is particularly true if the cause is eliminated by an intrusive medical procedure. Possible evidence of this kind of un-covering of a latent cause of death is the emergence of cancer as a principal cause of death as life expectancies have increased.

Table 2-8. *Projected Life Expectancy at Age Sixty-Five, United States, 2000–80*

Projection	Male	Female	Average
2000			
SSA intermediate	15.7	19.0	17.4
SSA low	15.7	19.0	17.4
2% improvement	15.7	19.0	17.4
2080			
SSA intermediate	20.4	23.4	21.9
SSA low	24.1	26.9	25.5
2% improvement			31.0
Increase 2000–80			
SSA intermediate	0.6	0.6	0.6
SSA low	1.1	1.0	1.0
2% improvement			1.7

Source: Office of the Chief Actuary, Social Security Administration, April 4, 2003.

The limited reliability model seems particularly compelling as a model of the human machine. However, the great complexity of the human system probably explains why mathematical models like that of Gompertz and Makeham only roughly model mortality patterns.

Alternative Projections

The authors explore an alternative assuming much greater increases in life expectancy than the Social Security Administration trustees' intermediate projection. The title of their chapter, "Our Uncertain Demographic Future," suggests that smaller increases might also be considered.

The alternative to the intermediate projection is a scenario that assumes (roughly) 2 percent annual reduction in death rates for the future (see table 2-9). This alternative scenario assumes mortality improvement over the next century that has not previously been approached for more than perhaps a decade at a time in this country. And the past century included major advances in public health, safety, and sanitation; general availability of primary and emergency medical care; adequate nutrition; revolutionary treatments for heart disease; and of course antibiotics. These advances cannot be replicated. Future progress may require interventions

Table 2-9. *Life Expectancy (Period Basis) at Birth, 2000–80*[a]

	2002 trustees' report		
Year	Intermediate	Low mortality	2 percent improvement
2000	76.5	76.5	76.5
2005	76.9	77.3	77.5
2010	77.4	78.1	78.7
2015	77.9	79.0	79.8
2020	78.4	79.8	81.0
2025	78.9	80.7	82.1
2030	79.4	81.5	83.2
2035	79.9	82.2	84.4
2040	80.3	83.0	85.5
2045	80.8	83.7	86.6
2050	81.2	84.4	87.7
2055	81.6	85.1	88.8
2060	82.0	85.7	89.9
2065	82.4	86.4	91.0
2070	82.8	87.0	92.2
2075	83.1	87.6	93.3
2080	83.5	88.2	94.4

a. All assumptions, with the exception of mortality, are the intermediate assumptions of the 2002 trustees' report. SSA Board of Trustees (2002).

that may not be such pure positives, as with improved sanitation, for example. Medical interventions like chemotherapy, furthermore, have negative side effects, which may increase frailty even as they postpone death.

The authors mention early in the chapter that they ignore the debilitating consequences of harmful behaviors that lead to, for example, obesity. It should, however, be noted that—given the consequences—achieving a sustained 2 percent annual improvement in mortality may be even more difficult than is suggested by considering historic periods alone. Speculation solely on the prospect of eliminating certain causes of death also ignores the challenge of maintaining even the effectiveness of the current antibiotics. Our biological enemies have proven adept in adapting and in some cases have developed resistance to all antibiotics.

There are other challenges to the proposition of greatly accelerated improvement in mortality. For example, many of the advances considered in support of possible rapid mortality improvement will be expensive to develop and potentially too expensive to apply to the population as a whole. Remedies for the few do little for general population mortality rates. While medicines generally become cheaper after introduction, labor-intensive procedures will continue to be expensive and therefore limited to a few. Even with the assumption by the Social Security trustees that health expenditures will grow 1 percent a year faster than overall gross domestic product, organ transplants and complex procedures are also likely to be limited to a few, particularly as the number of the aged increases.

Organ replacement does not, of course, fundamentally alter the aging process. In addition, the human body is of sufficient complexity that the technology for replacing parts will continue to be incomplete for a very long time. This probably means that, even with vital organ replacement, manifestations of aging will continue into the foreseeable future, and the end of our economically useful lives will remain between the ages of sixty and eighty. This prospect may restrict the investment required to pursue aggressive and expensive interventions. Some protocols already restrict some operations to individuals below a specified age. As scientific understanding and capabilities expand, rationing may become more common.

Projected life expectancy at birth under the alternative assumptions using the Social Security Office of the Actuary model concurs with the authors' calculations, indicating consistent methodologies (see table 2-9). Table 2-10 provides comparisons of life expectancy at age sixty-five. Both tables include the Social Security trustees' low-mortality projection, which reflects improvement at a considerably faster pace than over the past century and greatly faster than since 1982. Important questions are, What special circumstances existed over those years that slowed mortality improvement in the United States, and Why should we believe that these factors will not exist in the future?

Population Projections and Implications

The authors project populations using the Social Security trustees' intermediate projection, varying only the mortality assumptions. Because the intermediate projection reflects fertility at continued historically low rates, the population ages considerably in all scenarios. Table 2-11 provides standard aged dependency ratios to illustrate this. This is a purely demographic measure.

The authors use an adult dependency ratio, defined as the ratio between the population aged sixteen and over that is not in the labor force and the

Table 2-10. *Increase in Life Expectancy (Period Basis) at Age Sixty-Five, 2000–80*[a]

	2002 trustees' report		
Year	Intermediate	Low mortality	2 percent improvement
2000	17.4	17.4	17.4
2005	17.6	17.8	18.1
2010	17.9	18.4	18.8
2015	18.2	18.9	19.6
2020	18.5	19.5	20.3
2025	18.9	20.0	21.1
2030	19.2	20.6	21.9
2035	19.5	21.1	22.8
2040	19.8	21.6	23.6
2045	20.1	22.1	24.5
2050	20.3	22.7	25.3
2055	20.6	23.1	26.2
2060	20.9	23.6	27.1
2065	21.2	24.1	28.1
2070	21.4	24.6	29.0
2075	21.7	25.0	30.0
2080	21.9	25.5	31.0
Average increase per decade	0.6	1.0	1.7

Source: Office of the Chief Actuary, Social Security Administration, April 4, 2003.

a. All assumptions, with the exception of mortality, are the intermediate assumptions of the 2002 trustees' report. Board of Trustees (2002).

population of that same age group that is in the labor force. This ratio, which attempts to capture the economic burden of an aging population, has significant limitations. For example, if over time additional individuals enter the labor force and are paid for doing work that in the past was done without pay, like mowing lawns and caring for children, then measured economic activity and labor force participation increase, but the burden of caring for the elderly is not reduced. For this reason, this measure may appear to have risen less than has the actual burden of caring for "nonproductive" adults.

The authors consider scenarios with increased labor force participation rates in proportion to increases in the remaining portion of total life. This may be a solution with no ready means to achieve it. The authors appropriately indicate that, if the frailty model is correct, then such increases should

Table 2-11. *Aged Dependency Ratios, 2000–80* [a]

| | 2002 trustees' report | | |
Year	Intermediate	Low mortality	2 percent improvement
2000	0.212	0.212	0.212
2005	0.206	0.206	0.207
2010	0.212	0.213	0.213
2015	0.235	0.239	0.243
2020	0.270	0.278	0.284
2025	0.314	0.326	0.335
2030	0.352	0.370	0.383
2035	0.368	0.391	0.410
2040	0.369	0.399	0.424
2045	0.366	0.402	0.433
2050	0.370	0.411	0.451
2055	0.378	0.424	0.471
2060	0.391	0.442	0.496
2065	0.400	0.456	0.516
2070	0.412	0.472	0.540
2075	0.422	0.488	0.565
2080	0.431	0.504	0.591

Source: Office of the Chief Actuary, Social Security Administration, April 4, 2003.

a. All assumptions, with the exception of mortality, are the intermediate assumptions of the 2002 trustees' report. Board of Trustees (2002). Dependency ratio is the ratio of the population aged sixty-five and older to the population aged twenty to sixty-four.

not be expected. A further consideration is that the participation of the advanced elderly, even if achieved, may be part time and of low productivity. The adult dependency ratio does not capture this effect. In a world of increasing technology, the most desirable employees may be younger, not older. Even if frailty is diminished at higher ages in the future, the young will still be more flexible and will generally have more recent and more relevant education and training.

The authors also consider the possibility of increased legal immigration and its effect on population age distributions. Increasing immigration limits is largely a policy parameter and is thus a more controllable means to deal with population shifts than is increased labor force participation by the elderly. Moreover, young immigrants may better fill the service positions needed to assist an aging society. Policies rewarding the birth of a second or third child might have much the same effect in the long run as increased immigration limits.

Finally, the authors state that longer labor force participation would be likely only if increased life expectancy is accompanied by reduced age-specific morbidity. They state that recent trends indicate declining disability rates among the elderly. It should be noted that declines in the numbers of activities of daily living and instrumental activities of daily living among the elderly (noted by Ken Manton since 1982, based on the National Long-Term Care Survey) occurred at precisely the same time that mortality improvement of the elderly slowed (see table 2-6). If the slowdown in mortality improvement since 1982 is the result of less improvement in life extension among the frail during this period, then improving age-specific morbidity would be expected. If on the other hand mortality improvement for the aged accelerates to between three and four times the pace since 1982, as suggested in the alternative scenario (with an average 2 percent annual improvement), then increasingly frail populations will be more likely.

References

Aaron, Henry J., and Benjamin H. Harris. 2002. "Uncertainty and Pension Policy." Paper prepared for conference, Collaboration Projects (on Aging Issues), Tokyo, February 18–21.

Aaron, Henry J., and Robert D. Reischauer. 1998. *Countdown to Reform: The Great Social Security Debate.* New York: Century Foundation Press.

Ahlburg, Dennis A., and James W. Vaupel. 1990. "Alternative Projections of the U.S. Population." *Demography* 27 (4): 639–52.

Bell, Felicitie C., Alice H. Wade, and Stephen C. Goss. 1992. *Life Tables for the United States Social Security Area: 1900–2080.* Actuarial Study 107 (August).

Board of Trustees, OASDI (Board of Trustees, Federal Old-Age and Survivors Insurance and Disability Insurance Trust Funds). 2002. *The 2002 Annual Report of the Board of Trustees, Federal Old-Age and Survivors Insurance and Disability Insurance Trust Funds.*

Caselli, Graziella, and Alan D. Lopez. 1996. "Health and Mortality among the Elderly, Issues for Assessment." In *Health and Mortality among Elderly Populations,* edited by Graziella Caselli and Alan D. Lopez, 3–20. Oxford: Clarendon Press.

Costa, Dora L. 1999. Comments prepared for the first annual joint conference, Retirement Research Consortia, Washington, May 20–21.

Cutler, David M., and Ellen Meara. 2001. "Changes in the Age Distribution of Mortality over the Twentieth Century." Cambridge: National Bureau of Economic Research.

Fries, James F. 1980. "Aging, Natural Death, and the Compression of Morbidity." *New England Journal of Medicine* 303 (3): 130–35.

Gavrilov, L. A., and N. S. Gavrilova. 1991. *The Biology of Life Span: A Quantitative Approach.* New York: Harwood Academic Publishers.

Harris, John. 2000. "Intimations of Immortality." *Science* 288 (5463): 59.

Lee, Ronald D., and Lawrence R. Carter. 1992. "Modeling and Forecasting U.S. Mortality." *Journal of the American Statistical Association* 87 (419): 659–71.

Lee, Ronald D., and Ryan Edwards. 2001. "The Fiscal Impact of Population Aging in the U.S. Assessing the Uncertainties." Paper prepared for NBER meeting on tax policy and the economy, Washington, October 30.

Manton, Kenneth G., Eric Stallard, and James W. Vaupel. 1981. "Methods for Comparing the Mortality Experience of Heterogeneous Populations." *Demography* 18 (2): 389–410.

McNeil, Jack. 2001. *Americans with Disabilities.* Current Population Report (U.S. Census Bureau). February.

Olshansky, S. Jay, Bruce Carnes, and Aline Désesquelles. 2001. "Prospects for Human Longevity." *Science* 291 (5508): 1491.

Puca, Annibale A., and others. 2001. "A Genome-Wide Scan for Linkage to Human Exceptional Longevity Identifies a Locus on Chromosome 4." *Proceedings of the National Academy of Sciences USA* 98 (18): 10505–08 (www.pnas.org/cgi/doi/10.1073.181337598).

Quinn, Joseph F. 1999. "Has the Trend toward Early Retirement Reversed?" Paper prepared for the first annual joint conference, Retirement Research Consortia, Washington, May 20–21.

Schwartz, William B. 1998. *Life without Disease: The Pursuit of Medical Utopia.* University of California Press.

Vaupel, James W. 1988. "Inherited Frailty and Longevity." *Demography* 25 (2): 277–87.

Wilmoth, John R. 1996. "Mortality Projections for Japan: A Comparison of Four Methods." In *Health and Mortality among Elderly Populations,* edited by Graziella Caselli and Alan D. Lopez, 266–87. Oxford: Clarendon Press.

———. 2000. "Demography of Longevity: Past, Present, and Future Trends." *Experimental Gerontology* 35 (9–10): 1111–29.

ALAN M. GARBER
DANA P. GOLDMAN

3 | *The Changing Face of Health Care*

T HE CONSEQUENCES FOR human health of recent breakthroughs in fundamental biology, including the landmark
sequencing of the human genome, are impossible to predict with any certainty.
However, the biomedical research community is confident that unprecedented advances in its ability to prevent, detect, and treat disease are within
reach. If so, there will be striking changes in the health of the population—
perhaps distributed unevenly and occurring at different times for different
groups—and in the total resources devoted to medical care.

If there are no medical improvements, there will be very little change in
population health. Demographic changes alone will produce only modest
changes in the pattern of disease. Using a stylized model, we show that cures
for major diseases (or new ways to prevent them) could produce enormous
savings. Ways of preventing or curing illnesses that are not lethal but that
reduce the quality of life (roughly measured by disability) would also produce
large savings.

Our simulations assume that the new treatments would be inexpensive.
In the past, medical treatments have been costly. Because health insurance
pays for a substantial fraction of so many health care transactions and no
effective limit on total spending exists in the United States, insurance has
contributed in a fundamental way to the development and spread of costly
medical innovations. Many new treatments are so costly that only insured

105

or affluent patients can afford them. It is for this reason that health insurance critically influences which innovations are developed and come to market.

The nature of medical breakthroughs will have an important bearing on whether they raise or lower medical costs. Prospects for improved treatments of heart disease, diabetes, and Alzheimer's are excellent. Such breakthroughs would affect much of the population and could forestall expensive complications later. Genetic screening to better detect existing disease would have similar effects. Gene therapy and bioengineering are likely to lead to improved treatments for existing disease. Scientists might find new, dramatically effective ways to extend life span. Such advances could quickly increase the number of elderly Americans, particularly if new techniques forestall the onset of diseases such as cancer. A critical question is whether medical advances that extend life (perhaps through promotion of telomerase) also increase the likelihood of cancer. John Potts and William Schwartz, in their chapter in this volume, elaborate on these and other possibilities.

Some of these changes will be expensive. They will raise medical expenditures and hence the cost of health insurance. As a result, fewer people will be able to afford comprehensive coverage. With fragmented health insurance markets and incomplete health insurance coverage, the fruits of medical progress may be distributed unevenly. Even if insurance coverage becomes universal, the benefits that any socioeconomic group derives from innovations will depend on the prevalence of treatable disease in that group. If science finds cures for "rich people's diseases"—as cardiovascular disease once was—then the gap between the health of the rich and that of the poor will widen. Because molecular medicine holds the promise of significant breakthroughs, health policy will face a challenge—to encourage not only the development but also the widespread dissemination of these innovations. Whether it will be possible to ensure rapid diffusion of innovations and equal availability across population groups remains uncertain.

The Status Quo and Medical Miracles

Even without changes in medical technology, demographic and social forces will generate large changes in expenditures—and to a lesser extent in overall health. Many factors affect demand. Age, sex, functional status, disease, the price of care, living arrangements, and care from family and friends are the most notable.[1] These will generate important changes in the health care marketplace even in the absence of medical innovation.

New treatments will further complicate this future by affecting the cost and price of health care, particularly when the new technology makes it possible to treat conditions for which no effective treatment previously existed. Such treatments have usually both raised total expenditures and improved health. Before hemodialysis, for example, patients with severe kidney failure died rapidly. Now they can be kept alive indefinitely, although at considerable cost. Computerized tomography (CT) scans and magnetic resonance imaging (MRI) substitute for such alternatives as exploratory surgery that were so dangerous and costly that they were used relatively infrequently. Because CT scans and MRIs are safe and much less costly than previously available procedures, they not only substitute for older, less-effective, and higher-priced technologies but can also be used in far more diverse circumstances. As a result, they are used so often that they have increased total health expenditures even as the cost per procedure fell.

To illuminate how demographic change will affect health care spending, we project how many people of various demographic categories will be alive in each future year, and we estimate health care spending per person in each category. Two pieces of information are crucial: the size of the population and its health status. As mortality rates decline, health and functional status within age-sex categories can improve, worsen, or stay approximately the same. We assume, as do many actuarial models, that health within a given age-sex category remains constant. Given this assumption, only changes in the age composition of the population and general trends in spending that apply uniformly across age-sex categories influence future expenditures.

A growing body of research calls this assumption into question. Disease onset may be delayed in the future. According to one view, chronic conditions will manifest and health will fail at older and older ages. These changes in health will make it possible to extend the number of working years and to maintain or improve the quality of life in retirement. Significant morbidity, functional limitations, and costly care will become common only in the last few years of life. Extended longevity will tend to boost health spending because people have more years to consume health care, but compressed morbidity will tend to reduce health expenditures to the extent that disease and disability are postponed. On balance, savings are likely to predominate, and

1. This exogeneity assumption is not precisely correct. Medical breakthroughs may affect demographic factors by increasing longevity or by redefining what we mean by *disease*. The chapter by Henry Aaron and Benjamin Harris, this volume, considers the demographic factors. We return to the latter issue.

studies of specific diseases suggest that such savings are not negligible. Many factors—life-style changes, primary and secondary disease prevention, and dramatically improved treatments—have contributed to the decline in cardiovascular mortality, for example, and have also led to a postponement of disease and disability, which are major predictors of higher expenditures.[2] Thus declining mortality may not increase expenditures as much as predicted by models that assume unchanging age-specific health.

The apparent decline in the prevalence of disease and disability may reflect the effects of medical care as well as behavioral and life-style changes. For example, better control of blood pressure—largely achieved by use of medications—reduces the likelihood of stroke and other forms of cardiovascular disease, with their heavy burdens of morbidity and disability.[3] Better control of blood sugar and blood pressure in diabetics also reduces the incidence of kidney failure, neuropathy, retinopathy, and other serious complications in diabetics.[4] No consensus exists on why the prevalence of some diseases, such as asthma, has changed. Nor is it always possible to distinguish the relative contribution of life-style changes, preventive medical care, and treatment of disease to changes in mortality rates. These factors have helped reduce the toll of some diseases, but preventive care and treatment have had little effect on others, such as many common cancers. We explore the implications for medical costs if, on the one hand, disease incidence and treatment costs are unchanged and if, on the other hand, interventions can costlessly eliminate certain common diseases.

We use a microsimulation model to explore how future medical breakthroughs might affect health care spending on the elderly. We focus on the elderly not because they are the only ones likely to benefit but rather because they currently bear a disproportionately large burden of illness and these illnesses account for a large proportion of total medical spending. Furthermore, longitudinal data on the elderly are readily available. Conventional actuarial approaches are often constrained by their use of cell-based models in which each cell represents a subpopulation of interest. While it is theoretically possible to extend such models to support health care projections, practical shortcomings make it difficult to simulate changes in medical treatment. To characterize health status with any degree of complexity—for example, creating cells defined in part by sex and age group—the number of cells would need to be very large. The number of observations in each cell size would be

2. Hunink (1997).
3. See Collins and MacMahon (1994); Yusuf and others (2000).
4. DCCTRG (1993, 1995); UKPDSG (1998a, 1998b); DCCT/EDICRG (2000).

Figure 3-1. *Disease Prevalence among Medicare Beneficiaries, Ages Sixty-Five and Older, 2000–30*

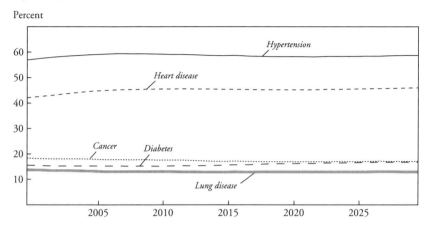

Percent

correspondingly small. As a result, it would be difficult or impossible to estimate transition probabilities among cells with precision. Microsimulation offers a conceptually and analytically superior alternative. Under this approach, we use extant data to simulate how the costs of treatment of a representative cohort of Medicare beneficiaries ages sixty-five or older will change from year to year. We also simulate how their health status changes, the diseases they get, their level of disability, and their eventual death. The model is 'refreshed' each year by bringing in a new cohort of sixty-five-year-olds who have just become eligible for Medicare.

Figures 3-1 and 3-2 display forecasts of prevalence rates for certain key diseases among all elderly (age sixty-five and older) and those turning age sixty-five each year between 2000 and 2030. The curves are relatively flat because these figures are based on the assumption that medicine will be practiced the same in each future year as it was between 1992 and 1998, when the data were collected. If no medical improvements occur, the prevalence of most major diseases will change little from now until 2030.

We then consider the impact of medical advances profound enough to eliminate some of the major diseases of the twentieth century. For example, as some advocates have only half-jokingly suggested, statins (or a more effective and less risky variant) might be added to the water supply—or more realistically, added to daily vitamins—to reduce the frequency of heart disease, much as fluoride was used to reduce tooth decay among children. In the second example, genetic profiling allows doctors to identify patients who will

Figure 3-2. *Disease Prevalence among Entering Medicare Beneficiaries, Age 65, 2000–30*

Percent

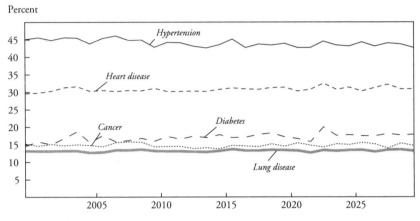

develop type 2 diabetes and start them on a prediabetes drug regimen that completely prevents the disease. Finally, a cancer vaccine tailored to each individual may both prevent the disease and cure existing cases starting in 2005.[5] Figure 3-3 shows how eliminating each of these diseases would affect total health care expenditures on the elderly population. These forecasts account for both direct and indirect effects, including reductions in morbidity and mortality from complications of disease that may not appear in death statistics and related aggregate figures. For instance, eliminating diabetes will reduce the likelihood of dying from heart disease and improve longevity; the estimates shown here account for that change. None of these forecasts takes into account the cost of providing the treatment. The first two examples— statins in the water and identification and treatment of prediabetes using off-the-shelf drugs—might not be costly. On the other hand, the genetic profiling of patients to tailor cancer vaccines individually might be quite expensive. This last treatment may be available to only a few privileged individuals, an issue we take up later.

Technologies that reduce morbidity could have similar effects. Most notably, disability dramatically increases the demand for medical services.

5. The relationship between other conditions and death is assumed unchanged. For example, this means that we mechanically eliminate diabetes among the existing cohort of Medicare eligibles as well as future entrants to Medicare but keep unchanged the transition hazard for all other conditions and functional states tracked by the model—hypertension, heart disease, cancer, death, and disability, for example.

Figure 3-3. *Health Expenditures by the Elderly, Four Scenarios, 2000–30*

Billions of U.S. dollars (1998)

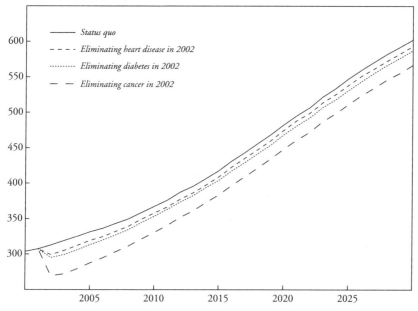

Disability among the elderly has fallen steadily in recent decades, suggesting that substantial cost savings will follow.[6] However, to forecast future disability, one must also consider the current health of tomorrow's Medicare beneficiaries—today's young and middle-aged adults. Remarkably little research has addressed trends in disability rates in these cohorts. Some trends are quite worrisome. Rates of obesity and diabetes are rising among the young. These trends raise doubts that reductions in disability rates will persist. Disability rates increased among the young between 1984 and 1996, a period when disability decreased among the elderly (see figure 3-4). Some of the improvement among the elderly can be attributed to better medical care.[7] Why disability rates are increasing among the young is not entirely clear, but evidence of deterioration in underlying health status is inescapable. In addition to increased obesity and diabetes, asthma has also become more prevalent.[8] It is important to note, however, that figures 3-1 and 3-2 account for these trends.

6. Singer and Manton (1998).
7. Singer and Manton (1998).
8. Lakdawalla, Goldman, and Bhattacharya (2001).

Figure 3-4. *Change in Disability Rates, by Age Group, 1984–96*[a]

Percent

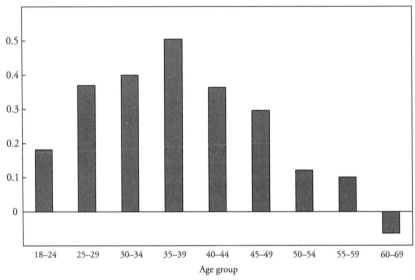

Age group

Source: Lakdawalla, Bhattacharya, and Goldman (2001), table 1.
a. Disability is defined as proportion of people who need assistance with routine needs.

The effect of disability on forecasted costs can be seen most clearly if we calculate the implications for costs of different disability scenarios, as in figure 3-5. The figure depicts three scenarios. The most costly shows per capita costs if disability rates are unchanged from levels assumed in this scenario and only the age and sex structure of the population changes over time. Aging is expected to reduce per capita costs somewhat between 2005 and 2020, with the influx of young-old people that will accompany the aging of the baby-boom cohort. By 2020, however, the continued aging of the baby boomers will start to raise per capita costs. (It is important to keep in mind that population aging consistently raises disability among the population as a whole, elderly and nonelderly combined.) The constant disability curve, however, makes clear that the vast majority of the projected decline in per capita costs owes itself to future declines in disability. The least costly shows costs if disability declines at the rate experienced from 1989 to 1994.[9] The intermediate case is based on the assumption that disability declines at the rate experienced from 1994 to 1999.[10]

9. Manton and others (1997).
10. Manton and Gu (2001).

Figure 3-5. *Monthly Medicare Costs, Three Projections, 2000–30*

1998 U.S. dollars

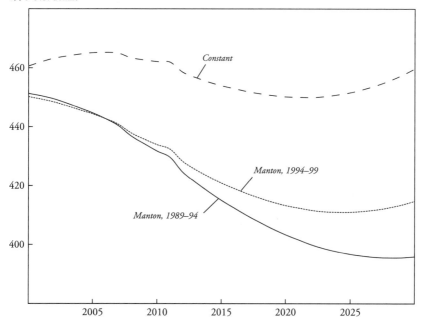

Source: Authors' calculations, Manton and others (1997).

This exercise rests on two latent facts. First, past reductions in disability were almost an incidental benefit of new medical care. Improvement in functional status by itself was not the primary objective of research. In contrast, the biomedical and public health communities now appreciate the importance of functional status as a measure of well-being among the elderly. Second, these communities are now more aware that functional status is an important determinant of health care costs and that the private and public rewards to reducing disability are tangible. As biomedicine turns its attention to ways to reduce the morbidity caused by certain diseases, either by eliminating the side effects of treatment or reversing the progression of disease, health care costs could fall substantially.

Demand for Medical Innovation

Although they are richer than most actuarial models used to project health expenditures, microsimulation models are silent about the critical effects of markets for medical innovations. They treat changes in disability and technology as exogenous events, driven by outside forces but not themselves influenced by changes in health care markets. Yet virtually all observers recognize that health care financing will undergo major changes in response to the cost pressures produced by population aging and technological advance. Plausible medical innovations could revolutionize several areas of medical care but only if it appears that they will attract enough revenue to justify investment in their development. Thus the demand for innovative forms of care is expected to drive their development and adoption.

The transitions from laboratory to approved product to dissemination into widespread practice cannot be understood without reference to the markets in which medical products and services are sold. These markets deviate in striking ways from idealized perfectly competitive markets, yet economic incentives predictably influence behavior in imperfect markets too.

The central feature is the pervasiveness of health insurance, which reduces the cost of medical care to patients: Patients pay for only a small fraction of charges at the time they are ill.[11] The increase in the use of services induced by this reduction in price is sometimes called *moral hazard.*[12] The RAND Health Insurance Experiment, which measured demand for care under various forms of health insurance, demonstrates that consumption of health services increases as the price to the consumer falls.[13] Just as health insurance tends to increase consumption, and hence expenditures, it increases demand for quality-improving technologies and thereby strengthens the incentives to develop them. Over the long term, incentives for technological innovation enrich the mix of medical products and services and boost growth of expenditures on health care.[14]

The market environment for new technologies will depend both on the number of people with health insurance and the characteristics of the insurance plans. Insurance policies that cover a broad range of services and/or providers or that have small deductibles and copayments are more likely to promote heavy use than are relatively constrained policies. Cost sharing has increased, and limits on coverage have narrowed in recent years as costs have risen. The uninsured, who pay the full price of medical care, are not even able to benefit from the discounted fees and medication prices that health plans negotiate. As health expenditures have grown as a percentage

11. Arrow (1963); Pauly (1968).
12. Pauly (1968).
13. Newhouse (1993).
14. Weisbrod (1991).

of gross domestic product, the number of Americans who are uninsured has reached 43.6 million.[15]

Changes in the number of uninsured are not independent of costs. At the same time that rising premiums make insurance less affordable, concern about health care spending has discouraged policymakers from considering measures to substantially extend comprehensive health insurance coverage, since they fear that such reforms would further stimulate health spending. Such concerns have impeded both the development of initiatives to extend insurance to the uninsured and the addition of new benefits, such as prescription drug coverage, to Medicare.

How successful are current efforts to control health expenditure growth, and how will such efforts affect the market for new technologies? Several approaches are commonly used. Medicare and some Medicaid programs directly regulate the prices paid to providers. Health maintenance organizations (HMOs) and other managed care plans intercede in the patient-provider relationship and provide an opportunity to control treatment and technology. Once viewed as the most promising way to slow expenditure growth, these efforts have not stemmed the rise in health expenditures, and both providers and patients have chafed at the controls imposed by HMOs. Such resistance has led to efforts to limit HMO oversight and to require some coverage for care outside of the HMO's network of doctors—so-called point-of-service plans. Thus capitation is unlikely to live up to its promise as the principal means of cost control. As capitation has fallen out of favor, interest in other forms of insurance has grown. Medical savings accounts and consumer-directed or self-directed plans pass financial responsibility and much decisionmaking authority back to the consumer.

Evidence on how each of these financing arrangements affects the demand for new technology is limited and inconclusive. It has long been known that the rate of rise in health expenditures is similar for HMOs and for traditional indemnity insurance, although more recent evidence suggests that managed care slows the adoption of some new procedures, such as laparoscopic cholecystectomy, and that markets with high managed care penetration are slower to adopt MRIs and other capital-intensive innovations.[16] At best, the long-run effects of such financing arrangements on the adoption of new technology appear to be modest. Furthermore, cost-sharing features that restrict the use of many health services and products usually phase out when

15. Mills and Bhandari (2003).
16. On the past similarity of cost increases, see Schwartz, (1987). On the adoption of new technology, see Escarce and others (1995); Baker (2001); Baker and Wheeler (1998).

total costs are high. Consequently, severely ill patients in intensive care units typically have little financial reason not to accept very costly treatments that promise any benefit, however small. Since health insurance is designed to protect patients from the potentially ruinous costs associated with severe illness, there is usually little cost sharing for very expensive procedures. The inevitable result is that, in the absence of external constraints on use of such procedures, benefits may be small relative to costs.

As consumers bear more of the costs of medical products and services, and as managed care plans and even less-restricted plans use bulk purchasing, managed pharmaceutical benefits, and other approaches to control expenditures, a large share of the market is becoming more price sensitive. As a result, cost-increasing medical innovations may find it more difficult in the future than they did in the past to find purchasers.

In addition, the scope of insurance coverage will be subject to great scrutiny. If researchers identify an anti-aging compound, it is unclear whether insurance would cover it. Current insurance contracts routinely limit reimbursement to cases of "medical necessity." Coverage is unlikely to be extended to such a compound if it is considered a life-style enhancement rather than a treatment for a disease.[17] For those whose genetic endowment elevates mortality risk, however, such a compound could directly treat a pathological condition. The compound would probably be covered in such cases. Insurers would then face a challenge to find ways to distinguish those for whom the compound would be covered from those for whom it would not be covered.

Restrictions imposed by managed care, increased cost sharing, and limits on coverage are creating the perception that demand for cost-increasing innovations will be weaker in the future than it was in the past, but how a particular technology will be received depends on the details of health insurance contracts. For example, medical savings account plans permit people to save a certain amount each year in a tax-sheltered account. Medical bills are paid first from accumulated balances in these accounts. Insurance covers all or most costs above high deductibles. Such coverage imposes few limits on very expensive technologies, particularly those targeted toward enrollees whose expenses exceed the deductibles. Paradoxically, such plans (which are frequently touted because they would lower costs) might create greater limitations on demand for low-cost innovations, because costs to use these innovations would be entirely out-of-pocket. Conversely, any plan with fixed copayments and no limit on out-of-pocket payments would strongly

17. Garber (2001); Bergthold (1995).

discourage the use of very expensive technologies. An increase in the number of the uninsured would effectively limit the market size for nearly all medical innovations. Because no single model of health insurance has emerged as dominant, it is premature to draw conclusions about the specific contours of future markets for medical innovations, beyond a continuation of the current trend toward greater price sensitivity.

Supply of Medical Innovation

As price sensitivity has increased, the traditional view of markets for medical products and services has lost much of its relevance. According to that view, the role of price competition for medical products and services is limited. Since consumers directly bear little of the cost of care, they are unlikely to search for the lowest-price alternative, choosing instead the highest-quality option. Pure quality competition characterizes a much smaller share of the market today than in the past.

As producers of medical innovations recognize these trends, their product development strategies are likely to respond accordingly. In a market characterized by little price sensitivity and a great willingness to pay for quality improvements, the dramatic innovations that are expected to result from the advances in molecular medicine would be expensive. When monopolists face demand that is insensitive to price, they tend to charge extremely high prices. In the traditional model of the indemnity insurance market, in which consumers pay perhaps 20 percent of the cost of a medical good or service, a profit-maximizing monopolist is unlikely to set the price so low that total spending falls. In fact, medical technology has driven large cost increases over the last several decades. To be sure, some innovations have been drugs that keep people out of the hospital and make them more productive at work; but prices are often set to reflect these benefits.

One of the most significant advances in molecular medicine may be more selective targeting of treatment. New tests, based on both genetic and nongenetic information, will help identify those patients most likely to benefit from a specific treatment. The concept of therapeutic targeting is not new. For many years, susceptibility tests have assisted in the treatment of bacterial infections by showing which antibiotics are most effective against the specific organism obtained from an infected patient. A current example of a targeted therapy is herceptin, which is effective only in women with breast cancer who carry a particular genetic abnormality.[18] From the point of view

18. Seidman and others (2001); Slamon and others (2001).

of the producers of such innovations, more precise targeting means that the population that benefits from the treatment will be smaller although their collective benefits could be greater than those for the larger but less-selected market. Investment in targeted therapies and in the tests used for targeting will surely depend upon producer expectations about insurance characteristics. The marketing divisions of pharmaceutical companies will often confront the question of whether they should seek high prices for a narrowly targeted therapy or accept lower prices in exchange for a larger market of patients whose average benefit from therapy is smaller.

Medical Innovation and Disease Prevention

Despite the difficulties imposed by rising health insurance costs and the likely increase in price sensitivity among insured patients, effective new technologies will be adopted by substantial fractions of the insured population. Some refer to the enthusiasm of American physicians and patients for new technology as a "technological imperative."[19] Furthermore, demographic changes will increase the potential market for medical innovations directed toward virtually all common chronic diseases. What kinds of change are we likely to see in the near term as innovations are adopted?

Improved preventive care, along with new and highly effective diagnostic tests and treatments, will lead to longer lives and enable Americans to spend more of their years free of pain and disability. As the science advances, the challenges of making these improvements widely available will grow. Drugs to lower cholesterol and blood pressure have already reduced the incidence of coronary heart disease and stroke. New treatments are on the horizon—selective estrogen receptor modulators to prevent cancer, new insulin-sensitizing drugs to prevent diabetes, and several ways to prevent Alzheimer's disease and Parkinson's disease. If these efforts are successful, the resulting breakthroughs have the potential to improve health outcomes at relatively low cost or even to be cost saving. For example, even before generic versions of statins and blood pressure drugs became available, the original and high-priced versions of these drugs were either cost effective or cost saving when used by patients who are most likely to benefit, in part because their costs compare favorably to the cost of treating the morbidity associated with the disease. However, at the lower price for generics, a larger segment of the population would be eligible for treatment, and cumulative drug cost

19. Fuchs (1974); Newhouse (1992).

may be high. Furthermore, any reductions in mortality could result in higher lifetime costs of treatment.

But in general, medical innovations will lead to better detection of early-stage disease, better treatment of established disease, and increases in life expectancy:

—Better detection of early-stage disease. Building upon the findings of the human genome project, scientists will increase our ability to create a genetic profile for each person in order to determine their susceptibility to disease. Such information could be used to learn who is prone to develop cardiovascular disease, depression, osteoporosis, diabetes, vision and hearing impairments, dementia, and urinary incontinence. Improved risk profiling will, in turn, lead to more effective targeting of therapies to ameliorate the morbidity and mortality associated with the disease. Even without better risk stratification through genomics, improved imaging techniques (CT scans, MRIs, functional MRIs, positron emission tomography scans) have improved the detection of disease before it causes symptoms. Either way, the cost of early treatment of chronic illnesses is likely to grow, even if such treatments forestall more costly treatment later.

—Better treatment of established disease. New treatments of established disease include gene therapy, cell or organ transplantation, and bioengineering. Scientists are exploring methods of encouraging the body to generate new blood vessels (angiogenesis) in patients with poor cardiac circulation. They are also working on ways to inhibit neovascularization (antiangiogenesis) associated with the growth of cancer. Stem cell transplants may relieve the symptoms of Parkinson's disease. Transplants from other species (xenotransplants), such as hearts from pigs, may extend the lives of people with failing hearts. Many of these treatments face large ethical and technological hurdles, and some are likely to remain very costly because they will not be amenable to economies of scale.

—Increases in life expectancy. A striking implication of studies of the mechanisms of aging is that it might be possible to manipulate our biology to extend life span. Hundreds of nonhuman studies have shown that caloric restriction significantly slows the rate at which animals age. In addition to the general slowing of aging, caloric restriction tends to prevent or reduce the frequency of many specific diseases. Calorie-restricted animals live as much as 40 percent longer on the average than do control animals. These studies, and the linking of certain genes to caloric intake, have led to speculation that it may be possible to manipulate life span in humans through caloric restriction. Yet another example involves telomeres, the repeated sequences of DNA located at the ends of chromosomes. Each time a normal cell divides, the telomeres shorten; when they reach a certain short length, cell division halts and the cell enters a state known as senescence, or aging. The enzyme telomerase, when introduced into normal cells, is capable of restoring telomere length—or resetting the clock and increasing the life span of cells. Thus telomerase could be used to extend life span.[20]

These examples of some of the advances in biology give tantalizing hints of the way that medicine might evolve, eventually leading to far more effective treatments. Yet whether a scientific finding turns into an effective treatment is not solely a matter of scientific knowledge, determination, and serendipity. The size of the market—the potential sales revenue—must be large enough to justify the investment necessary to develop, test, and earn approval for the innovation. The rate of diffusion of new technologies, therefore, depends heavily on the characteristics of the markets in which they are to be introduced.

Health Disparities across Socioeconomic Groups

Up to now we have said little about how different socioeconomic groups might be affected by medical advances. With fragmented health insurance markets and incomplete health insurance coverage, the fruits of medical progress will be distributed unevenly. Furthermore, the benefits that any socioeconomic group derives from innovations will depend on the prevalence of treatable disease in that group. In addition, technology tends to widen health disparities by lowering the quality-adjusted price of health care, to the disproportionate benefit of the better educated. While new treatments may seem expensive in nominal dollars, they often lower the quality-adjusted price of health care. A novel treatment for a previously untreatable disease provides the extreme example. This treatment makes available at a certain cost a health improvement that was previously unavailable at any price. Essentially, it has reduced what was previously an infinite price to something that, while expensive, is affordable to some. And just as a discount on apples saves

20. Telomerase is not present or significant in most normal cells and tissues, but during tumor progression, telomerase is abnormally reactivated in all major cancer types. Its presence enables cancer cells to maintain telomere length and hence provides them with indefinite replicative capacity. This link between cancer and telomerase generates skepticism about its promise as an antiaging compound. In fact, telomerase inhibition in cancer patients holds promise as a novel way to cause cancer cells to age and ultimately die.

the most money for people who eat lots of apples, so reductions in the price of health care disproportionately benefit, all else equal, the heaviest health care users (who are the more highly educated patients). This finding is counter to the intuition of many people, including policymakers, who assume that lower prices will benefit the poor.

There is an important countervailing force. Certain innovations change the nature of health production by making patient inputs much less productive. Just as price reductions disproportionately benefit the educated—who are the heaviest health investors—reductions in productivity disproportionately hurt the educated. For example, the typhoid vaccine made it much easier to prevent typhoid without spending a great deal of time boiling water, washing fresh vegetables, and maintaining a high level of hygiene. Thus it made it easier to prevent typhoid even for the less educated. Therefore, the advent of the typhoid vaccine—and many other vaccines for infectious disease—have narrowed health disparities. As another example, the development of stem cell transplants to treat diabetes would, if they work as promised, regenerate healthy pancreatic cells that effectively cure the disease. This development would disproportionately benefit the less educated, who do not manage this illness with existing technology as well as the highly educated.[21]

Policy Challenges and Open Questions

Our simulations show that the benefits of costless reductions in disease or disability are large. Such breakthroughs, of course, would not be costless. Instead, they will result from large public and private investments in research and development. Furthermore, they are likely to be produced monopolistically and sold at high prices, at least when first introduced. In fact, without other treatment options, a monopolist could extract profits that would transfer much of the benefit from the new innovation from consumers.

The well-off and the well-insured will be the first to benefit from the new technologies. Both the quality and length of their lives should improve. Expensive new technologies will necessitate either higher insurance premiums or increased cost sharing, possibly narrowing the group of people who will be able to absorb the costs of and benefit from the new technologies. As time passes after the introduction of the technologies, other forces will mod-

21. This differential in self-management has been shown even in the context of a randomized clinical trial for type 1 diabetes. Results from the Diabetes Control and Complications Trial demonstrate that the less educated benefited more from intensive disease management, mainly because they were not doing as well at controlling the illness upon trial entry. Goldman and Smith (2002).

erate prices. The introduction of effective substitutes will promote competition and, potentially, lower prices. Monopoly pricing will end when patents expire. As the technologies mature, the challenge of finding appropriate financing will diminish.

Not all innovations will affect expenditures in the same way. Some advances in the early detection of disease will increase treatment of subclinical disease, which would increase short-term expenditures. Yet some forms of screening that lead to highly effective, inexpensive prevention could, on net, reduce future health care costs. Perhaps the greatest challenge comes from setting new standards of care for technologies that are more expensive and *somewhat* more efficacious. Such technologies will make health insurance and health care less affordable. Some people will get better, albeit more costly, care. Others may lose access to the older, lower-cost care. The fundamental problem is not technological progress but the way that health insurance deals with it.

On the supply side, the challenges are several. The fixed costs of bringing new medical technology to market are high. For medications, hundreds of millions of dollars are required for clinical trials. Despite advances that might lower the costs of discovering and screening drugs that might eventually be marketed, trials will need to be performed for the foreseeable future, and there is little potential to decrease their costs substantially, unless the designs and sizes of the trials are changed. Some advances in molecular medicine, by improving the identification of individuals who have great potential to benefit from an intervention, may make it possible to conduct clinical trials with smaller numbers of participants. Yet even with such advances, the revenue needed to support the investment in bringing a product to market will remain high.

It is the balance between the need for revenue on the supply side and the sensitivity to price on the demand side that will determine the rate of adoption. Pricing strategies will thus be critical. The history of nonionic contrast media used in X-ray studies is illustrative. The new injectable chemicals had some advantages over drugs previously used for the same purposes for most patients who needed a contrast agent for their imaging studies. But the older, hyperosmolar contrast agents were much less costly. As a result, many hospitals and health plans developed guidelines to limit use of the newer, more expensive agents to patients who were at particularly high risk of reacting adversely to the older agents. At a lower price, the nonionic agents might have completely displaced the older agents and generated more revenue for the producers. Instead, their use was limited. Producers of new drugs and devices face similar pricing issues, knowing that revenues will decline if prices are set too high. Although their ability to price discriminate may allow them to recover greater revenues, their ability to charge different niches different prices may erode over time. The rise of multitiered copayments for prescription medications is evidence that the niche of price-insensitive purchasers is shrinking.[22] The net effect is that, at least until the innovations become available at low cost, they will go unused by some Americans who might benefit from them. Yet policies intended to reduce the prices of innovations have the potential to discourage the introduction of the innovations at all. The challenge for policy will be to encourage the rapid development and widespread dissemination of medical innovation; uneven rates of diffusion may be an unavoidable price of rapid technological innovation in health care.

22. Joyce and others (2002).

References

Arrow, Kenneth J. 1963. "Uncertainty and the Welfare Economics of Medical Care." *American Economic Review* 53 (5): 941–73.

Baker, Laurence C. 2001. "Managed Care and Technology Adoption in Health Care: Evidence from Magnetic Resonance Imaging." *Journal of Health Economics* 20 (3): 395–421.

Baker, Laurence C., and Susan K. Wheeler. 1998. "Managed Care and Technology Diffusion: The Case of MRI." *Health Affairs* 17 (5): 195–207.

Bergthold, Linda. 1995. "Medical Necessity: Do We Need It?" *Health Affairs* 14 (4): 180–90.

Collins, Rory, and Stephen MacMahon. 1994. "Blood Pressure, Antihypertensive Drug Treatment, and the Risks of Stroke and of Coronary Heart Disease." *British Medical Bulletin* 50 (2): 272–98.

DCCTRG (Diabetes Control and Complications Trial Research Group). 1993. "The Effect of Intensive Treatment of Diabetes on the Development and Progression of Long-Term Complications in Insulin-Dependent Diabetes Mellitus." *New England Journal of Medicine* 329 (14): 977–86

———. 1995. "The Effect of Intensive Diabetes Therapy on the Development and Progression of Neuropathy." *Annals of Internal Medicine* 122 (8): 561–68.

DCCT/EDICRG (Diabetes Control and Complications Trial/Epidemiology of Diabetes Interventions and Complications Research Group). 2000. "Retinopathy and Nephropathy in Patients with Type 1 Diabetes Four Years after a Trial of Intensive Therapy." *New England Journal of Medicine* 342 (6): 381–89.

Escarce, José J., and others. 1995. "Falling Cholecystectomy Thresholds since the Introduction of Laparoscopic Cholecystectomy." *Journal of the American Medical Association* 273 (20): 1581–85.

Fuchs, Victor R. 1974. *Who Shall Live? Health, Economics, and Social Choice.* Basic Books.

Garber, Alan M. 2001. "Evidence-Based Coverage Policy." *Health Affairs* 20 (5): 62–82.

Goldman, Dana, and James Smith. 2002. "Can Patient Self-Management Help Explain the SES Health Gradient?" *Proceedings of the National Academy of Sciences USA* 99 (16): 10929–34.

Hunink, Maria G. 1997. "The Recent Decline in Mortality from Coronary Heart Disease, 1980–1990. The Effect of Secular Trends in Risk Factors and Treatment." *Journal of the American Medical Association* 277 (7): 535–42.

Joyce, Geoffrey F., and others. 2002. "Employer Drug Benefit Plans and Spending on Prescription Drugs." *Journal of the American Medical Association* 288 (14): 1733–39.

Lakdawalla, Darius J., Dana Goldman, and Jay Bhattacharya. 2001. "Are the Young Becoming More Disabled?" Cambridge, Mass.: National Bureau of Economic Research.

Manton, Kenneth G., and Xi Liang Gu. 2001. "Changes in the Prevalence of Chronic Disability in the United States Black and Nonblack Population above Age 65 from 1982 to 1999." *Proceedings of the National Academy of Sciences USA* 98 (11): 6354–59.

Manton, Kenneth G., and others. 1997. "Chronic Disability Trends in Elderly United States Populations: 1982–1994." *Proceedings of the National Academy of Sciences USA* 94 (6): 2593–98.

Mills, Robert J., and Shailesh Bhandari. 2003. *Health Insurance Coverage in the United States: 2002.* Current Population Report (U.S. Census Bureau). September.

Newhouse, Joseph P. 1992. "Medical Care Costs: How Much Welfare Loss?" *Journal of Economic Perspectives* 6 (3): 3–21.

———. 1993. *Free for All? Lessons from the Rand Health Insurance Experiment.* Harvard University Press.

Pauly, Mark V. 1968. "The Economics of Moral Hazard." *American Economic Review* 58 (3): 531–37.

Schwartz, William B. 1987. "The Inevitable Failure of Current Cost-Containment Strategies: Why They Can Provide Only Temporary Relief." *Journal of the American Medical Association* 257 (2): 220–24.

Seidman, Andrew D., and others. 2001. "Weekly Trastuzumab and Paclitaxel Therapy for Metastatic Breast Cancer with Analysis of Efficacy by HER2 Immunophenotype and Gene Amplification." *Journal of Clinical Oncology* 19 (10): 2587–95.

Singer, Burton H., and Kenneth G. Manton. 1998. "The Effects of Health Changes on Projections of Health Service Needs for the Elderly Population of the United States." *Proceedings of the National Academy of Sciences USA* 95 (26): 15618–22.

Slamon, D. J., and others. 2001. "Use of Chemotherapy Plus a Monoclonal Antibody against HER2 for Metastatic Breast Cancer that Overexpresses HER2." *New England Journal of Medicine* 344 (11): 783–92.

UKPDSG (UK Prospective Diabetes Study Group). 1998a. "Intensive Blood-Glucose Control with Sulphonylureas or Insulin Compared with Conventional Treatment and Risk of Complications in Patients with Type 2 Diabetes (UKPDS 33)." *Lancet* 352 (9131): 837–53.

———. 1998b. "Tight Blood Pressure Control and Risk of Macrovascular and Microvascular Complications in Type 2 Diabetes: UKPDS 38." *British Medical Journal* 317 (7160): 703–13.

Weisbrod, Burton A. 1991. "The Health Care Quadrilemma: An Essay on Technological Change, Insurance, Quality of Care, and Cost Containment." *Journal of Economic Literature* 29 (2): 523–52.

Yusuf, Salim P., and others. 2000. "Effects of an Angiotensin-Converting Enzyme Inhibitor, Ramipril, on Cardiovascular Events in High-Risk Patients: The Heart Outcomes Prevention Evaluation Study Investigators." *New England Journal of Medicine* 342 (3): 145–53.

GARY BURTLESS

4 | *Labor Market Effects of Dramatic Longevity Improvement*

D EMOGRAPHERS AGREE THAT life spans will improve in the next century. There is less agreement on the likely extent of improvement. In this chapter I consider the labor market effects of accelerated improvement in human life spans. If life spans increase dramatically, the main labor market effects will occur as a result of changes in the age profile of the labor force, increases in the length of typical careers, or modification of current arrangements for financing consumption in old age.

I focus first on how longer life spans would shift the age distribution of the working population. Such a change will occur if a larger number of people survive to work at older ages, even if labor force participation rates and retirement decisions do not change. This change would be magnified if surviving adults respond to longer life spans by delaying retirement. I next consider whether increased longevity is likely to change the timing of retirement. I also consider how consumption in old age will be financed or reformed if retirements are not delayed.

My conclusions can be summarized briefly. Accelerated improvement in longevity will have only a small direct effect in altering the age structure of the work force. Survival rates in age groups with high labor force participation rates are already so high that further mortality improvements cannot much affect the size and composition of the work force under age sixty-five.

Among older age groups the labor force participation rate is so low that further mortality improvements will have little impact on the average age of the work force. It follows that increased longevity can change the age profile of the work force significantly only if it causes people to change the lifetime pattern of their labor force participation.

There is no theoretical reason that accelerated increases in longevity should cause workers to retire earlier or later than they would if life spans continue to change at their historical pace. In part, the response to longer life spans depends on changes in work capacity and attitudes toward retirement that accompany the improvement in longevity, and these are difficult to predict. Career workers have greatly extended the portion of their adult lives spent in retirement. Past gains in longevity would have added to the length of a typical retirement, even if the average retirement age had not changed. However, the average retirement age has fallen in all industrial countries, adding even more years to retirement.

The historical and cross-national evidence strongly suggests that retirement is a "superior" good, which means that workers consume more of it as their lifetime incomes rise. Real wages and lifetime incomes are likely to rise along with increased longevity. The gain in lifetime wealth can be spent on longer retirement, and this will be true whether or not mortality reductions accelerate in the future.

The more profound effects of increased longevity are likely to result from induced changes in the compensation system and in public and occupational pension systems. As life spans lengthen, pension programs will have to be reformed to preserve financial solvency. Cross-national evidence suggests that the incentives embodied in pension systems powerfully influence labor force behavior of adults between the ages of fifty-five and seventy. This evidence implies that policy reforms induced by population aging are likely to have a bigger effect on age-specific participation rates—and hence on the age profile of the working population—than the direct effect of mortality reductions themselves.

Mortality Rates and the Age Composition of the Work Force

Life spans in developed countries have increased dramatically in the past 150 years. Between 1850 and 2000, the period life expectancy of a 20-year-old white American male increased 15.5 years, rising from 40 years of remaining life to 55.5 years.[1] Among white women, expected life spans grew even more—from 40.0 years to 60.8 years for a 20-year-old white woman. Much of this improvement resulted from reduced mortality among older people. A 60-year-old white female could expect to live an additional 17.0 years in 1850 but an additional 23.3 years in 1998, an increase of nearly 40 percent. Life expectancy for 60-year-old men increased from 15.6 to 19.7 years, a gain of about one-fourth.

When life expectancy rises continuously, cohort life expectancy provides a more meaningful indication of probable life span than the more familiar period life expectancy.[2] Cohort life expectancies are calculated using death rates not from a single year but from the series of years in which an individual will actually reach succeeding ages if he or she survives. Chulhee Lee has calculated cohort life expectancies for American men attaining age twenty in successive decades between 1850 and 1990.[3] His calculations are based on historical mortality experience through 1990 and Social Security Administration projections for later years. (The Social Security Administration projections were made in 1992.) Lee finds that cohort life expectancy for 20-year-old American males increased by one-third between 1850 and 1990, from 43.7 to 57.8 years.

The increase in average life span has two obvious effects on the labor market. Reductions in mortality at younger ages increase the percentage of working men who attain advanced years. Even if participation rates are unchanged, increased longevity raises the average age of the potential work force. At the same time, reduced mortality rates increase the fraction of workers who reach ages when retirement is common, lifting the number of years that a worker will spend in retirement. If age-specific retirement rates remain unchanged, the percentage of a worker's life spent in retirement will increase. The expected age at death for a twenty-year-old male in 1850 was slightly less than sixty-four years, while the expected age at death for a twenty-year-old man today is seventy-eight years. Because labor force participation is much lower among men past age sixty-four than among men under sixty-four, a rise in average life spans must increase the percentage of life past age twenty devoted to retirement unless the average age at retirement also increases. The impact of accelerated mortality decline on the age profile of the work force will be small, however, if age-specific retirement rates are unchanged.

1. U.S. Census Bureau (1975, 1998). Period life expectancy is calculated for a given year using the actual or expected death rates at each age for that year.
2. See Henry Aaron and Benjamin Harris, this volume, for definitions of cohort and period life expectancy.
3. Lee (1998, chap. 3).

Figure 4-1. *Percent of Labor Force Age Sixty-Five or Older under Four Mortality and Labor Force Participation Assumptions, 1890–2075*[a]

Labor force (percent)

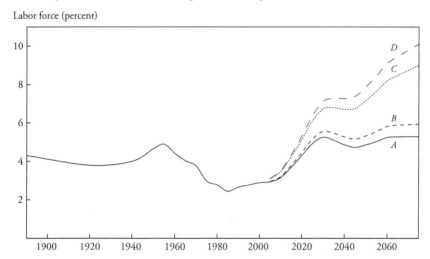

Source: Author's tabulations of data from U.S. Census Bureau (1975, 1998); U.S. Bureau of Labor Statistics (www.bls.gov).

[a]Assumptions about future mortality improvement and participation rate changes:
—A. Current rate of mortality improvement and constant labor force participation rates after 2000.
—B. Accelerated mortality improvement and constant labor force participation rates after 2000.
—C. Current rate of mortality improvement and gradual labor force participation increase at older ages after 2000.
—D. Accelerated mortality improvement and gradual labor force participation increase at older ages after 2000.

To estimate the effect of sharply lower mortality rates on the age structure of the work force, I make two forecasts of the age structure of the U.S. labor force. One is based on the assumption that future reductions in mortality rates will follow the predictions of the Social Security Administration.[4] The second is based on the assumption of accelerated reductions in future mortality along the lines described in the appendix to the chapter by Henry Aaron and Benjamin Harris in this volume. Their projections imply much faster future increases in the percentage of the American population that is past age sixty-five. The actuary's prediction shows that approximately 22 percent of the Social Security area population in 2075 will be age sixty-five or older. The alternative assumption is 29 percent.

If the age profile of labor force participation remains constant, accelerated reductions in the mortality rate will not noticeably affect the age distribution of the U.S. labor force. Figure 4-1 shows the impact of accelerated mor-

4. Board of Trustees (2001).

tality reductions on the percentage of the U.S. work force that is at least sixty-five years old. According to Census Bureau statistics, between 1890 and 1960 the fraction of labor force participants who were past age sixty-four remained relatively constant at about 4 percent. Although the percentage of all people past age fifteen who were at least sixty-five years old increased, the labor force participation rate of Americans past age sixty-five declined fast enough so that the proportion of older labor force participants remained relatively constant. The fraction of older participants in the labor force fell from 1960 through 1985, when it began to rise as both the numbers and the participation rates of older people started to climb. This trend will accelerate as the large baby-boom generation reaches age sixty-five, even if labor force participation rates of older workers do not rise any further. After 2030 the fraction of labor force participants who are sixty-five or older will remain roughly constant at 5.3 percent of the work force (assumption A, figure 4-1).

Under the more optimistic assumption regarding mortality improvement, the fraction of older labor force participants will be about one-half percentage point higher, or 5.9 percent of the total work force (assumption B). This is a very small impact. The American labor market would have little difficulty accommodating so modest an increase in the proportion of aged workers in the labor force.[5] These calculations imply that, if age-specific labor force participation rates remain unchanged, even dramatic improvements in survival rates at middle and advanced ages will not increase substantially the percentage of workers who are past ages fifty-five or sixty-five. Of every 1,000 Americans who reach age twenty, 815 can be expected to reach age sixty-five even if there are no further improvements in age-specific mortality rates. Dramatic improvements in mortality would increase the proportion of workers who attain age sixty-five, modestly increasing the number of surviving sixty-five-year-olds who are available to work. Labor force participation rates past age sixty-five are now so low, however, that even a large increase in the aged population would negligibly raise the percentage of the total work force that is sixty-five or older.

A rise in the labor force participation rate of older Americans would have a much bigger impact on the age profile of the work force. The potential effects of changes in older Americans' activity rates on the share of the labor force that is elderly are shown in assumptions C and D in figure 4-1. Under

5. I have also examined two trends resulting from the sharp reduction in the mortality rate that began in 2000: the percentage of the work force that is fifty-five or older and the percentage that is forty-five or older. These trends show even smaller proportional effects of a drop in mortality. This should not be surprising, because a sharp drop in the mortality rate will have a proportionately larger effect on the number of survivors past age sixty-five than it will on the number past ages fifty-five or forty-five.

the alternative assumption about future mortality improvements, mortality rates will decline much faster after 2000 than in assumption B. And if the work force participation rates of older Americans increase, the age profile of the work force would change much more drastically (assumptions C and D).

Assumption C is based on the assumption that mortality rates will improve as predicted in the 2001 Social Security Administration's trustees' report. But assumption C does not assume that labor force participation rates will remain constant, as in assumption A, but that they will gradually rise above the age-specific rates observed in 1950. The Census Bureau estimates that participation rates of sixty-five-to-sixty-nine-year-olds fell from 35 percent in 1950 to 24 percent by 2000. Under assumption C, this rate will climb steadily between 2000 and 2075, returning to the 1950 rate by 2050 and continuing to rise thereafter until it reaches 41 percent by 2075, 17 percentage points higher than the rate observed in 2000. The proportion of the work force that is sixty-five or older would reach 9 percent by 2075, two-thirds greater than if activity rates remain unchanged.

Assumption D is calculated under the assumption that mortality improvements will occur at an accelerated pace beginning in 2000 and that the work force participation rate for older people will rise. The pace of mortality improvement is the same as that assumed in assumption B, and the rate of increase in labor force participation is the same as the rate assumed in assumption C. Under these assumptions, workers at least sixty-five years old would slightly exceed 10 percent of the work force by 2075, compared with a rate of less than 6 percent under the baseline assumptions regarding mortality improvement and labor force participation and slightly less than 3 percent today.

These forecasts show that increased life spans will not materially increase the proportion of the labor force that is elderly unless labor force participation rates among the elderly also increase.

Labor Force Participation at Older Ages

Increased longevity can change the age pattern of employment either directly or indirectly. A worker who expects to live longer than his father might choose to retire at an older age than his father did in order to hold approximately constant the proportion of life after age twenty that is devoted to retirement. This shift would be a direct behavioral response to increased longevity. A reduction in pension generosity caused by the increased costs resulting from increased longevity might also cause workers to delay retirement. This would be an indirect effect of longer life spans on labor force behavior. This section considers whether longer life spans have *directly* influenced the age pattern of the labor force. In the following section, I consider indirect effects.

Theory

Increases in expected life spans have ambiguous implications for the age pattern of employment and retirement. Suppose workers can earn E every year they work. Each worker must decide at what age to retire. I disregard years before people are capable of working and assume that they are continuously employed from the age at which they enter the labor market until they retire at age R. After retiring, workers remain out of the labor force until they die. If workers have S years to divide between work and retirement, then the years they devote to retirement leisure, L, is

$$L = S - R$$

For simplicity, I ignore the fact that workers can lend or borrow at a positive interest rate and assume instead that the interest rate is zero. Regardless of how workers choose to divide their labor earnings among consumption during successive periods, they face a trade-off between lifetime, average annual consumption, C, and the number of years they devote to retirement. The budget constraint is defined by

$$C = (R/S)\,E,$$

where R/S is the fraction of the workers' potential life span that is spent in paid employment.

In this stylized model, each worker's retirement choice can be described in terms of a simple trade-off between the level of annual consumption and the duration of retirement. The top panel of figure 4-2 illustrates the trade-off. Annual consumption is represented on the vertical axis, and the number of years spent in retirement,

$$L = S - R$$

is indicated on the horizontal axis. Suppose initially that the expected life span is S_0 while the annual wage rate is E_0. The lifetime budget constraint describing the trade-off between years spent in retirement and annual average consumption is the straight line $E_0 S_0$. Workers are assumed to prefer more consumption each year, holding work lives fixed, and longer retire-

Figure 4-2. *Years of Retirement and Annual Consumption, Two Wage Assumptions*

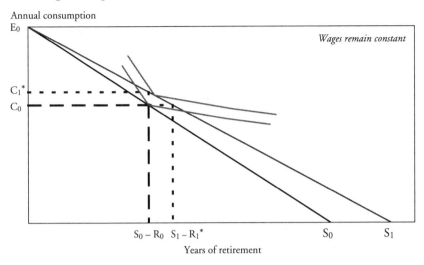

Annual consumption

E_0

Wages remain constant

C_1^*
C_0

$S_0 - R_0$ $S_1 - R_1^*$ S_0 S_1

Years of retirement

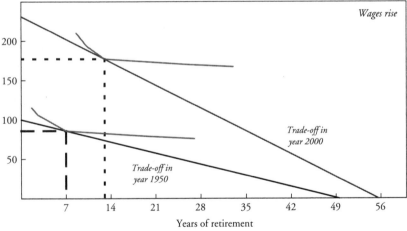

Annual consumption index

Wages rise

200

150

100

50

Trade-off in
year 2000

Trade-off in
year 1950

7   14   21   28   35   42   49   56

Years of retirement

ments, holding consumption fixed, but they can boost consumption only by working longer and can boost the duration of retirement only by consuming less. Each worker's problem is to select the best possible combination of average consumption and years of retirement in light of his or her preferences and the trade-off shown in the figure. The most desirable combination occurs if workers retire at age R_0 and consume their lifetime earnings at an average rate of C_0 a year.

If the potential life span increases from S_0 to S_1, workers are better off, even if the annual wage rate remains unchanged. The new lifetime budget constraint is the straight line E_0S_1. In principle, the retirement age could rise, fall, or stay the same. Theory offers no guide as to whether it will change or how much, if any, of the added life expectancy will be devoted to retirement. If workers postpone retirement by 100 percent of added life expectancy, annual consumption can rise to C_1^* because a larger percentage of their life span would be devoted to employment. On the other hand, if workers wish to maintain annual consumption at the old rate C_0, they must retire at R_1^*, which exactly maintains the original percentage of potential life span that is devoted to employment:

$$R_1^* \big/ S_1 = R_0 \big/ S_0 .$$

Economic theory provides no guidance on which of these outcomes is most likely.[6]

Neither can historical evidence shed much light on this question. Most improvements in the human life span have been accompanied by rising average incomes and wages. In fact, rising real income is probably the most important single reason for the increase in average life spans, since it helped bring about improvements in shelter, diet, public health, medical technology, and health care spending. In addition to enjoying longer life spans, workers also earn much higher annual wages than were available in the past. The lower panel of figure 4-2 illustrates the combined effects of longer American life spans and higher average wages over the half century since 1950 on the consumption-retirement trade-off. In 1950 typical male workers had a remaining life expectancy of slightly more than forty-nine years and, given then-prevailing labor force participation rates, could expect to spend about seven years in retirement.[7] Between 1950 and 2000 real wage rates climbed 131 percent (1.7 percent a year for fifty years). During the same half century, male life expectancy at age twenty increased 5.1 years, or 12.3 percent. The higher budget constraint in the figure illustrates the new trade-off between annual consumption and years spent in retirement. Changes in age-specific

6. In this section I treat retirement as an individual decision. However, most workers are married, and the decision of when to retire depends in part on the work history and retirement decision of a spouse. A full-blown model of retirement would take account of the joint decision of family members regarding the choice of retirement ages. Since this chapter focuses on the impact of longer life spans, however, most of the main issues are addressed by considering the effects of lower mortality rates on a single worker. Since both husbands and wives are expected to enjoy longer life spans as result of lower mortality, this simplification seems defensible.

7. This estimate, as well as the estimates of expected years in retirement, is taken from estimates of period life expectancy for U.S. men in Lee (1998, chap. 3).

labor force participation rates imply that the expected number of years spent in retirement increased by six years, or by a little more than the total increase in males' expected life span. In sum, improvements in average wages and longevity and changes in retirement behavior substantially increased both average consumption and the expected duration of retirement. Annual consumption more than doubled, and the number of years devoted to retirement increased by about 85 percent.

Because both life spans and average wages increased at the same time, it is difficult to determine how much of the change in retirement behavior can be attributed to longer life spans and how much to higher wages. As noted earlier, there is no theoretical reason to assume that longer life spans will automatically produce delays in the average retirement age, even when wages remain constant. Because a longer life span makes workers wealthier, they may choose to use some or all of their added years of life to extend the duration of their retirement. When wages rise at the same time that life spans grow longer, the increase in lifetime wealth offers even greater potential for workers to improve their well-being by spending more of their lives in retirement while boosting annual consumption.

Pensions and the Age Profile of Earnings

This analysis of longevity, retirement, and consumption is based on a highly stylized description of workers' choices. The real choices are more complicated than those implied in figure 4-2. Earnings vary over the life cycle. Figure 4-3 shows the pattern of lifetime earnings for U.S. men born in the early 1930s who survived to age sixty-two without becoming disabled and who earned wages covered by Social Security during at least ten years between ages twenty-two and sixty-one, the minimum earnings period required for Social Security old-age pension eligibility at age sixty-two.[8]

The top panel of figure 4-3 shows the average wage at each year of age measured as a ratio of the economywide average wage in the same year. The top line shows the average wage received by men who earned taxable wages in a year; the bottom line shows the average wage received by all men in the sample, including men who did not earn any taxable wages at a given age. For example, men in this sample who earned wages at age twenty-four received an annual wage that was 81 percent of the U.S. average wage. Only about 80 percent of the sample earned taxable wages when they were twenty-four years old, however (see lower panel of figure 4-2). Including the zero earnings

8. These estimates reflect tabulations of individual Social Security earnings records of men interviewed in the 1990–93 Survey of Income and Program Participation (SIPP).

Figure 4-3. *Career Earnings Pattern of Men Born 1931–35*

Ratio of wages to average economywide wage

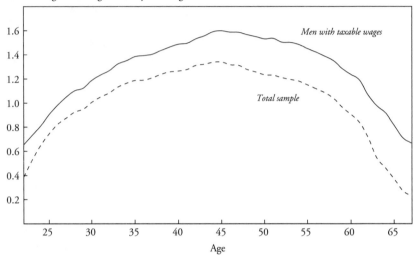

Percent of men who earn wages covered by Social Security

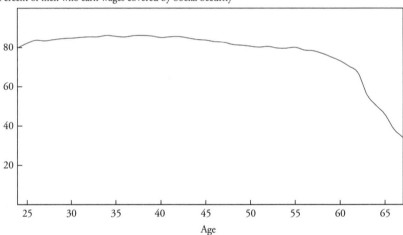

Source: Author's tabulations of 1990–93 Survey of Income and Program Participation files matched to Social Security Administration earnings records.

amounts received by workers who did not earn any taxable wages reduces the average wage of twenty-four-year-old workers to 65 percent of the economy-wide wage.

These tabulations show that past age forty-five men earn progressively lower wages relative to the economywide average. The decline in labor force participation as men grow older partially explains the drop in average wages, but relative earnings also decline by progressively larger annual amounts among men who remain steadily employed. Clearly, wage rates are not constant over workers' careers. It follows that the trade-off between consumption and time spent in retirement varies at different ages.

The Trade-Off When Wages Fall in Old Age. The earnings pattern displayed in figure 4-3 can be used to calculate the trade-off between consumption and retirement faced by a typical male. If one assumes that a twenty-year-old male can expect to survive for sixty years, that he can earn the relative wages displayed in the top panel of figure 4-3, and that economywide average wages will remain constant over his career, it is straightforward to calculate the annual consumption he can afford in an average year after his twentieth birthday if he retires at successively younger ages.[9] The dark, solid line in the top panel of figure 4-4 shows the trade-off between annual consumption, measured as a percentage of the worker's lifetime average wage, and the number of years spent in retirement. Note that the slope of the budget constraint is quite small when years of retirement are low. This shape reflects the very low wages available to men at advanced ages. If a seventy-five-year-old can earn just 25 percent of his average lifetime wage, he sacrifices little lifetime consumption by retiring at age seventy-five. In contrast, as the number of years in retirement increases from twenty to fifty, the slope of the lifetime budget constraint is very steep. Workers who wish to retire between ages thirty and sixty must sacrifice considerable consumption for each additional retirement year.

The shape of the lifetime budget constraint provides a simple explanation for the drop in labor force participation at older ages. Men who are older than sixty-five on the average can earn a potential wage that is less than half the relative wages they earned at age forty-five. The sharp falloff in earnings capacity at older ages makes it progressively less expensive for workers to "buy" a year of retirement as they grow older. In a very poor society, of course, older workers might not be able to afford retirement, even at advanced ages, because average incomes are very close to the margin of survival. That is one

9. If the average economywide wage rises steadily over the worker's career, the lifetime budget constraint will be more steeply sloped but will still have the same general shape shown in figure 4-4.

Figure 4-4. *Trade-Off between Years in Retirement and Annual Consumption*

Average annual consumption as a percent of average lifetime wage

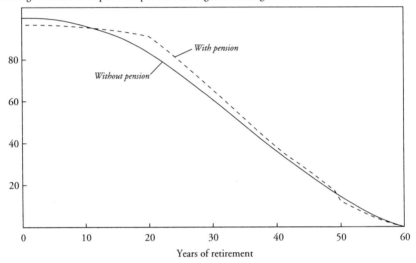

Years of retirement

Average annual consumption

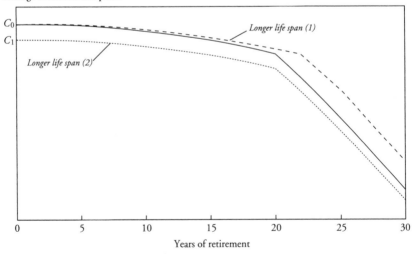

Years of retirement

explanation for the higher labor force participation rates among the elderly early in the twentieth century. In a rich society, retirement in old age is not only possible but quite attractive, because a year of retirement necessitates only a small drop in consumption.

Retirement and Pensions. Public and private pension schemes introduce additional complications in the choice of retirement age. Pensions provide dependable income to workers who have reached pensionable age, such as age sixty, but many systems provide benefits only to workers who have substantially withdrawn from the labor force or ceased working in their career job. These pension systems effectively reduce the net wage for workers who continue to work past the pensionable age. Workers who are eligible for pensions equal to two-thirds of their annual wage at age sixty and who lose their pension if they postpone retirement after age sixty in effect are adding just one-third of their annual wage to lifetime income for each year they continue to work past their sixtieth birthdays.

The broken budget constraint in the top panel of figure 4-4 shows how a simple pension system affects workers' lifetime consumption possibilities. In comparison with the budget constraint when there is no pension, the pension budget constraint provides more lifetime income to workers who devote at least twelve years but no more than fifty years to retirement. I assume that workers must work for at least ten years to qualify for a pension. Workers who contribute for fewer years lose all of their contributions. As workers' pension contributions increase, they become entitled to larger retirement pensions, which boost their lifetime incomes. If workers postpone their retirement after age sixty, however, they forfeit some or all of the pension they could receive if they ceased working. Compared with the no-pension budget constraint, workers who spend between twelve and twenty years of their potential careers in retirement receive higher lifetime incomes and pay a smaller price in lost consumption for each additional year of retirement they buy. The pension scheme shown in figure 4-4 should discourage workers from retiring very late in life and encourage retirements around or shortly before the pensionable age.

Many of the world's pension systems have the features just mentioned. Thus they provide financial incentives for workers to retire around the pensionable age and inflict large financial penalties on workers who retire long after the pensionable age. Not surprisingly, these features strongly influence retirement behavior. They have almost certainly contributed to the trend toward earlier retirement in the world's industrialized countries.[10]

10. See Gruber and Wise (1999).

Longer Life Spans When Added Years Are Productive. The top panel
of figure 4-4 shows the lifetime trade-off between years of retirement and
annual consumption when the expected life span is held constant. If life
expectancy increases unexpectedly, the worker's choices will change. The
lower panel of figure 4-4 shows some of the possible consequences of such
a shift. One option is that workers will earn the same average wage over their
longer potential life span. If life expectancy at age twenty rises by 5 percent—
from sixty to sixty-three years, for example—workers' earnings capacity
at each age past their peak earnings year might improve by just enough
to leave their average lifetime wage unchanged. If so, workers who devote
their entire life to employment would enjoy the same annual consumption
before and after the improvement in life expectancy. The shift in their lifetime budget constraints is illustrated as the move from the solid line to the
broken line (longer life span 1) in the lower panel of figure 4-4. Note that
average consumption when the worker devotes zero years to retirement is
exactly the same before and after the improvement in longevity because
average wages are not affected by a longer life. The discontinuity in the old
and new budget constraints results from the pension formula, as explained
above. Workers who postpone their retirements past the pensionable age
give up part of the pension wealth they have accumulated earlier in their
careers.

The figure plainly shows that changes in the pension formula in response
to increased life expectancy can be crucial in determining how many additional retirement years are consumed following an increase in life spans. If
the pensionable age is left unchanged, many workers will continue to retire
around the pensionable age. In that event, the fraction of their life devoted
to retirement would increase. If the pensionable age is raised, workers will tend
to delay their retirement, partially or fully offsetting the impact of increased
longevity.

Longer Life Spans with Additional Unproductive Years. The lowest budget constraint in the bottom panel of figure 4-4 illustrates an alternative
possibility. If additional years at the end of a worker's life are completely
unproductive, then average annual consumption must fall. That is, if life
spans increase by 5 percent while workers' lifetime earnings capacity remains
unchanged, workers must find a way to divide a constant level of lifetime
income over a longer life, reducing their average flow of consumption by
almost 5 percent. The budget constraint labeled longer life span (2) represents
this shift as an almost proportional reduction in average consumption at

each duration of retirement.[11] Whether workers choose to devote five, ten, or twenty-five years to retirement, they must accept reduced annual consumption to make it possible for them to survive during the added years of (unproductive) life. To simplify matters, the bottom panel of figure 4-4 is drawn on the assumption that the pensionable age increases by the full increment in workers' life spans. If the pensionable age increased less than the increase in life spans, the discontinuity in the lifetime budget constraint would occur further to the right, encouraging some workers to buy somewhat longer retirements. If workers wish to maintain the same annual flow of consumption before and after the improvement in life spans, they must reduce the duration of retirement. In the lower panel of figure 4-4, for example, the workers who initially choose to devote twenty years to retirement would need to reduce the retirement span to fourteen years if they wish to maintain the same average consumption level after longevity improved. Workers who initially plan to retire before the pensionable age would not need to reduce retirement as much to preserve their annual consumption.

The two possibilities considered are obviously extreme. They have different implications for retirement behavior. If the added years of workers' life represent years in which people have no capacity to earn wages, the small minority of workers who originally intend to devote all their life to paid employment will be forced to accept a longer retirement. On the other hand, the much larger fraction of workers who initially plan to devote some of their potential work life to retirement will have a powerful reason to delay retirement in order to maintain consumption. Alternatively, workers' lifetime earnings capacity may increase more or less in proportion to the improvement in longevity. In that event, increased longevity enriches workers, in the sense that they can now achieve previously unattainable combinations of consumption and retirement. Under these circumstances, workers are likely to use at least some of their added lifetime wealth to buy added retirement. How increased longevity affects participation rates will depend crucially on the change in workers' earnings capacity. In addition, changes in the structure of the pension system that follow life span improvements can affect how the increase in life expectancy is divided between extra retirement and added years of paid employment.

11. The consumption loss is not strictly proportional. The budget constraint labeled Longer life span (2) must eventually intersect the original budget constraint, because workers with long life spans can obviously purchase more years of retirement than workers with short life expectancy. Workers who initially planned to spend nearly all their lives in retirement are clearly better off with longer than with shorter life spans, but this is not an interesting case because few workers devote most of their potential careers to retirement.

Longer Life Spans and Pension Solvency. Pension funds face a budget constraint. If life spans increase significantly and no change is made in the pensionable age or in the formula determining benefits, a fund that was previously in balance must either increase contribution rates or face insolvency. This is true in both capital-funded and pay-as-you-go pension systems, if pensions are calculated under a standard defined-benefit formula. The rise in average life spans increases the expected duration of retirement and boosts the liabilities of both kinds of systems. The funding imbalance can be eliminated in one of two ways: through an increase in contributions or taxes, which reduces workers' incomes while they are in the labor force; or through reductions in monthly pensions, which reduce workers' incomes after they have retired.[12]

Figure 4-5 shows average earnings and average consumption by age, to illustrate the impact of population aging on Social Security outlays and aggregate tax burdens. Social Security is a pay-as-you-go, defined-benefit pension program that supports benefits largely from current contributions of active workers. Because most nations use this financing method, these estimates are relevant for most rich industrialized countries. Not surprisingly, the estimates displayed in the figure show that average consumption is higher than average earnings until workers reach their early twenties. Then average earnings far exceed consumption until workers reach age sixty. As wages fall after age sixty, consumption exceeds earnings by ever larger margins. The consumption of retired workers past age sixty is largely financed out of taxes or contributions paid by workers between twenty and sixty years old.

As long as the population age distribution is stable and the ratio of pensions to earnings is fixed, the pay-as-you-go contribution rate imposed on active workers can remain constant. If the ratio of retirees to active workers increases, resulting increases in contribution rates imposed on the working population can discourage employment and effort and thereby undermine the solvency of the pension system. Instead of encouraging workers to delay

---

12. A capital-funded pension system is one that builds up financial reserves in anticipation of the pension liabilities it faces when workers retire. A pay-as-you-go system does not maintain financial reserves, instead relying on the contributions of active workers to pay for the benefits received by pensioners. A defined-benefit pension system is one that calculates pensions based on a formula linking each worker's monthly pension to his or her average wage and duration of employment in jobs covered by the pension system. In contrast, a defined-contribution system specifies an annual contribution requirement (usually a fixed percentage of wages) but does not promise a specific monthly retirement benefit. The monthly pension is determined by the value of the investment accumulation and the worker's age when he or she begins to claim retirement benefits. Obviously, an increase in expected life spans will reduce the monthly pension payable under a defined-contribution system if workers in successive generations continue to retire at the same age.

Figure 4-5. *Age Profiles, Consumption and Labor Earnings, 1987*

Thousands of U.S. dollars

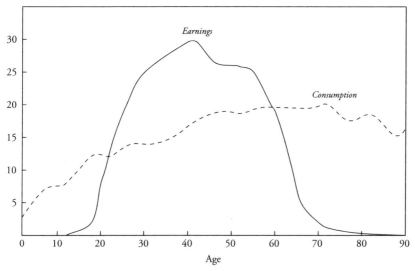

Source: Lee and Tuljapurkar (1997).

their retirement in order to maintain lifetime consumption, some kinds of
pension reform can actually reduce the willingness of working-age adults to
remain employed. Workers cannot indefinitely consume more than they produce. If longevity increases, the pension system must eventually be reformed
to preserve solvency. How these reforms are designed can powerfully affect the
proportion of the life span that workers will choose to spend in employment.

Evidence

What is the evidence for changes in the age pattern of labor force participation in response to changes in average life spans? I first consider evidence
from the United States and then some cross-national evidence from rich and
poor countries.

Historical Evidence for the United States

Three major trends in the life-cycle labor market behavior of American workers have characterized the past century. Entry into full-time work has been
postponed, as potential workers have spent longer and longer periods enrolled
in formal schooling. Full-career workers have left the active labor force at

younger ages, devoting a growing share of their expected life spans to retirement, a once uncommon status. The life-cycle employment profiles of both
women and men have converged. Both men and women typically enter the
labor force after twelve to twenty years of formal schooling and then work
for pay relatively continuously until disability or full retirement, sometime
between ages fifty-five and seventy. Men have retired at progressively younger
ages, while women have participated in the paid labor force in progressively
larger proportions.[13] I focus on the age profile of male labor force participation. Long-term historical trends among women are more difficult to describe.
Female retirement patterns early in the last century are hard to measure
because most women worked primarily within the home—and without pay—
during most of their adult lives.

In the middle of the nineteenth century, retirement was uncommon.
Three of four American men past age sixty-five were employed.[14] Retirement
became more common throughout the first half of the twentieth century.
Fewer than half of men sixty-five and older held a job in 1950. By 1985 the
proportion at work had declined still further. Just 16 percent of men over age
sixty-five were employed or actively seeking a job; 84 percent were outside
the active labor force. (People are considered to be labor force participants if
they hold jobs or are actively seeking work.) The percentage of women past
age sixty-five who were employed or looking for work also shrank during the
first four decades following World War II, mainly because the average age of
women past sixty-five was rising. The reduction in women's employment was
far smaller than among men because the percentage of older women who
worked outside the home had never been high.

Figure 4-6 depicts the drop in work among older men. In each calendar
year, the participation rate is lower among men in successively older age
groups. Complete withdrawal from the labor force was less common in the
early years of the twentieth century than at the end. Even at age seventy, for
example, the male participation rate in 1910 was over 60 percent. By the
1980s, the participation rate at age seventy had fallen by two-thirds, to just
20 percent. Although participation rates have fallen at all ages, declines in participation rates at the oldest ages began sooner and were larger. A striking feature of figure 4-6 is that men's participation rates, which fell steadily up to
the mid-1980s, have stabilized or even increased modestly since then.

---

13. In addition to these shifts in the life-cycle profile of market work, the workweek and the
work year have shrunk for typical workers, although these two trends probably ended in the United
States in the early 1970s.

14. Costa (1998, pp. 28–31).

Figure 4-6. *Male Labor Force Participation Rates at Selected Ages,*
1910–2001[a]

Percent

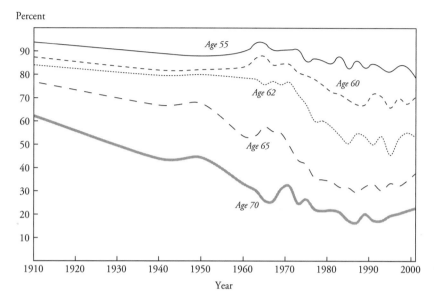

Source: Ransom, Sutch, and Williamson (1991); Munnell (1977); author's tabulations of March
Current Population Survey files for 1963 through 2001.
a. Labor force participation rates for 1910, 1940, and 1970 are based on responses to employment
questions in the decennial censuses. Rates for 1963–99 are the arithmetic average participation rates. Participation rates based on the census differ somewhat from those measured by the *Current Population Survey*, partly because the main goal of the *CPS* is to obtain reliable labor force statistics. Adjusting the
decennial census statistics to make them strictly comparable to the *CPS* estimates would have only a slight
effect on the patterns displayed in the figure.

The story for older women is different. Their participation rates in the
post–World War II era reflect two partly offsetting phenomena: the early
retirement trend of older workers in general and the increasing labor force
participation of married women. As a result of the latter, the participation
rates of older women did not exhibit the dramatic postwar declines seen
among men. Instead, as shown in table 4-1, age-specific female labor force
participation rates generally increased. Between 1950 and 2000–01, the
female participation rate rose 38 percentage points at age fifty-five and smaller
percentages at older ages.

What is similar to the male experience is the shift in trends after 1985. As
with men, there is a noticeable break from the earlier trend in older women's
labor force participation. Between 1970 and 1985, labor force participation
rates of women age sixty-two or older barely increased at all or declined. Since
1985 participation rates of both older men and women rose. The similarity

Table 4-1. *Labor Force Participation, by Age and Gender, 1940–2001*

Percent of population

Gender and year	Age				
	55	60	62	65	70
Men					
1940	90	82	80	67	44
1950	88	82	80	68	45
1960	90	83	79	54	33
1970	89	81	73	47	27
1984–85	83	69	50	32	17
2000–01	79	70	53	38	23
Women					
1940	20	17	15	12	6
1950	28	23	21	16	8
1960	43	35	29	20	12
1970	50	43	36	22	11
1984–85	52	44	32	17	10
2000–01	66	50	40	24	12

Source: Munnell (1977, p. 70); author's tabulations of March *Current Population Survey* files for 1984, 1985, 2000, and 2001.

of the break points in the male and female time series is striking.[15] Women's participation rates at older ages have risen strongly since 1985, while among older men the long-term decline in participation rates has ended and may even have reversed.

Historical information about participation rates can be used to trace the long-term trend in the average age at retirement. If we define the average retirement age as the youngest age at which fewer than half of men in an age group remain in the work force, the average male retirement age fell from seventy-four years in 1910 to sixty-three years in 2000–01, a drop of about 1.2 years a decade. Note, however, that the recent stability or slight upward trend in older men's participation rates means the trend toward earlier male retirement in the United States has slowed and may even have ceased.

The decline in the average male retirement age occurred in an environment of rising life expectancy among older Americans. Chulhee Lee has calculated the combined effects of longer life spans and earlier labor market withdrawal on the number of years in an average American male lifetime that

15. See Quinn (1999).

is devoted to labor force participation and retirement.[16] Lee's calculations were performed using estimates of both period and cohort life expectancy for males attaining age twenty between 1850 and 1990. As noted above, Lee used historical labor force participation rates to estimate retirement patterns for each cohort and Social Security Administration projections of age-specific participation rates after 1990.

If participation rates at older ages increased in line with the improvement in life expectancy, the percentage of remaining life expectancy devoted to retirement might remain unchanged. As shown in figure 4-6, however, precisely the opposite occurred. Labor force participation at older ages declined as life spans lengthened. Figure 4-7 shows Lee's estimates of cohort life expectancy as well as the division of remaining life expectancy between work and retirement. His tabulations imply that cohort life expectancy increased by slightly more than fourteen years—almost one-third—between 1850 and 1990 (see top panel of figure 4-7). Virtually all of the increase was devoted to added years in retirement. The expected duration of a working career after age twenty increased by only six months. The percentage of life after age twenty devoted to retirement rose from 6 percent to over 28 percent of remaining life expectancy, a fourfold increase.

The average number of years that American men devote to paid employment has remained almost unchanged over the 150 years studied. Using cohort life expectancies, Lee estimates that the average twenty-year-old in 1850 spent slightly more than forty-one years of his remaining life in gainful employment. The average twenty-year-old in 1990 can expect a working career lasting forty-one and a half years, assuming the Social Security Administration's 1992 projections of labor force participation and mortality improvement turn out to be valid. The duration of male working lives has remained virtually constant because mortality improvement has just about offset reductions in labor force participation at older ages. The typical twenty-year-old man is more likely now than in the past to survive until age sixty, a period during which the probability of employment is high. The reduction in mortality between ages twenty and sixty has been large enough to slightly increase the expected duration of a man's working career. Because labor force participation rates have fallen sharply after age sixty, however, all of the gains in longevity after age sixty have taken the form of longer retirements.

Male life expectancy has improved at uneven rates, and the trend toward earlier labor force withdrawal was even more erratic. Table 4-2 contains estimates of period and cohort life expectancy and of labor force participation rates for older men over a 140-year period, divided into three periods,

16. Lee (1998).

Figure 4-7. *Remaining Life Expectancy, Twenty-Year-Old Men,*
1850–1990

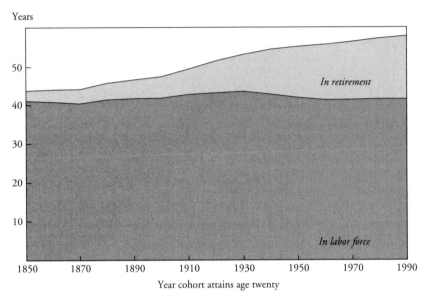

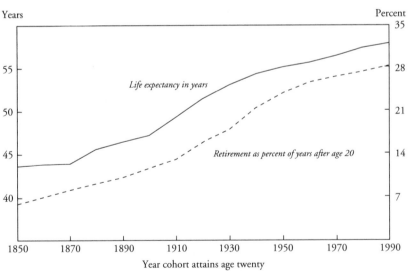

Year cohort attains age twenty

Source: Lee (1998), p. 14.

Table 4-2. *Trends in Male Life Expectancy at Age Twenty and Labor Force Participation at Older Ages, 1850–1990*

Year	Life expectancy (years)		Labor force participation (percent)	
	Period	Cohort	Age 55–64	Age 65+
Year				
1850	38.4	43.7	92.2	76.6
1900	41.7	47.3	91.0	65.4
1950	49.0	55.0	88.1	47.0
1990	53.0	57.8	67.0	18.4
Change				
1850–1900	+3.3	+3.6	–1.2	–11.2
1900–50	+7.3	+7.7	–2.9	–18.4
1950–90	+3.9	+2.7	–21.1	–28.6
Change (percent)				
1850–1900	+8.6	+8.2	–1.3	–14.6
1900–50	+17.4	+16.3	–3.2	–28.1
1950–90	+8.0	+5.0	–24.0	–60.9

Sources: Lee (1998, p. 14); Costa (1998, p. 29).

1850–1900, 1900–50, and 1950–90. The greatest gain in life expectancy occurred between 1900 and 1950, when cohort life expectancy increased about 7.7 years (16 percent). Labor force participation fell faster in this period than it did in the previous fifty years but much more slowly than in the next forty years. This rate fell dramatically between 1950 and 1990, but life expectancy increased only moderately during this period.

The pattern of decline in labor force participation cannot be explained by variations in the rate of wage improvement. Although authoritative data on U.S. wage levels before World War I are unavailable, output growth suggests that per capita incomes rose at approximately the same rate in each of the three periods covered by table 4-2.[17] If wages grew at about the same rate as real incomes, gross wage rates increased by similar amounts in each period. Clearly, these work force participation rates did not change by similar amounts in each period. One possibility is that the introduction of Social Security pensions in 1941, the liberalization of Social Security benefits between 1951 and 1974, and the widespread adoption and liberalization of employer-

---

17. Per capita income growth has been approximately constant since 1850, with U.S. real incomes doubling every thirty-five years. See Parente and Prescott (2001, p. 12).

sponsored pensions in the four decades after 1940 encouraged workers to leave employment at progressively younger ages. Even if gross wage rates were improving at a stable rate, an increased percentage of wages was devoted to paying for pensions and insurance benefits that are mainly available to workers who leave the active work force. In 1935 virtually none of the labor compensation paid to U.S. workers consisted of employee or employer contributions for retirement. In 1997 employee and employer contributions to Social Security and employer-sponsored pension plans accounted for slightly more than 15 percent of average hourly compensation.[18]

The financial incentives in Social Security and employer-sponsored pensions explain some of the reduction in male labor force participation after 1940. Social Security is now the main source of cash income of most households headed by someone sixty-five or older. The program provides slightly more than 40 percent of the total cash income received by the aged. Among aged households in the bottom 60 percent of the elderly income distribution, Social Security provides over three-quarters of cash income. Until 1941 Social Security provided no income at all to the aged. Today the program replaces about 42 percent of the final wage earned by a full-career single worker who earns the average wage and claims a pension at the normal retirement age (NRA).[19] If the worker has a nonworking dependent spouse, the benefit replaces 63 percent of the worker's final wage. Benefits are clearly large enough so they can be economically significant in influencing the choice of retirement age.

While this evidence seems to suggest that the introduction and liberalization of Social Security and employer-sponsored pensions is responsible for most of the postwar decline in male activity rates, there are some reasons to be cautious about this interpretation. Workers are much wealthier today than they were at the beginning of the twentieth century. The increase in wealth would have led workers to retire earlier than previous generations, even in the absence of Social Security and private pensions. Social Security, Medicare, and employer-sponsored retirement plans were established and expanded in part to help workers achieve the popular goal of living comfortably without work in old age. If these programs had not been developed,

18. U.S. Census Bureau (1998, p. 439).

19. The NRA is the youngest age at which insured workers can claim "unreduced" retirement pensions, not the age at which most workers normally claim benefits or retire. During most of the history of the Social Security program, and for all workers attaining age sixty-five before 2003, that age was sixty-five. Under a law passed in 1983, the NRA was raised gradually to sixty-six for workers who attain age sixty-six in 2009 and to sixty-seven for workers who attain age sixty-seven in 2027. See Board of Trustees (2001, p. 96). The estimated replacement rate at the NRA is reported in Social Security Administration (1993). Most workers claim benefits before age sixty-five (more than two-thirds in 2002).

it is likely that workers and employers would have found other ways to pursue the same goal. The details of pension eligibility and incentives in the pension benefit formulas have surely encouraged workers to retire at some ages rather than others, but it is probably more accurate to say that pensions accelerated a trend toward earlier retirement that was occurring before most workers had access to them. Depending on the details of a pension plan, workers may be encouraged to retire earlier or later in life. Even in the absence of pensions, workers would likely have found ways to pay for earlier retirement.

The activity rates displayed in table 4-1 and figure 4-6 suggest that the trend toward earlier male retirement may have ended in the United States in the mid-1980s. Trends in neither wages nor longevity can explain this shift, as both wages and longevity have continued to increase since 1985. One important change since the early 1980s is that the nation's main pension program, Social Security, is no longer growing more generous. Between 1950 and 1980 Social Security benefits rose both absolutely and in relation to average earnings. Most workers received pensions that were higher than those they would have obtained if their Social Security contributions had been invested in safe private assets. After 1985 fewer retirees received windfalls from the program. The Social Security amendments of 1977 and 1983 trimmed retirement benefits modestly in order to keep the program solvent, ending four decades of benefit expansion and liberalization.

Congress has changed Social Security rules and the pension formula to increase the attractiveness of work after the normal retirement age. The amount of income a recipient can earn without losing any Social Security benefits has been increased for workers between sixty-two and the normal retirement age; and after the full-benefits age, benefits are not reduced regardless of earnings. In the 1977 and 1983 Social Security amendments, Congress also increased the reward that workers receive for delaying initial benefit receipt past the full-benefits age (the NRA). For workers attaining age sixty-two after 2004, benefits for workers who delay receipt will be increased by an actuarially fair amount, which means that retirees on the average will receive benefits over their lifetimes with approximately the same present value regardless of the age at which they initially claim benefits. By 2004 the Social Security system will provide approximately age-neutral pensions.

Important changes have also occurred in private pensions. The relative importance of defined-contribution pension plans has increased dramatically, while the importance of old-fashioned defined-benefit plans has fallen. Defined-contribution plans are age-neutral by design. They have none of the age-specific work disincentives that are common in traditional defined-benefit plans. As a growing percentage of workers reaches retirement age under defined-contribution plans, fewer workers will have reason to leave their jobs to avoid a loss in lifetime retirement benefits.

Some changes in the U.S. environment are the result of policy initiatives specifically intended to encourage work at older ages. For example, mandatory retirement has been nearly eliminated. In the early 1970s employer rules that required workers to leave their jobs no later than a particular age, usually age sixty-five, covered about half of all American workers. In 1978 the earliest legal age of mandatory retirement was raised from sixty-five to seventy, and in 1986 mandatory retirement provisions were outlawed altogether for most workers. The increase and eventual elimination of mandatory retirement ages not only increased the options open to older employees who wanted to remain on their jobs but also sent a powerful message to Americans about the appropriate age to retire.

This message was reinforced by a provision of the 1983 Social Security amendments that is gradually raising the NRA in Social Security from sixty-five to sixty-seven. The higher NRA will become fully effective for workers who reach age sixty-two in 2022. This amendment did not change the age of initial entitlement—age sixty-two—but the benefit reduction reduces the lifetime consumption path that workers can sustain if they retire at the same age as they would have done under prior law. This reduction in lifetime wealth reinforces the retirement-delaying incentives of the benefit increase offered for deferring the age at which the workers claim benefits.

I have so far focused on retirement of men. It is worth remembering, however, that increased labor force participation among women has more than offset the employment reductions of older men. Women's labor force participation has increased at every age between twenty-two and seventy (see figure 4-8). Between the late 1950s and the 1990s the percentage of thirty-year-old women who earned Social Security–taxable earnings increased from 30 percent to 75 percent. The percentage of older women who earn taxable wages increased by smaller but still impressive amounts. Although some scholars believe that women in career jobs now retire at an earlier age than their counterparts of three or four decades ago, the jump in the proportion of women who work in career jobs has increased the percentage of women who are employed, even at ages far above the pensionable age. The massive shift in the composition of U.S. labor supply, resulting from trends in female labor force participation, was accommodated by American employers and labor market institutions. If participation rates of older Americans should begin to rise as a direct or indirect result of future mortality improvement, it is hard to see why employers and labor market institutions would be unable to accommodate a large shift in the age profile of the work force.

Figure 4-8. *Women Earning Wages Covered by Social Security,*
by Birth-Year Cohort, 1926–1965

Percent of women in birth cohort

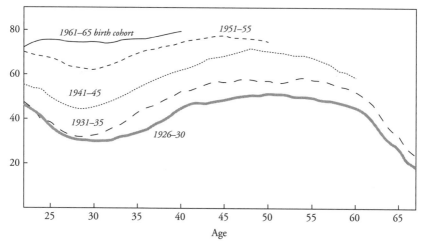

Age

Source: Author's tabulations of 1990–93 Survey of Income and Program Participation files matched
to Social Security Administration earnings records.

Cross-National Evidence

The decline in labor force participation rates at older ages has not been confined to the United States. Participation rates among men age fifty-five and
older have fallen in all industrialized countries. As expected life spans in rich
countries have increased, men have devoted ever smaller fractions of their adult
lives to paid employment. The overall pattern of decline in activity rates has
been similar in many of the industrial countries. Figure 4-9 shows the relation of male life expectancy and labor force participation among men age
sixty-five and older in Germany, the United Kingdom, France, and the
United States. Between 1910 and 1995, for example, life expectancies of
fifteen-year-old German males rose from slightly less than forty-eight years to
fifty-nine years, while the participation rate of German men age sixty-five and
older fell from slightly above 50 percent to less than 5 percent. All four countries display similar patterns.

The long-term trend toward earlier retirement in the United States has
therefore been matched by equivalent trends in other rich countries. In a
recent survey of the determinants of retirement in rich countries, economists from the Organization for Economic Cooperation and Development
(OECD) estimated the average age at which men and women withdrew from

Figure 4-9. *Male Period Life Expectancy at Age Fifteen and Labor Force Participation, Men Age Sixty-Five and Older, Four Countries, 1900–98*

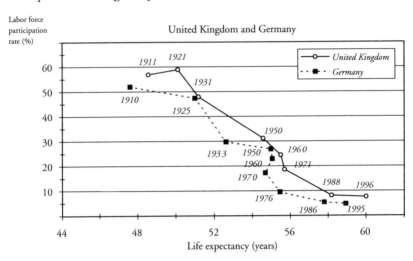

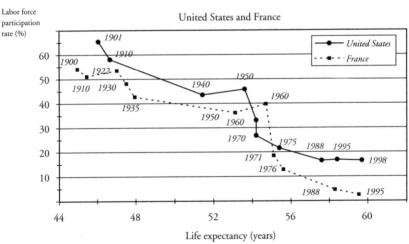

Source: United Nations (1949), table 6; UN (1979), table 8; UN (1992), table 22; UN (1999), table 22; Costa (1998); OECD (2002).

the active work force for selected years between 1950 and 1995 in twenty-four high-income nations.[20] Average retirement ages have declined in nearly all of the countries since 1950. In 1950 the average retirement age for men was sixty-five or higher in almost all twenty-four countries. Between 1950 and 1995 male retirement ages had fallen everywhere except in Iceland. In most countries the drop in the average retirement age was at least three years. In a quarter of the countries, an average male now retires before his sixtieth birthday. The average retirement age of women with working careers has fallen even faster. (Note, however, that a much higher percentage of women now have lengthy careers in paid employment than was the case in 1950.)

Differences in countries' average incomes alone cannot explain cross-national differences in the average retirement age. As one of the richest OECD countries, the United States might be expected to have one of the lowest retirement ages. Instead, it has one of the highest. In 1950 its average retirement age placed the United States in the middle of the twenty-four countries in the OECD survey. By 1995 it had one of the highest average retirement ages. Only four of the twenty-four countries had a higher male retirement age (Iceland, Japan, Norway, and Switzerland), and only five had a higher female retirement age (Iceland, Japan, Norway, Sweden, and Turkey). In the seven largest OECD economies, the average retirement age of both men and women has fallen over time. But the decline has been smaller in the United States and especially in Japan than in the other five countries.

Cross-national comparisons that include the world's poorest countries shed light on the effect of extremely low income on labor force participation at older ages. Robert Clark, Elizabeth Anne York, and Richard Anker collected participation rate and per capita income data for 134 countries.[21] They divided the sample of countries into low-, middle-, and high-income categories and then calculated the mean work participation rate within each age group and income category. In all countries, whether rich or poor, participation rates of male workers decline as they grow older, more in rich than in middle-income and poor countries (see figure 4-10). Since most young men work, this pattern implies that participation rates at the oldest ages are significantly lower in rich than in the middle-income and poor countries. Greater wealth allows older workers to retire at an earlier age. Rich countries' participation rates are also lower at younger ages, but the gap in male activity rates between rich and poor countries is relatively modest at ages below sixty.

20. Blöndal and Scarpetta (1998).
21. Clark, York, and Anker (1997). Countries with low incomes had 1990 per capita incomes below $610 a year; middle-income countries had per capita incomes between $611 and $7,620 a year; high-income countries had incomes above $7,620 a year.

Figure 4-10. *Labor Force Participation at Older Ages, 134 Countries, by Income, 1990*

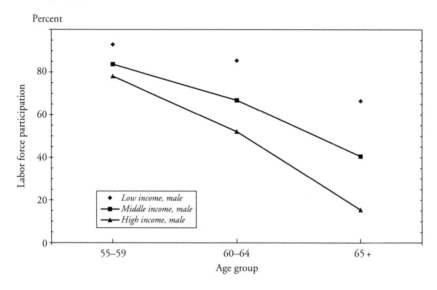

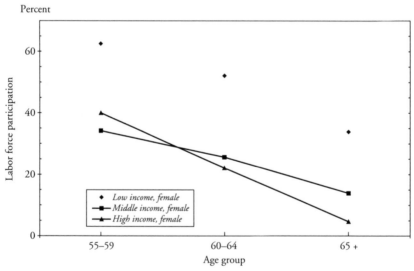

Source: Clark, York, and Anker (1997).

Figure 4-11. *Income and Labor Force Participation, Men Aged Sixty-Five and Older, 1990*

Labor force participation rate (percent)

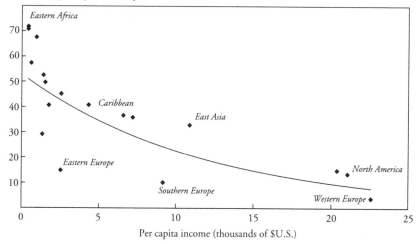

Per capita income (thousands of $U.S.)

Source: Clark, York, and Anker (1997).

Workers live longer in rich than in poor countries. For example, life expectancy at birth is approximately 10 percent higher in countries in the top one-fifth of the world income distribution than it is in countries in the middle one-fifth of the world income distribution and more than one-third higher compared with countries containing the poorest one-fifth of the world's population.[22] Earlier retirement and longer average life spans in the rich countries mean that men in those countries consume significantly more retirement leisure than do males in less affluent countries. Tabulations of activity rates within geographical regions and subregions also reveal a strong negative association between average income levels and participation rates (see figure 4-11). The poorest regions and subregions have significantly higher labor force participation rates than wealthy regions. These tabulations strongly reinforce the conclusion that retirement is a superior good, one that workers consume more of as their lifetime incomes improve.

The case for believing that male activity rates fell partly as a result of improved living standards is strengthened by the results of time series and cross-sectional regression that show the effects of income growth on partic-

22. Author's tabulations based on World Health Organization longevity data.

Table 4-3. *Effect of Life Expectancy and per Capita Income on Older Males'*
Activity Rates, Twelve Countries[a]

Independent variable	LFP age 55–64[b]		LFP age 65+[b]	
	1	2	3	4
Constant	311.11	317.18	263.31	260.69
Male life expectancy at age 15	−0.42	...	0.31	...
	(2.67)	...	(1.53)	...
Male life expectancy at age 65	...	0.02	...	−0.28
	...	(1.37)	...	(3.38)
Log (per capita income)	−24.24	−25.60	−27.04	−24.50
	(11.18)	(9.85)	(11.69)	(14.79)
Adjusted R^2	0.288	0.288	0.275	0.275
N	24	24	18	18

a. For each country included, one observation is included from the early 1970s and a second observation from the middle 1990s. Labor force participation rates are from OECD (2002); life expectancy
estimates are from United Nations (1979, 1992, 1999).

b. Dependent variable is labor force participation rate (LFP) of males aged 55–64 (columns 1 and 2)
and of males aged 65 and older (columns 3 and 4).

ipation rates in the rich countries. I was able to assemble consistent data on
labor force participation rates, real income levels measured in constant international dollars, and life expectancy for the early 1970s and the mid-1990s
for twelve industrialized countries. The data consist of observations at two
points in time of the relation among income, life expectancy, and male labor
force participation. The regression results in table 4-3 suggest that a nation's
per capita income level has a significant, powerful, and negative effect on the
work force participation rates of both fifty-five-to-sixty-four-year-old men
and men sixty-five and older. In contrast, male life expectancy has a small
and very imprecisely estimated effect on male activity rates.

Pension System Incentives

Differences in the state of the overall job market explain some of the differences in retirement trends across rich countries. Economies with low
unemployment rates and tight labor markets offer more attractive work
opportunities to older workers. Cross-country differences in old-age and disability pensions, unemployment benefits, and health insurance coverage also

have tended to push European workers into early retirement and to keep older American and Japanese workers in the labor force. Jonathan Gruber and David A. Wise, in their examination of pension systems and retirement incentives in eleven industrialized countries, identified large differences in the treatment of labor earnings once workers reach the pensionable age.[23] Some countries, like the United States, provide relatively modest public pensions and do not penalize workers for delaying their retirement beyond the age of pension eligibility. Other countries, like France and the Netherlands, provide much more generous public pensions and impose heavy financial penalties on workers who remain employed after the pensionable age. Gruber and Wise find a strong correlation between national retirement patterns and the labor supply incentives embodied in national pension systems. People between fifty-five and seventy years old work at relatively high rates in countries that offer modest pensions and treat earned income after the pensionable age generously. Countries that offer generous pensions and penalize earnings after the pensionable age have relatively low participation rates at older ages.

These findings imply that national retirement systems powerfully influence the trend in labor force participation at older ages. One implication of this finding is worth noting. If increases in longevity should accelerate, pension systems will become insolvent unless the contribution rate or the pensionable age is increased or annual benefit payments are reduced. The Gruber and Wise findings imply that future retirement patterns can be shaped by the details of pension reform plans that will be adopted to avoid insolvency. If voters and policymakers wish to increase labor force participation after age sixty-five, the age of pension eligibility and the benefit formula can be designed to make retirement after those ages more attractive. If instead they wish to maintain a low participation rate at age sixty-five, a less generous pension system can still be designed that encourages retirement before workers reach sixty-five.

Conclusion

Increases in average income and expected life spans have dramatically improved workers' well-being over the past century and a half. Workers have responded to higher wages and the prospect of a longer life by devoting an increased share of their adulthood to retirement.

23. See Gruber and Wise (1999).

Should medical advances accelerate increases in the average life span, it is reasonable to ask how work behavior and labor market institutions will respond. The direct impact of lower mortality rates on the U.S. labor market will be small. Assuming that current life-cycle patterns of labor supply persist, most of the addition to future life spans will occur at ages when few people work. The age structure of the future work force is much more likely to be affected by changing birth rates and immigrant flows than by speedier reductions in the mortality rate. Increased longevity can significantly influence labor markets through its direct or indirect effects on the age profile of labor force participation. There is little reason to think the direct effects on labor force participation will be large. For a century and a half, life expectancies of career workers rose and labor force participation rates of workers past age sixty fell. If workers aimed to remain employed for a constant proportion of their adult lives, participation rates at older ages should have risen rather than fallen as average life spans got longer.

The long-term rise in the percentage of adulthood devoted to retirement has been driven mainly by rising incomes, not by the increase in expected life spans. Increased wages and unearned incomes have added to the lifetime wealth of successive generations of workers. Some of the increase in wealth has been used to purchase a longer retirement. If average life spans had remained unchanged over the past two centuries, but wages and incomes had risen at the same pace, the average age at retirement would have fallen and the average length of retirement increased. This scenario is far-fetched, however. Average life spans grew longer *because* wages and incomes improved. At the same time, the average health and work capacity of the adult population improved. Career workers now withdraw from paid employment in their fifties and early sixties rather than their late sixties and early seventies because they can afford to do so, not because poor health or strenuous job requirements push them into a longer period of enforced idleness.

The most likely effect of increased life expectancy is to induce reform of a nation's pension system. Such reform will in turn affect labor force participation rates in old age. Even now, major industrial countries, including the United States, must confront sharply growing public pension costs. If increases in longevity accelerate, this challenge will increase, intensifying pressure on lawmakers to reform the pension system.

No one can be sure how pensions will be reformed. However, there are only four ways to eliminate pension deficits: increase pension contributions, reduce benefits, raise the pensionable age, and introduce new funding from outside the pension system. So far, the United States has reformed Social

Security by raising payroll taxes, cutting benefits, and strengthening incentives for workers to work past the traditional retirement age.[24] Some critics of Social Security think we should replace the existing system in whole or in part with a system of individual defined-contribution retirement accounts. Although reductions in pensions as longevity increases are not inevitable, they are likely. A higher age of entitlement for benefits is another possible result. Both kinds of reform will encourage workers to delay retirement, at least modestly, boosting the employment rate of older Americans. Participation rates of Americans ages sixty-two and older are already rising slowly. Curtailing public retirement benefits would reinforce this trend.

24. Although the 1983 Social Security amendments gradually raised the NRA from sixty-five to sixty-seven, they left the early entitlement age unchanged at age sixty-two. For workers who claim pensions between ages sixty-two and sixty-seven, the rise in the NRA is equivalent to a benefit cut.

COMMENT
Dora L. Costa

Gary Burtless convincingly shows that the impact of any dramatic improvements in longevity on older men's and women's labor force participation rates will be slight. Very few men or women work at older ages. Men's participation rates at older ages have been declining for more than a century despite increase in life expectancy and improvements in health. Much of the rise in retirement rates is attributable to rising incomes, whether income in the form of higher wages, higher private pensions, or higher Social Security benefits. Forty percent of the decline in participation rates of men older than sixty-four occurred before the establishment of Social Security and before the growth of private pensions. Most studies find that the impact of changes in Social Security benefit levels is modest.

Are there then any scenarios under which we could expect dramatic labor force effects of increases in longevity? Perhaps. These scenarios would need to incorporate the political pressures that would arise from a severe financial crisis in Social Security. A reduction in the age at which reduced Social Security benefits are first payable (currently, age sixty-two) and a reduction in disability benefits is certainly plausible under the economic pressure of dramatic increases in longevity. The immediate effect of such a policy change would be to lower retirement rates among the poor, who have little in the way of savings. The long-run effect of such a policy might be to change social norms about when to retire to a later age. A financial crisis in Social Security will put political pressure on employers to accommodate older workers by increasing job flexibility and by actively recruiting older workers.

Burtless mainly examines the direct effects of increased life expectancy on labor force participation rates at older ages. But increases in longevity that affect the entire life cycle can have important indirect effects on retirement rates and can differentially affect different types of worker. Although quantifying these effects may not be possible, history can help guide our speculations. My speculations focus on the potential effects of differential longevity increases by education, changes in molecular medicine that allow more women to achieve careers, and interactions between increases in longevity and the structure of work.

The twentieth century has been both the health capital century and the human capital century. First high school education became the norm. Now college is becoming the norm. Although there have been cycles in health, in the long run rising longevity has been accompanied by improvements in health. Burtless emphasizes that increased incomes have improved health, but increases in health have undoubtedly improved productivity and therefore the income available for retirement. While further increases in health and in education may raise retirement rates by raising the income available for retirement, there are some countervailing trends as well.

Retirement begins in school. The college-educated remained in the labor force longer both in 1940 and in 1990. Census tabulations reveal that the percentage of college-educated men older than sixty-four who were out of the labor force doubled between 1940 and 1990. The percentage of men of the same age group with less than a high school education who were retired almost tripled between those years. Social Security replaced a greater portion of their wages; their jobs were more physically demanding and much less interesting; and switching to another job has always been harder for workers without a general education. College graduation rates for both men and women have been increasing rapidly, beginning with cohorts born in 1920. Only 14 percent of white men born in 1920 graduated from college compared to 30 percent of those born in 1955, at the height of the baby boom. Increases in education may slow the rate of increase in retirement rates, outweighing any income effects. Advance in molecular medicine may increase the disparity in retirement rates by education. Ever since the germ theory of disease was first accepted, the better educated and their children have traditionally had better health outcomes, and this cannot be explained by their higher income levels. Knowing your genetic predisposition may well require the elimination of environmental risks, and the better educated are more successful in modifying their health habits and in seeking the best treatments.

The twentieth century has also been the century of women. Burtless discusses the rise in married women's labor force participation since 1950. Beginning in the 1970s, women's enrollment in graduate programs has increased dramatically, from minimal percentages to almost half of the students in law and medical schools. Advances in molecular medicine that increase the period of fertility may lead to even greater general and firm-specific human capital skill investment on women's parts. As more women enter the labor force, particularly in career jobs, we will no longer be able to think of men's or women's retirement decisions but will need to think of the joint retirement decision. Among couples in which the husband was age sixty-two to sixty-nine, the correlation in couples' retirement status controlling for education and for demographic characteristics was negative in 1940 but rose over time to become 0.4 by 1998.[1] This correlation may well increase as spouses become

---

1. Calculated from the census microsamples and the *Current Population Survey*.

more similar in career aspirations. Because the evidence thus far suggests that women's retirement affects men's but not vice versa, the entry of women into careers may lower men's retirement rates.

Last, I consider interactions between increases in longevity and changes in the structure of work. The labor markets that we are familiar with are generally characterized by long-term contracts between workers and firms. To reduce turnover, firms offer workers higher salaries as prizes at older ages but then introduce incentives in the form of pensions to induce retirement when workers are paid more than their marginal product. This was not always so. Nineteenth- and early twentieth-century labor markets have been characterized as spot markets, in which workers were paid their marginal product and firms viewed the mainly unskilled workers as readily interchangeable. Technological change led firms to invest in their workers' firm-specific human capital but to want to hire workers when they are young. Our world may be changing once more. The move away from defined-benefit plans and toward defined-contribution plans may be symptomatic of broader changes. If we are moving away from long-term contracts and toward short-term contracts with educated free agents, firms may become much more willing to hire older workers.

One of the major accomplishments of the twentieth century has been the growth of leisure. Retirement has given individuals time for self-fulfillment. Molecular medicine promises to expand this period of self-fulfillment by extending disability-free life at older ages. If it can also improve health and therefore productivity at older ages, this will ease the financial strains on Social Security. The big question that we will face is how we will finance the treatments that molecular medicine will offer.

References

Board of Trustees, OASDI (Board of Trustees, Federal Old-Age and Survivors Insurance and Disability Insurance Trust Funds). 2001. *The 2001 Annual Report of the Board of Trustees, Federal Old-Age and Survivors Insurance and Disability Insurance Trust Funds.*

Blöndal, Sveinbjörn, and Stefano Scarpetta. 1998. "The Retirement Decision in OECD Countries." Working Paper 202. Paris: Organization for Economic Cooperation and Development.

Clark, Robert L., Elizabeth Anne York, and Richard Anker. 1997. "Economic Development and Labor Force Participation among Older Persons." Working paper, College of Management, North Carolina State University.

Costa, Dora L. 1998. *The Evolution of Retirement: An American Economic History, 1880–1990.* University of Chicago Press.

Gruber, Jonathan, and David A. Wise, 1999. "Introduction and Summary." In *Social Security and Retirement around the World,* edited by Jonathan Gruber and David A. Wise. University of Chicago Press.

Lee, Chulhee. 1998. "The Expected Length of Retirement in the United States, 1850–1990." Ph.D. diss., University of Chicago; also available as a working paper, Division of Economics, Seoul National University.

Lee, Ronald, and Shripad Tuljapurkar. 1997. "Death and Taxes: Longer Life, Consumption, and Social Security." *Demography* 34 (1): 67–81.

Munnell, Alicia H. 1977. *The Future of Social Security.* Brookings.

OECD (Organization for Economic Cooperation and Development). 2002. *OECD Statistical Compendium.* Paris.

Parente, Stephen L., and Edward C. Prescott. 2001. "International Income Levels: Past, Present, and Future Differences." Working paper, University of Minnesota.

Quinn, Joseph. 1999. "Has the Early Retirement Trend Reversed?" Paper prepared for Retirement Research Consortium and Boston College, Chestnut Hill, Mass., May.

Ransom, Roger L., Richard Sutch, and Samuel H. Williamson. 1991. "Retirement: Past and Present." In *Retirement and Public Policy,* edited by Alicia H. Munnell, 45–46. Dubuque, Iowa: Kendall/Hunt.

Social Security Administration. 1993. "The Notch: What It Is . . . And What It Isn't." Publication 05-10042.

United Nations. 1949. *Statistical Yearbook 1948.*

———. 1979. *Demographic Yearbook.*

———. 1992. *Demographic Yearbook 1990.*

———. 1999. *Demographic Yearbook 1997.*

U.S. Census Bureau. 1975. *Historical Statistics of the United States from Colonial Times to 1970.*

———. 1998. *Statistical Abstract of the United States.*

JOHN B. SHOVEN

5 The Impact of Major Improvements in Life Expectancy on the Financing of Social Security, Medicare, and Medicaid

THREE PROGRAMS ALONE—Social Security, Medicare, and Medicaid—account for almost 43 percent of all federal budget outlays, or $954 billion in fiscal year 2004.[1] Most of Medicare's beneficiaries are over the age of sixty-five, although Medicare also covers younger people who are disabled and victims of end-stage renal disease. Approximately 83 percent of Social Security's outlays are payments received by retirees, their families, and widows and widowers.[2] Medicaid, designed to provide health insurance for the poor, pays roughly 29 percent of its benefits to the poor elderly, particularly the very elderly poor in the form of nursing home and long-term care.[3] The federal government supports certain of

The author is Charles R. Schwab Professor of Economics, Wallace R. Hawley Director of the Stanford Institute for Economic Policy Research, Stanford University. The author would like to thank Jay Bhattacharya, Victor Fuchs, Alan Garber, Dana Goldman, Dan Kessler, and Tom MaCurdy for data and also for helpful discussions. Stephen Goss and Jason Schultz of the Social Security Administration provided essential assistance. The author would also like to thank Colleen Flaherty and Shujing Li for outstanding research assistance.

1. Office of Management and Budget (2003, table 11.3).
2. Board of Trustees, OASDI (2002, table III.A.7). The 83 percent number is the sum of the monthly benefits for retired workers and auxiliaries and the monthly benefits of aged widows and widowers divided by total monthly OASDI benefits.
3. In 1998, 4 million aged Medicaid beneficiaries received payments for services averaging $9,700. Total payments for services from Medicaid in 1998 were about $142 billion. HCFA (1998).

the elderly with such additional programs as veteran's pensions, civil service pensions, and Supplementary Security Income.

Each of the three big programs—Social Security, Medicare, and Medicaid—is thought to face major long-run financial challenges because of population aging, the insufficiency of taxes earmarked to finance them (in the case of Medicare and Social Security), and the probable high cost of new medical technologies (in the case of Medicare and Medicaid). This chapter examines how the financial future of these three major federal programs would be affected by possible dramatic improvements in age-specific mortality rates in the next seventy-five years. The optimistic mortality scenario of this chapter is the "2 percent case" described in the chapter by Henry Aaron and Benjamin Harris, this volume.

The impact of rapid mortality improvements on Social Security is the most straightforward to predict. As longevity increases, the program's costs go up accordingly. If Social Security benefits are not scaled back, the optimistic mortality improvement scenario will boost the cost of Social Security by 16 percent by 2050 and by 26 percent by 2080.[4] Sufficient increases in the age of eligibility for full Social Security benefits could offset or eliminate these cost increases.

The impact of rapid mortality improvements on Medicare and Medicaid is less obvious. It depends on how health at different ages changes as mortality improves. If the age-specific health status remains roughly constant, the increased life expectancy that accompanies mortality improvement will add to the number of high medical maintenance years that the average person experiences toward the end of life. Under this scenario, the more rapid the increase in longevity, the faster the growth of Medicare and Medicaid costs. Alternatively, health status might depend on the number of years until death rather than the number since birth. Under this scenario, age-specific health status improves as mortality rates fall. The number of high medical cost years before death remains roughly constant, and the costs of Medicare and Medicaid do not increase drastically even when mortality improves dramatically. This scenario, which I contend is plausible, suggests that the financial consequences of rapid mortality improvement for Medicare and Medicaid may not be as daunting as commonly believed.

---

4. Author's calculations based on data from the Office of the Actuary, Social Security Administration.

> **Box 5-1.** *Computation of Social Security Retirement Benefits*
>
> Benefits are based on the primary insurance amount (PIA). If a single worker claims benefits at the full benefit age—commonly called the normal retirement age—the monthly benefit equals the PIA. Workers who claim benefits before the full benefit age receive a smaller benefit; those who claim later receive a larger benefit. The PIAs of Social Security participants depend on their average indexed earnings over the best thirty-five years of employment. One needs at least ten years of covered work history to qualify for an inflation-indexed retirement annuity. Married couples receive either the larger of both spouse's benefits based on their own work records or 150 percent of the higher PIA (assuming both spouses have reached the age of eligibility for full PIA benefits when benefits are initially claimed). This latter feature, termed *spousal benefits,* sharply favors one-earner households. Widows and widowers receive the benefit based on their own work record or on that of their deceased spouse, whichever is larger.

Social Security

Social Security is the largest single federal budget expenditure. The program actually comprises a package of social insurance programs, indicated by the acronym OASDI, which includes old-age, or long-life, insurance, consisting of inflation-indexed life annuities that covered workers receive upon retirement; survivors insurance, which provides benefits for widows and widowers of covered workers as well as children of deceased participants; and disability insurance, which partially replaces the lost income of disabled workers.[5] Retirement benefits for participants and their survivors account for the bulk of OASDI expenditures. (The way in which benefits are calculated is sketched in the box.)

People can begin to collect Social Security retirement benefits as early as age sixty-two. However, monthly benefits are increased for each month after age sixty-two that eligible workers delay claiming benefits. The increase averages 0.53 percent of the primary insurance amount (PIA) for every month that one

5. The full acronym is OASDHI, which includes not only Old-Age, Survivors, and Disability Insurance, but also Hospital Insurance (Medicare part A), which provides hospital insurance for elderly Social Security participants over the age of sixty-five, the disabled, and patients suffering from end-stage renal disease. Medicare part B includes physician and other benefits and is separately financed by general revenues and premiums. I follow the standard practice of considering OASDI separately from Medicare (HI).

delays collecting benefits from age sixty-two to the age of full PIA eligibility.[6] Monthly benefits continue to increase above the PIA for those who retire at ages older than the age of eligibility for full benefits by a roughly actuarially fair percentage.[7] For example, people born in 1941 who chose to start receiving Social Security on their sixty-second birthday (in 2003) received 76.67 percent of the amount given by the PIA calculation. If the same people delayed receiving benefits until they were seventy (2011), their monthly benefits would be 132.5 percent of the PIA, or 72.8 percent more than if they had retired at age sixty-two. The age of eligibility for full PIA is scheduled to increase to sixty-six for those reaching age sixty-two in 2005 and to sixty-seven for those reaching 62 in 2022 and later. Raising the age for full PIA lowers initial monthly benefits regardless of the age at which benefits are claimed.

Most OASDI income comes from a 12.4 percent payroll tax on the first $87,000 of annual earnings. The 12.4 percent figure is legally fixed, but the earnings cutoff automatically increases each year at the same rate as average earnings. Income tax revenue from the portion of Social Security benefits that is subject to personal income tax is recycled into the Social Security and Medicare programs. Finally, Social Security and Medicare receive interest payments from the rest of the federal government on the special issue government bonds in their trust fund.

Current projections indicate that the present value of taxes earmarked for Social Security is significantly less than the present value of future benefits. The OASDI Board of Trustees calculates the seventy-five-year outlook for OASDI under high-cost, intermediate-cost (or "best guess"), and low-cost assumptions. The key assumptions for relevant demographic and economic variables are shown in table 5-1.

The rates of mortality improvement shown in table 5-1 are the age-and-sex-weighted average rate of mortality improvement and include the more rapid improvement expected at younger ages. The corresponding age-and-sex-adjusted rates of mortality improvement for those age sixty-five and over are 0.70 percent for the intermediate-cost assumption and 0.30 and 1.23

---

6. Technically, monthly benefits are decreased by five-ninths of 1 percent for each of the first thirty months that one retires before the age of eligibility for full PIA and five-twelfths of 1 percent for each additional month over and above thirty-six months prior. When sixty-five was the retirement age for full benefits, those retiring at sixty-two received 80 percent of their PIA. When sixty-seven becomes the retirement age for full benefits (for those born in 1960 and later), those retiring at sixty-two will get 70 percent of the PIA.

7. The delayed retirement credit is 7.5 percent a year (prorated monthly) for those born in 1941. The PIA is multiplied by one plus the delayed retirement credit to determine monthly benefits. The delayed retirement credit will be 8.0 percent a year for those born after 1942 (www.ssa.gov/oact/cola/benefits.html).

Table 5-1. *Values of SSA Demographic and Economic Variables,*
Three Cost Assumptions

Variables	Intermediate cost	Low cost	High cost
Demographic			
Fertility (children per woman)	1.95	2.20	1.70
Mortality improvement (percent a year)	0.73	0.35	1.29
Annual net immigration (thousands)	900	1,210	655
Economic			
Increase in consumer price index (percent)	3.0	2.0	4.0
Increase in covered wage (percent)	4.1	3.6	4.6
Average unemployment (percent)	5.5	4.5	6.5
Trust fund interest rate (percent)	6.0	5.7	6.2

Source: Board of Trustees, OASDI (2002).

percent for the low-cost and high-cost assumptions.[8] These rates of mortality improvement are projected for the years 2026 to 2080. The intermediate projection is based on the assumption that mortality improvement for the elderly will gradually accelerate from an annual rate of 0.50 percent to 0.70 percent over the first twenty-five years of the century.

I employ the intermediate OASDI set of assumptions and examine the impact of changing the assumed rate of mortality improvement. While rapid reductions in the mortality rate likely affect other variables—inflation and immigration, for instance—I ignore these possible effects. The low-cost and high-cost assumptions shown in table 5-1 are similarly not mutually coherent. Each assumption underlying the low-cost and high-cost assumptions set is chosen because it either lowers costs (in the former case) or increases costs (in the latter). The lack of coherence can be illustrated by noting that the higher fertility rate in the low-cost scenario might be expected to reduce the rate of growth of real wages. However, the low-cost assumption set includes faster growth in real wages than does the intermediate-cost assumption set.

Because inflation-adjusted life annuities are the single most important benefit financed by the OASDI system, it is not surprising that its financial outlook is sensitive to the evolution of mortality rates. Table 5-2 and figure 5-1 show the income and expenditures of OASDI as a percentage of aggregate

8. For points of reference, the geometric average rate of mortality improvement over the twentieth century was 0.84 percent a year for those between sixty-five and sixty-nine and 0.75 percent a year for those between seventy-five and seventy-nine.

Table 5-2. *OASDI Income and Cost Rates, Three Intermediate-Cost Assumptions, 2002–80*

Percent

Year	Intermediate cost		Intermediate cost with 2 percent mortality improvement		Intermediate cost with 2 percent mortality improvement plus 1 month/year increase in age of full benefits	
	Income	Cost	Income	Cost	Income	Cost
2002	12.70	10.84	12.70	10.84	12.73	10.84
2005	12.70	10.46	12.70	10.51	12.73	10.51
2010	12.75	11.04	12.75	11.19	12.78	11.19
2015	12.87	12.36	12.89	12.66	12.91	12.66
2020	12.99	14.24	13.01	14.72	13.03	14.72
2025	13.09	16.02	13.13	16.76	13.15	16.75
2030	13.18	17.24	13.23	18.32	13.25	18.21
2035	13.22	17.77	13.30	19.25	13.31	18.97
2040	13.24	17.77	13.34	19.72	13.34	19.22
2045	13.25	17.78	13.37	20.20	13.36	19.42
2050	13.26	17.92	13.41	20.78	13.38	19.66
2055	13.29	18.24	13.46	21.50	13.40	19.97
2060	13.31	18.60	13.50	22.21	13.42	20.26
2065	13.34	18.98	13.55	22.93	13.44	20.55
2070	13.36	19.38	13.59	23.72	13.46	20.88
2075	13.38	19.76	13.64	24.55	13.48	21.25
2080	13.40	20.11	13.69	25.40	13.50	21.61
Actuarial balance		−1.87		−3.40		−2.78

Source: Author's calculations based on data from Office of the Actuary, Social Security Administration.

covered earnings (the aggregate payroll tax base) under Social Security's intermediate-cost assumption set and if mortality improves 2 percent annually for the next seventy-five years.

Table 5-2 and figure 5-1 show that Social Security already has a serious financial imbalance in the intermediate-cost assumption case and that this imbalance substantially worsens if mortality improves according to the 2 percent scenario. In 2002 Social Security actuaries reported that the program faces a projected deficit over seventy-five years under its intermediate-cost

Figure 5-1. *Income and Cost of OASDI as a Percentage of Covered Payroll, Three Forecasts, 2002-72*

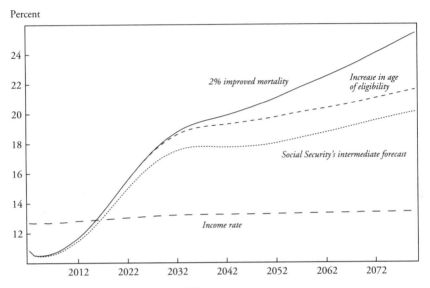

Source: Social Security Administration, Office of the Actuary.

assumption equal to 1.87 percent of covered payroll. That means that an immediate and permanent increase in the payroll tax by 1.87 percentage points (from 12.4 percent to 14.27 percent) would bring the seventy-five-year present value of OASDI income up to the seventy-five-year present value of costs.[9] Figure 5-1 shows that under the intermediate-cost assumption, Social Security's payroll and income tax revenues exceed costs until 2017.[10] The program's costs as a percentage of covered payroll are projected to start rising sharply in 2008 and to continue going up until 2032. They are projected to remain on a plateau between 17.6 and 18.0 percent of covered payroll between 2032 and 2052, when cost increases resume.[11] Costs over this period are projected to be about 35 percent greater than income. By 2080 the OASDI system's projected costs are 20.11 percent of covered payroll, while income is only 13.40 percent. The costs in figure 5-1 show what

9. Alternatively, an immediate and permanent decrease in benefits by slightly more than 13 percent eliminates the seventy-five-year actuarial deficit.

10. Income includes only the proceeds of the payroll tax and the recycled personal income tax receipts received by the OASDI Trust Fund. Thus it excludes the interest transfer from the rest of the government. This is the standard presentation of the Board of Trustees.

11. The plateau in the cost rate between 2032 and 2052 is one final echo of the baby boom in the aftermath of World War II and the Great Depression.

the payroll tax rate (ignoring income tax revenues) would have to be to run the system on a true pay-as-you-go basis so that annual expenses exactly match currently legislated benefits.

Improved mortality has little effect on projected revenues. The income numbers for the intermediate-cost case with 2 percent mortality improvement are slightly higher than for the standard intermediate-cost case because increased longevity means that total benefit payments increase and more personal taxes are therefore recycled into the OASDI system. Though gradual, the impact on program cost is much larger than it is on revenues, largely because increasing longevity extends the average payout period for inflation-adjusted Social Security annuities. Improved longevity boosts the gap between tax revenues and costs in 2020—1.25 percent of payroll under the simple intermediate-cost case and 1.71 percent for the intermediate-cost plus 2 percent mortality improvement case—and by even more with the passage of time. With rapidly improving mortality, program costs do not flatten out in the 2030s and 2040s as they do under the standard intermediate-cost case. By 2050 the deficit is 4.66 percent of payroll for the standard intermediate case and 7.37 percent for the 2 percent improvement case. By 2080 the gap between expenditure and tax revenue in the 2 percent case is 11.71 percent of covered payroll, almost twice the 6.71 percent gap for the standard intermediate-cost case. An immediate increase in the payroll tax rate of 3.40 percentage points in the 2 percent mortality improvement case would be necessary to achieve a seventy-five-year actuarial balance, compared with the 1.87 percentage point increase under the intermediate-cost projection. With the passage of time, successive seventy-five-year actuarial deficits tend to increase because each successive projection contains fewer relatively low-cost early years and more high-cost later years.

The projections in table 5-2 and figure 5-1 are not worst-case scenarios but result from maintaining the intermediate-cost assumptions for everything other than mortality. Things could turn out better or worse. If fertility or immigration or growth of real covered wages are lower than assumed in the intermediate-cost projection, the financial outlook for OASDI would be poorer than shown for both mortality scenarios. Conversely, higher fertility, immigration, or real wage growth would improve prospects, although there is little prospect that even very favorable developments could eliminate projected deficits.

My interpretation of the data is that leaving the age of full PIA eligibility at age sixty-seven after 2022 in the face of rapidly improving mortality of the elderly is not financially viable and that other measures to keep the system in balance—drastic reductions in monthly benefits or sharply increased payroll taxes—are inferior alternatives. In one scenario, the age of full PIA is increased by one month a year beginning in 2023. That is, instead of stopping at age sixty-seven, the age of full PIA continues to go up by one month a year. This in effect lowers initial monthly benefits at any particular age of retirement by roughly 0.5 percent of the PIA. Of course, participants could offset their lower benefits at any particular age of retirement by working longer and delaying retirement.

Raising the age of full benefit eligibility by one month a year perceptibly improves OASDI's financial prospects. The pay-as-you-go deficit (again, ignoring income taxes) in 2080 is 8.11 percent of covered payroll, compared to 11.71 percent under the 2 percent case with the full-benefit age frozen at age sixty-seven, and 6.71 percent under the intermediate-cost projection. Raising the full-benefit age by one month a year offsets about 72 percent of the added deficit that increased longevity otherwise generates. In fact, adjusting the age of full-benefit eligibility one month a year appears to be even more powerful than this comparison suggests. If mortality improves according to the 2 percent scenario and the age of eligibility for full PIA is increased one month a year, program costs increase at roughly the same rate as in the intermediate-cost forecast. The enlarged deficit under the 2 percent scenario, relative to the intermediate-cost assumption, is due to the fact that the new adjustments in the age of eligibility for full benefits do not begin until 2023, more than twenty years after the assumed improved mortality begins to increase the costs of Social Security. The one-month-a-year adjustment appears to be about right in the event of a 2 percent mortality improvement. The projections do suggest that if the age of eligibility for full benefits is increased before 2023, the annual cash flow deficit is reduced. Of course, other adjustments are necessary to close the remaining substantial solvency gap.

There is an issue of whether increasing the normal retirement age is equivalent to cutting benefits. I am on record as saying the two policies are identical in terms of their effect on a participant's monthly benefit for any particular retirement age.[12] However, in terms of lifetime benefits, raising the age of eligibility for full PIA is not cutting benefits at all, simply offsetting some or all of the automatic lifetime benefit increases that occur with improvement in mortality.[13] These longevity-based increases in lifetime benefits are so substantial in the 2 percent mortality improvement scenario that they almost certainly need to be offset by increasing the age of eligibility for a full PIA.

12. Aaron and Shoven (1999).
13. With a 2 percent mortality improvement, life expectancy at the age of eligibility for full PIA continues to increase even if that age is adjusted upward at the rate of one month a year.

Medicare

The second largest government social insurance program for the elderly is Medicare, which is divided into two parts, hospital insurance (HI), also known as Medicare part A, and supplementary medical insurance (SMI), or Medicare part B. HI helps pay for hospital, home health, skilled nursing, and hospice care for the aged and disabled. It is financed primarily by a 2.9 percent payroll tax paid by workers and employees. Its only other source of revenue, other than trust fund interest, is its share of the recycled tax payments on Social Security benefits. Unlike the OASDI payroll tax, the 2.9 percent HI tax is payable on an unlimited amount of earnings. SMI pays for physician, outpatient hospital, home health, and certain other services for the aged and disabled. Three-fourths of SMI's funding comes from the general fund of the U.S. Treasury, with the other one-fourth coming from insurance premiums and copayments paid by participants. General revenue support for SMI has increased sharply from when Medicare was introduced in the mid-1960s, when premiums accounted for about half of income. Under the Balanced Budget Act of 1997 general revenues will continue to cover 75 percent of SMI costs, while participants cover the remaining 25 percent.

The long-run financial problems of Medicare are more difficult to assess but appear to be worse than those of OASDI. The future costs of Medicare are more uncertain than those of OASDI because they depend not only on an increase in the elderly population but also on whether per capita health care spending on the elderly rises faster or slower than per-worker earnings. The per capita cost of health care, in turn, depends on the age composition of the elderly population (since health spending differs by age), on changes in the age-specific health status of the elderly, and on the relative price of health care. The intermediate-cost projections of Medicare trustees rest on the assumption that the age-specific per capita cost of medical care rises 2.0 percent a year faster than overall prices.[14] These and other assumptions lead to a projected seventy-five-year actuarial deficit of the HI program of 2.02 percent of taxable payroll, slightly more than the projected 1.87 percent OASDI deficit. That is, the current 2.9 percent HI payroll tax would have to be immediately and permanently increased to 4.92 percent to bring about a seventy-five-year balance.[15]

The time pattern of cash surpluses and deficits is similar for HI and OASDI. According to intermediate-cost projections, Medicare part A is

14. Board of Trustees, Medical Insurance (2002).
15. The HI and the OASDI tax bases are not the same due to the $87,000 cutoff for covered earnings for OASDI taxes.

expected to run small cash-flow surpluses until 2015 and then incur increasingly large deficits—an estimated 0.38 percent of payroll in 2016, rising to 2.84 percent by 2040, to 4.84 percent by 2060, and to 7.19 percent by 2080. Cash-flow balance requires that the current 2.9 percent payroll tax rate rise to 10.09 percent by 2080.[16] The combined OASDI and HI payroll tax rates in 2080 are 30.20 percent, nearly double today's 15.3 percent. This increase does not include the effects of more rapid mortality improvement than assumed in the intermediate-cost projections.

The costs of SMI (part B of Medicare) are also projected to increase greatly over the next seventy-five years. The SMI program does not face the same solvency problems as the HI program because general revenues and participant premiums are increased by statute to match rising expenses. According to the intermediate-cost projection, SMI's expenditures will rise as a fraction of gross domestic product (GDP), from 1.04 percent in 2002, to 2.10 percent by 2030, and to 3.22 percent by 2065. Should the cost of medical services rise by more than 2.0 percent a year faster than prices and 1.0 percent a year faster than wages, the growth is even greater.

The 2002 *Annual Report* contains two types of data that portray the magnitude of SMI cost increases.[17] The first shows out-of-pocket expenses of SMI participants as a fraction of the projected average Social Security retirement benefit (see figure 5-2). Those reaching age sixty-five in 2050 need to devote 20.5 percent of their Social Security benefit to cover the SMI monthly premium and copayments. Twenty years later, these costs absorb 32.7 percent of the average Social Security monthly benefit. In contrast, SMI bills for today's sixty-five-year-olds average about 14 percent of their Social Security benefits and about 20 percent for today's eighty-five-year-olds. The other source of finance for SMI, payments from general revenues, is projected to require almost 23 percent of the combined income tax revenues in 2070, up from about 6 percent today (see figure 5-3).

I estimate the impact of the alternative mortality scenarios on the costs of Medicare by examining per enrollee age- and gender-specific Medicare costs in recent years and then superimposing assumed changes in the age structure of the population and in the cost of health care. The data on expenditure per enrollee for males and females are shown in the appendix to this chapter. The expenditures are for Medicare part A and part B combined and are thus financed by a combination of payroll taxes, general government revenue, and premiums. Figures 5-4 and 5-5 graph the age-specific total Medicare expen-

---

16. Once again, this projection omits income tax revenues earmarked to HI.
17. Board of Trustees, Medical Insurance (2002).

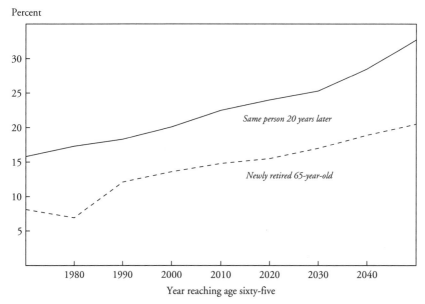

Figure 5-2. *Out-of-Pocket Supplemental Medical Insurance Expenses as a Percentage of Average Social Security Benefit, 1970–2050*

Percent

Same person 20 years later

Newly retired 65-year-old

Year reaching age sixty-five

Source: Board of Trustees, Medical Insurance (2002), table II.C14.

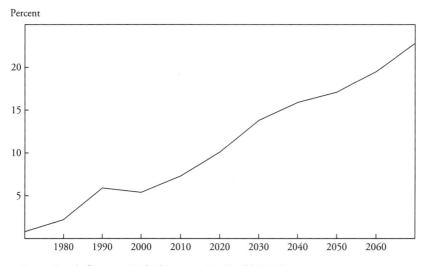

Figure 5-3. *Projected General Revenue Requirement for Supplemental Medical Insurance as a Percentage of Total Personal and Corporate Tax Revenues, 1970–2070*

Percent

Source: Board of Trustees, Medical Insurance (2002), table II.C15.

Figure 5-4. *Average Expenditure, Male Medicare Enrollee,*
Aged Sixty-Five to One Hundred, 1989 and 1997[a]

2003 dollars

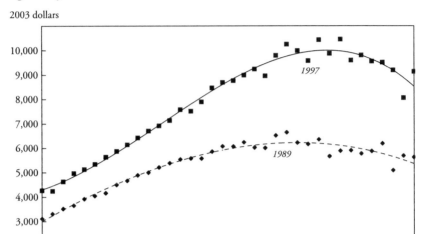

Source: Large sample of Medicare claims records compiled by Tom MaCurdy, Stanford University.
a. The polynomial equations are
   Costs in 1989 = −17,337 + 237.67age + 3.44age^2 − .036*age^3.
   Costs in 1997 = 149,505 − 6,175age + 84.64age^2 − 3.71*age^3.

Figure 5-5. *Average Expenditure, Female Medicare Enrollee,*
Aged Sixty-Five to One Hundred, 1989 and 1997[a]

2003 dollars

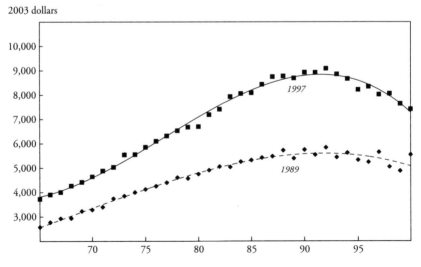

Source: See figure 5-4.
a. The polynomial equations are
   Costs in 1989 = 24,344 − 1,223.45age + 19.85age^2 − .096*age^3.
   Costs in 1997 = 158,782 − 6,458.51age + 87.35age^2 − .096*age^3.

Figure 5-6. *Annual Rate of Real Expenditure Increase per Enrollee, Aged Sixty-Five to One Hundred, 1989–97*[a]

Percent

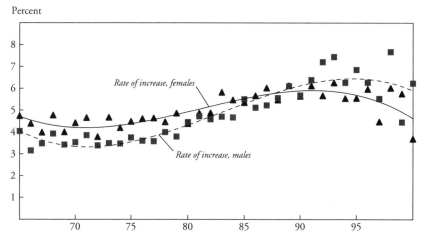

a. The polynomial functions are
Rate of per capita expenditure increase for males = 2.145 − .080age + .0010age^2 − .0000041age^3.
Rate of per capita expenditure increase for females = 2.592 − .096age + .0012age^2 − .0000048age^3.

diture data for 1989 and 1997 for both males and females and include a fitted three-degree polynomial. The figures illustrate the very rapid increase in real per capita Medicare expenditure for all ages experienced over this eight-year interval. Figure 5-6 shows the geometric average percentage rate of increase in Medicare real expenditures by age for each sex. Once again, three-degree polynomial approximations to the data are shown. The average real rate of increase between 1989 and 1997 is around 4 percent a year for people between the ages of sixty-five and eighty and approximately 6 percent a year for people in their eighties and nineties.

Clearly, if Medicare expenses increase at this pace for long, they will consume an enormous fraction of the government budget—and the country's output, for that matter. Perhaps surprisingly, per-enrollee costs peak at age ninety-two or ninety-three for both men and women and then fall noticeably. Exactly why is unclear. Perhaps patients and physicians choose less aggressive treatments for the very elderly. Perhaps the very elderly are likely to be in long-term-care facilities, which are financed more by Medicaid than by Medicare. Finally, figures 5-4 and 5-5 indicate that Medicare spends far more on men than on women at all ages.

To project future Medicare costs under different life expectancy scenarios, one must project future age-specific health status, health care prices, and the population-age structure. One approach is to assume that the pattern of age-specific Medicare expenditures persists. Under that approach, all one need do is extend the graphs to higher ages, multiply the age-specific spending by the number of people predicted to be alive at the various ages, and then multiply the aggregate result by the assumed compounded rate of price increase for health care services. Such an "age-based forecast" is used by Medicare trustees.

It is not clear, however, whether the age-specific health status of the elderly should be expected to improve or worsen as mortality improves. Medical technology might keep alive a growing fraction of very sick old people who otherwise would have died. In that event, the average health status of ninety-year-olds could worsen. While this is imaginable, it seems unlikely to me. Furthermore, it is not consistent with the trends in age-specific disability data or the declining age-specific incidence of functional impairments.[18] The age-based model implicitly holds age-specific health status constant. Even that is not consistent with the trend evidence, which strongly suggests that average age-specific health status is improving.

There is considerable evidence that age by itself is not associated with increasing Medicare spending at all, once functional status and years until death are taken into account.[19] Tim Miller uses the data from James Lubitz, J. Beebe, and C. Baker to show convincingly that years-until-death is a far better predictor of Medicare costs than age is.[20] Lubitz, Beebe, and Baker gathered information on 129,166 deaths occurring in 1989 and 1990 of people age sixty-five and over and then matched their death certificates to their Medicare administrative data. Table 5-3 reproduces Miller's presentation of the data. Medicare costs of people four or more years before death are similar, whether they die at seventy-five, eighty-five, or ninety-five. For fewer than four years until death, the spending is greater for younger individuals. David Cutler and Ellen Meara also conclude that years-until-death predicts medical costs better than age in regression analyses.[21] While these data are for particular individuals, they suggest another way of forecasting future Medicare expenses under different demographic scenarios.

The alternative to the age-based approach is to plot total Medicare spending by remaining life expectancy rather than by age. The remaining life expectancy by age and sex for 1997 can be found in the United States Life Tables.[22] The data in the appendix tables can then be expressed in terms of remaining life expectancy. The results of taking such an approach are illus-

18. For disability data, see Manton, Corder, and Stollard (1997).
19. Cutler and Meara (2001); Lubitz, Beebe, and Baker (1995).
20. Miller (2001); Lubitz, Beebe, and Baker (1995).
21. Cutler and Meara (2001).
22. Anderson (1999).

Table 5-3. *Annual Medicare Costs per Enrollee by Years before Death*[a]
Dollars

	Age at time of death		
Years before death	75	85	95
0	13,500	10,700	7,000
1	8,600	6,900	4,900
2	5,100	4,600	3,700
3	4,200	4,000	3,200
4	3,400	3,600	3,300
5	3,000	3,300	3,000
6	3,000	2,800	2,800
7	2,400	2,800	2,500
8	2,400	2,500	2,400
9	1,900	2,200	2,100
10 or more	n.a.	1,700	1,800

Source: Miller (2001), table 1.
a. Based on 129,166 deaths in 1989 and 1990.

trated in figures 5-7 and 5-8. Medicare spending increases as remaining life expectancy declines until reaching a peak, with remaining life expectancy at roughly four years. One interesting result of expressing per capita Medicare costs in this manner is that the difference between Medicare spending on men and women essentially disappears. The spending on the two sexes with remaining life expectancies of six or eight or ten years is almost identical. Peak spending with a remaining life expectancy of about four years is somewhat higher for men. This remaining difference may be due to the fact that most very elderly men are married whereas most very elderly women are not. Marital status is likely an influence on the aggressiveness of treatment. Figures 5-7 and 5-8 suggest that women are effectively younger than men of the same age or at least that they have a higher remaining life expectancy.

The alternative to assuming that the pattern of age-specific Medicare spending will remain constant (the Medicare trustees' approach) is to assume that the pattern of Medicare spending will remain unchanged with respect to remaining life expectancy. The difference is important; take, for instance, what would happen if the remaining life expectancy of ninety-year-old women increased from 4.7 years today to 8.0 years some time in the next fifty years. The age-specific approach would hold constant the health status and therefore the relative Medicare spending of ninety-year-old women. In contrast, the remaining-life-expectancy approach would assign to ninety-year-old

Figure 5-7. *Average 1997 Medicare Expenditure, Male Medicare Enrollee, and Remaining Life Expectancy*

2003 dollars

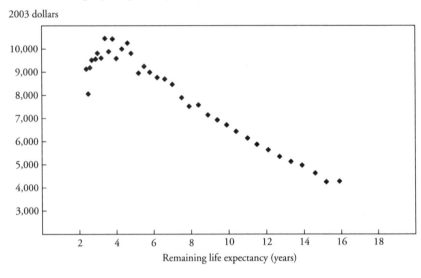

Remaining life expectancy (years)

Figure 5-8. *Average 1997 Medicare Expenditure, Female Medicare Enrollee, and Remaining Life Expectancy*

2003 dollars

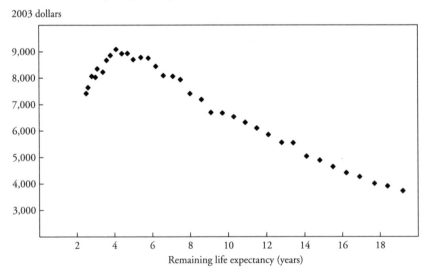

Remaining life expectancy (years)

Figure 5-9. *Estimated Total Medicare Expenditures as a Percentage of GDP,*
2000–70[a]

Percent

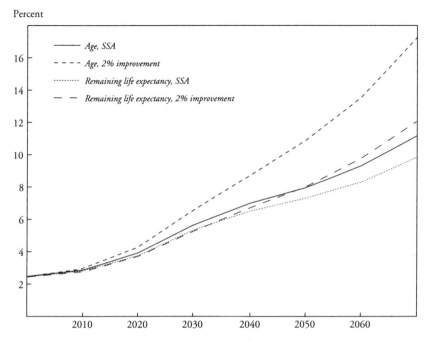

a. Given a 2 percent annual real increase in price of health services.

women the relative Medicare spending characteristics of women today with
eight years of remaining life expectancy (who are eighty-two years old). The
remaining-life-expectancy method basically treats people in the future at any
given age as younger than people today of the same age—that is, healthier and
in need of fewer health care services than people today of the same age. The
exception is people over the age of ninety-two or ninety-three. If they or their
doctors choose more aggressive treatments as their remaining life expectancy
increases, the cost of their medical care may rise relative to that for younger
people.

The results of the two approaches (holding the pattern of age-specific or
remaining-life-expectancy-specific spending fixed) for the two mortality scenarios are shown in figure 5-9, where total Medicare costs are reported as a
fraction of GDP.

Figure 5-9 indicates clearly that Medicare costs will increase dramatically
under all four alternatives—from 2.44 percent of GDP in 2000 to between
9.8 and 17.1 percent of GDP by 2070. If the Medicare trustees' assumption

about the 2 percent per year relative increase in the cost of health care is valid, then Medicare spending is likely at least to quadruple as a fraction of GDP over the next seventy years.

Figure 5-9 also shows that differences between the model that holds the age-specific pattern of per capita Medicare expenditures fixed and the model that holds the remaining-life-expectancy pattern constant are large. Total costs for the age-specific model are far more sensitive to improvements in mortality rates. For instance, with the age-specific model, total Medicare costs in 2070 rise from 11.1 percent of GDP (for the official intermediate-mortality forecast) to 17.1 percent (for the 2 percent annual improvement case). The more optimistic mortality scenario adds a full 6.0 percent of GDP to the cost of Medicare. The range of cost outcomes is far narrower with the remaining-life-expectancy model—ranging from 9.8 to 12.0 percent of GDP. While even this range indicates that Medicare costs will quadruple as a fraction of GDP, the consequences of rapid mortality improvement on Medicare costs are significantly smaller.

It is impossible to know which of these two models is more reasonable. I tend to favor the remaining-life-expectancy model, but the recent data of rising age-specific Medicare spending while age-specific measures of health status improved cause me to be cautious. David Cutler and Ellen Meara reconcile most of the divergence between rising costs and improving health by showing the extremely rapid growth in postacute care (rehabilitation) spending by Medicare participants.[23] This trend, presumably, will not continue indefinitely. The official Medicare forecasts use the age-based model, while Tim Miller argues that the remaining-life-expectancy model is more plausible.[24]

To oversimplify somewhat, the issue is whether per capita Medicare spending peaks for people in their early nineties because of age or relatively brief remaining life expectancy. Under all scenarios, the number of people in their early nineties is going to grow enormously. What we do not know is whether the health of ninety-year-olds tomorrow will resemble the health of ninety-year-olds today or the health of people of younger ages. Health spending per person is likely to continue to rise as death nears. What is less certain is whether the number of these high maintenance years will increase as mortality improves.

The remaining-life-expectancy approach is itself an intermediate case. It rests on the assumption that the number of years during which medical expenditures are high will stay roughly constant. Two alternative assumptions bound

23. Cutler and Meara (2001).
24. Miller (2001).

a range of possibilities. At one extreme is the possibility that improved mortality greatly increases the period of high morbidity. This is the assumption implicit in Medicare's age-based forecasts. At the other extreme is the assumption that the period of heightened morbidity and high medical costs will be compressed as people increasingly remain in good health until very near death.[25] The remaining-life-expectancy approach is intermediate in keeping relatively constant the period of high health costs and morbidity. I believe that this intermediate approach should be part of our best-guess forecast.

Medicaid

Title XIX of the Social Security Act (known as Medicaid) was established in 1965 as a federal-state entitlement program that pays for medical assistance for people with low incomes and few assets. Unlike Social Security and Medicare, Medicaid varies from state to state. States set varying eligibility standards and rules regarding the breadth and depth of services. Federal guidelines and regulations set minimums and specify certain groups who must be covered, but states set policy on additional benefits. Medicaid is aimed at the poor, not explicitly at the elderly. Nonetheless, the elderly receive substantial Medicaid benefits, particularly the very old who cannot afford Medicare's cost sharing and who need services not covered by Medicare, including extensive acute care or nursing home care. Medicaid expenditures totaled $194.7 billion in 2000, approximately 2 percent of GDP, of which the federal government provided $111.1 billion.

Figure 5-10 shows Medicaid expenditure per person for different age categories of the elderly in 1998. To say that the need for and utilization of Medicaid is sharply increasing with age is probably an understatement. Average Medicaid payment goes up rapidly with advancing age. Unlike Medicare, there is no sign that expenditures fall above any age: The older enrollees are, the more likely they will need long-term care, which they cannot afford without financial aid, and outpatient prescription drugs, which Medicare does not cover.

While my data for Medicaid are more limited than those for Medicare, I use the same technique to project spending. That is, I convert expenditure as a function of age to expenditure as a function of remaining life expectancy. The resulting pattern of per capita Medicaid expenditure as a function of remaining life expectancy is shown in figure 5-11.

25. Fries (1980).

Figure 5-10. *Per Capita 1998 Medicaid Expenditures, by Age Group*

2003 dollars

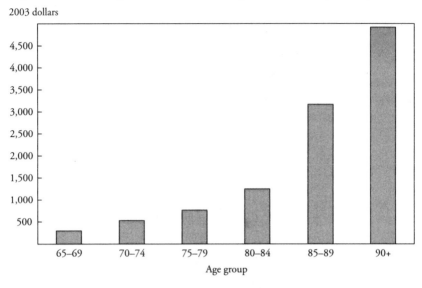

Age group

Figure 5-11. *Per Capita 1998 Medicaid Expenditure and Remaining Life Expectancy*

2003 dollars

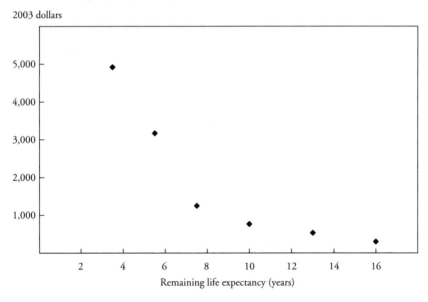

Remaining life expectancy (years)

Figure 5-12. *Estimated Total Medicaid Expenditures on Persons over Age Sixty-Five as a Percentage of GDP, 2000–70*[a]

Percent

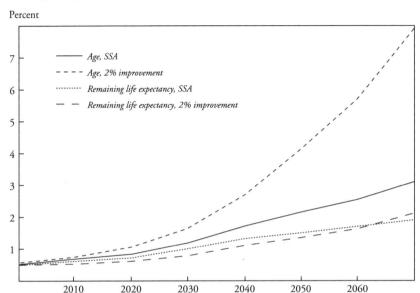

a. Given a 2 percent annual real increase in price of health services.

These estimates permit me to examine the future costs of Medicaid under different mortality scenarios with an age-based and a remaining-life-expectancy model. We know that per capita Medicaid expenses rise rapidly with age and we know that there are going to be many more very elderly people by 2050. The unresolved question is whether their need for Medicaid is better represented as a function of their age (years since birth) or their remaining life expectancy. Once again, my conjecture is that the remaining-life-expectancy model is more accurate. One reason for this view derives from the impression that many long-term-care stays begin when a married elderly person becomes a widow or widower. This death of the first spouse will typically occur at progressively older ages as mortality improves. The remaining-life-expectancy model accounts for this shift; the age-based model does not.

Figure 5-12 shows the Medicaid expenditures of people over the age of sixty-five as a percentage of GDP. Two patterns are apparent. First, Medicaid costs for the elderly increase dramatically as a percentage of GDP in all four cases. Second, the results of the age-based model differ greatly from those of the remaining-life-expectancy model. The age-based model combined with the 2 percent mortality improvement scenario leads to a conclusion that Medicaid costs of the elderly will increase fourteenfold as a share of GDP by 2070. At that point, Medicaid costs alone will account for almost 8 percent of GDP. The remaining-life-expectancy model effectively assumes that long-term care and nursing home stays occur when remaining life expectancy is short and therefore assumes that those stays typically start at progressively older ages. Projected Medicaid spending on the elderly increases, but only to less than one-third the level suggested by the age-based approach. Furthermore, projections of Medicaid costs as a fraction of GDP are essentially independent of the assumed rate of mortality improvement. The intuition of this result is that, under the remaining-life-expectancy model, roughly the same fraction of the elderly requires assistance and the duration of that assistance remains roughly constant.

Conclusions

The financial impact of dramatic mortality improvement is easiest to forecast for Social Security. Social Security has long-term financial problems even with best-case mortality assumptions. Increasing longevity will boost Social Security expense, in the absence of any change in its benefits. An obvious policy change is an increase in the age of eligibility for full PIA by a significant fraction of the increased life expectancy. The extra budget cost of significantly increased life expectancy is largely avoided if the age for full benefits is adjusted and workers are encouraged to remain employed to older ages.

Medicare and Medicaid costs increase more proportionately than do those of Social Security, at least if the relative cost of health care increases as the Medicare trustees predict. Whether and how much the optimistic mortality scenario examined in this book exacerbates the long-run budget costs imposed by Medicare and Medicaid depends crucially on whether the health service demands of the elderly are a function of age or of remaining life expectancy—that is, whether on average the elderly become healthier or sicker at any given age. I believe that it is most likely that the age-specific health status of the elderly will improve and that Medicare and Medicaid costs depend more on years until death than on years since birth. If so, then sharply increased longevity will not add materially to the already large projected increase in the cost of these programs.

There is no doubt that the health costs of the elderly will consume an increasing share of GDP and the federal government budget. However, if it turns out that health service demands are best described as a function of remaining life expectancy, these health care costs will be considerably more manageable than if health care demands simply rise with age. The remaining-life-expectancy approach offers some good news: In terms of health care costs, maybe we can afford to live longer.

Appendix 5A

Medicare Costs per Enrollee, by Age and Gender, 1989–97

Table 5A-1. *Males*[a]

2003 dollars

Age	1989	1990	1991	1992	1993	1994	1995	1996	1997
65	3,112	3,189	3,347	3,485	3,506	3,666	3,858	3,961	4,273
66	3,314	3,362	3,580	3,733	3,647	3,921	4,038	4,279	4,247
67	3,525	3,586	3,708	3,992	3,949	4,114	4,316	4,595	4,633
68	3,655	3,821	3,947	4,084	4,213	4,312	4,448	4,592	4,973
69	3,921	4,034	4,141	4,302	4,396	4,491	4,773	4,844	5,131
70	4,049	4,146	4,376	4,560	4,550	4,684	4,899	5,190	5,346
71	4,163	4,413	4,623	4,742	4,745	4,915	5,136	5,368	5,633
72	4,498	4,623	4,904	4,985	5,024	5,121	5,462	5,769	5,870
73	4,665	4,842	4,975	5,194	5,223	5,494	5,682	5,810	6,139
74	4,891	5,036	5,285	5,361	5,349	5,650	5,843	6,151	6,427
75	4,997	5,307	5,305	5,831	5,646	5,717	6,081	6,509	6,709
76	5,214	5,401	5,574	5,817	5,894	6,093	6,273	6,699	6,920
77	5,385	5,351	5,950	6,187	6,091	6,485	6,619	7,014	7,135
78	5,539	5,626	5,912	6,353	6,363	6,656	6,921	7,315	7,579
79	5,579	5,816	6,040	6,208	6,627	6,677	7,183	7,481	7,515
80	5,571	5,631	6,151	6,331	6,557	7,131	7,347	7,648	7,893

81	5,853	5,881	6,307	6,631	6,773	7,146	7,552	7,922	8,463
82	6,070	5,983	6,323	6,793	6,978	7,439	7,825	8,169	8,690
83	6,063	5,985	6,664	6,677	6,990	7,596	7,803	8,800	8,760
84	6,238	6,298	6,788	6,982	7,419	7,783	8,290	8,631	8,986
85	6,020	6,501	6,699	7,144	7,094	8,143	8,449	8,651	9,243
86	6,005	6,174	6,905	7,136	7,623	7,840	8,334	9,032	8,953
87	6,518	6,374	7,162	7,425	7,653	8,096	8,754	9,375	9,800
88	6,649	6,345	6,780	7,175	7,784	8,206	8,678	9,284	10,253
89	6,217	6,277	7,025	7,010	7,476	7,889	8,961	8,970	9,992
90	6,158	6,327	6,704	7,052	7,663	8,642	8,793	9,507	9,582
91	6,355	6,544	6,501	7,408	7,447	8,446	8,887	9,462	10,432
92	5,662	6,443	6,932	7,368	7,839	8,396	9,250	9,938	9,880
93	5,887	6,079	6,027	7,212	7,869	8,736	8,810	9,234	10,455
94	5,904	5,537	6,454	7,735	7,948	7,980	8,968	9,707	9,600
95	5,772	6,886	7,159	7,133	7,442	8,097	9,276	8,629	9,807
96	5,874	6,776	5,966	7,361	6,953	8,562	8,463	9,150	9,556
97	6,184	7,275	8,078	6,661	6,910	7,577	7,542	9,896	9,513
98	5,088	4,929	6,859	6,351	6,275	9,153	8,632	9,522	9,189
99	5,686	5,087	6,490	6,279	8,297	5,355	7,902	10,717	8,057
100	5,626	6,001	5,944	5,279	7,794	7,193	5,668	8,212	9,129
Average	5,331	5,497	5,877	6,110	6,389	6,761	7,103	7,668	7,910

Source: Data based on a sample of actual Medicare claims compiled by Tom MaCurdy of Stanford University. Numbers have been updated to 2003 dollars using the consumer price index.

a. Expenditures are for Medicare part A and part B and are financed by a combination of payroll taxes, general government revenue, and participant premiums.

Table 5A-2. *Females*[a]

2003 dollars

Age	1989	1990	1991	1992	1993	1994	1995	1996	1997
65	2,573	2,748	2,866	2,995	2,983	3,292	3,346	3,594	3,727
66	2,771	2,752	2,970	3,188	3,170	3,364	3,615	3,802	3,906
67	2,930	3,041	3,022	3,181	3,365	3,504	3,720	3,975	4,005
68	2,939	3,069	3,246	3,349	3,363	3,714	3,864	3,997	4,266
69	3,226	3,271	3,394	3,466	3,605	3,820	4,024	4,366	4,416
70	3,286	3,414	3,564	3,693	3,811	4,006	4,147	4,441	4,646
71	3,398	3,608	3,768	3,867	3,972	4,189	4,502	4,672	4,889
72	3,742	3,728	3,960	4,034	4,209	4,362	4,694	5,079	5,037
73	3,849	3,859	4,163	4,297	4,321	4,665	4,869	5,201	5,544
74	4,001	4,017	4,265	4,379	4,595	4,908	5,187	5,373	5,558
75	4,126	4,211	4,478	4,627	4,729	4,921	5,352	5,583	5,858
76	4,254	4,320	4,663	4,883	4,945	5,303	5,480	6,038	6,102
77	4,397	4,526	4,796	5,116	5,175	5,435	5,634	6,038	6,319
78	4,607	4,720	5,008	5,069	5,369	5,574	5,990	6,192	6,533
79	4,568	4,757	4,887	5,340	5,377	5,744	6,155	6,397	6,678
80	4,753	4,897	5,100	5,393	5,641	6,042	6,383	6,702	6,699
81	4,914	4,907	5,295	5,433	5,778	6,233	6,655	7,007	7,189
82	5,062	5,264	5,431	5,811	5,923	6,382	6,872	7,339	7,412
83	5,048	5,215	5,585	5,932	6,202	6,556	7,243	7,552	7,937

84	5,264	5,245	5,779	6,139	6,231	6,712	7,333	7,712	8,062
85	5,330	5,444	5,667	6,103	6,580	6,841	7,416	7,872	8,090
86	5,430	5,616	5,841	6,264	6,512	7,051	7,508	8,056	8,438
87	5,483	5,666	5,993	6,374	6,837	6,880	7,915	8,334	8,751
88	5,729	5,584	6,049	6,335	6,655	7,325	8,106	8,327	8,775
89	5,403	5,718	6,155	6,375	6,787	7,282	7,973	8,449	8,696
90	5,756	5,557	6,177	6,520	6,616	7,251	7,957	8,385	8,931
91	5,547	5,384	5,689	6,449	6,696	7,379	7,966	8,299	8,922
92	5,845	5,594	5,983	6,208	6,885	7,145	8,215	8,340	9,086
93	5,448	5,578	5,943	6,489	7,033	7,226	7,853	8,347	8,854
94	5,631	5,646	6,143	6,517	6,523	7,679	7,811	7,870	8,670
95	5,337	5,338	5,264	6,151	6,906	7,16	7,781	8,257	8,223
96	5,250	5,393	5,635	5,792	6,981	6,813	7,372	7,661	8,347
97	5,657	5,241	5,689	6,269	6,281	7,209	6,901	7,503	8,026
98	5,054	4,731	5,544	5,514	6,672	6,359	7,496	8,053	8,064
99	4,883	4,231	4,715	4,803	5,764	6,234	6,117	8,231	7,641
100	5,552	4,034	5,041	5,061	5,347	5,482	7,321	7,154	7,420
Average	4,640	4,620	4,938	5,206	5,496	5,835	6,299	6,672	6,937

Source: See table 5A-1.

a. See table 5A-1.

COMMENT
William G. Gale

It is by now commonplace to observe that the long-anticipated aging of the population—due to declining birth rates, lengthening life spans, and the imminent passage of the baby boomers into retirement—will place significant pressure on the government budget generally and on Social Security, Medicare, and Medicaid in particular. It would be natural to also suppose that biological and medical advances that significantly increase life span would exacerbate these problems and prove to be unambiguously bad news for the public finances. The surprising conclusion of John Shoven's thoughtful chapter is that this need not be the case.

His chapter presents three sets of results. First, under the baseline projections made by the Social Security and Medicare trustees, the federal government faces significant long-term financing problems. This standard and uncontroversial finding implies that there is a fundamental (that is, large, persistent, growing) imbalance between projected tax revenues and spending commitments, even before considering potential improvements in projected mortality.

Second, and also consistent with conventional wisdom, improved mortality will (in the absence of other changes) adversely and significantly affect Social Security finances. The projected shortfall in the year 2080 under standard mortality assumptions is 6.7 percent of payroll but under the 2 percent mortality improvement scenario is 11.7 percent (for an explanation of the 2 percent mortality improvement scenario, see the chapter by Henry Aaron and Benjamin Harris, this volume).

Third, and most intriguing, the effects of improved mortality on Medicare and Medicaid finances hinge on whether medical expenditures depend on people's age since birth or on their years until death. Currently, the bulk of lifetime expense for each person under Medicare and for the elderly under Medicaid is associated with high-cost events in the last few years of life. If expenditures depend on remaining life expectancy, improved mortality would delay the onset of those high-cost events but would not add much to lifetime expenses per person. In contrast, if expenditures depend on age since birth, improved mortality would lengthen the high-cost period and increase per person expenditures.

Shoven makes the case, cautiously and plausibly, that expenditures are likely to depend on remaining life expectancy. This in turn implies that improved mortality has almost no effect on projected expenditures in

Medicare and Medicaid. A few numbers highlight the main points here. In 2000 Medicare spending and federal and state Medicaid spending on the elderly totaled less than 3 percent of gross domestic product. By 2080, under baseline assumptions for mortality and using the age-since-birth model, expenditures will rise to 14 percent of GDP. These numbers indicate the severity of the underlying problem. If mortality rates improve by 2 percent annually and if age since birth determines costs, expenditures will rise to almost 25 percent of GDP in 2080, showing that improvements in mortality would have disastrous consequences for Medicare and Medicaid finances. On the other hand, if costs depend on remaining life expectancy, expenditures in 2080 will equal 12 percent of GDP under standard mortality assumptions and 14 percent under the 2 percent improvement scenario, showing that future Medicare and Medicaid finances are not particularly sensitive to mortality improvement if expenditures depend on years until death.

It must be noted that an enormous amount of uncertainty surrounds the long-term estimates upon which projections rest. The uncertainty relates to demographic issues, which are discussed elsewhere in this volume; to underlying economic trends and productivity growth; and to behavioral and policy responses to improved mortality.

Shoven also provides perspectives on the fundamental issue of the extent to which increased life expectancy translates into more "good health" years versus more "bad health" years. More bad health years imply added burdens on the rest of the population. More good health years put less pressure on health expenses and could mean longer careers–which would boost GDP and improve the ability of society to pay for already promised public services. Problems caused by increased life span do not show up in cash flow until well into the twenty-first century—and really well into the second half of the century. The back-loaded nature of the problem will make it more difficult to deal with politically. Shoven implicitly raises the issue of shortfalls, breaking them into the portion stemming from the baseline projections and the portion attributable to increased longevity.

Policy changes could make a big dent in the problems created by increased longevity. As noted above, Shoven shows that increased longevity will hurt Social Security's financial status, other thing equal. He also shows that 70 percent of the deterioration in the long-term finances due to increased longevity could be eliminated if the normal retirement age—the age at which full benefits can be obtained—were raised by one month a year starting in 2023. Such an adjustment would raise the normal retirement age to seventy-two years by 2083. If there really is a 2 percent annual improvement in mortality, as modeled by Aaron and Harris, such an increase in the retirement age does not seem particularly burdensome.

Household behavior may also change in response to lengthening longevity. Labor supply could increase due to a change in normal retirement age and to improved age-specific health. Both labor supply and saving could rise to account for the fact that a longer life span would require added saving for retirement.

While precise calculations are beyond the scope of this comment, it is clear that the induced changes in labor supply and saving could be large enough to offset a significant part of the 30 percent of the shortfall that would not be offset by a later retirement age. For example, as a rough calculation, if the retirement age rose by five years, average career length would rise by about 15 percent. Suppose that aggregate wages rise by about 10 percent (since elderly workers earn less than average), average adjusted gross income rises by 7 percent (since wages are about 70 percent of adjusted gross income), and average income tax revenues rise by 3–5 percent (since elderly households have lower than average income). Income tax revenues would increase by 0.3–0.5 percent of GDP (since the tax currently raises about 10 percent of GDP), or 0.75–1.25 percent of taxable payroll. Half or more of the 1.5 percent of the projected taxable payroll gap in 2080 would thus be closed (see table 5-2).

Needless to say, these are imprecise estimates. Their purpose is only to show that changes in the normal retirement age as modeled by Shoven, coupled with changes in labor supply due to some combination of changes in policy rules, health, and retirement saving needs, could significantly offset the added burdens that improved mortality would place on the Social Security system.

That finding—along with the fact that increased mortality may, but need not, make Medicare and Medicare financing problems worse—is the good news. The bad news is that, even without assuming any change in projected mortality, the underlying baseline is still a major problem for fiscal sustainability. Addressing that issue is beyond the scope of Shoven's chapter, and of this volume, but it remains a key issue looking forward.

References

Aaron, Henry J., and John B. Shoven. 1999. *Should the United States Privatize Social Security?* MIT Press.

Anderson, Robert N. 1999. "United States Life Tables, 1997." In *National Vital Statistics Reports,* vol. 47. Hyattsville, Md.: National Center for Health Statistics.

Board of Trustees, Medical Insurance (Boards of Trustees of the Federal Hospital Insurance and Federal Supplementary Medical Insurance Trust Funds). 2002. *The 2002 Annual Report of the Boards of Trustees of the Federal Hospital Insurance and Federal Supplementary Medical Insurance Trust Funds.*

Board of Trustees, OASDI (Board of Trustees, Federal Old-Age and Survivors Insurance and Disability Insurance Trust Funds). 2002. *The 2002 Annual Report of the Board of Trustees, Federal Old-Age and Survivors Insurance and Disability Insurance Trust Funds.* Government Printing Office.

Cutler, David M., and Ellen Meara. 2001. "The Concentration of Medical Spending: An Update." In *Themes in the Economics of Aging,* edited by D. Wise, 217–34. University of Chicago Press.

Fries, J. F. 1980. "Aging, Natural Death, and the Compression of Morbidity." *New England Journal of Medicine* 303 (3): 130–35.

HCFA (Health Care Financing Administration). 1998. "Medicaid: A Brief Summary."

Lubitz, James, J. Beebe, and C. Baker. 1995. "Longevity and Medicare Expenses." *New England Review of Medicine* 332 (3): 999–1003.

Manton, Kenneth, Larry Corder, and Eric Stallard. 1997. "Chronic Disability Trends in Elderly United States Populations: 1982–94." *Proceedings of the National Academy of Sciences USA* 94 (6): 2593–98.

Miller, Tim. 2001. "Increasing Longevity and Medicare Expenditures." *Demography* 38 (2): 215–26.

Office of Management and Budget. 2003. *Budget for Fiscal Year 2004.* Historical tables.

ALEXANDER M. CAPRON

6 *Ethical Aspects of Major Increases in Life Span and Life Expectancy*

THIS CHAPTER EXAMINES ethical issues raised by molecular medicine and the increase in life spans that it may enable. These questions are quite different from those considered in other contributions to this volume, most of which focus on established scientific, economic, and demographic data and analytical models. They explore the implications of the lengthened life spans that new preventive and curative interventions emerging from molecular medicine will produce. To be sure, these projections and interpretations are subject to error and may be controversial: Just how rapidly will science advance? Will physicians and patients accept new medical technologies? Will third parties pay for them? How will employers and employees react to various incentives? What changes in life patterns will be sought by individuals and families? How will educational institutions, merchants, developers of private housing, vacation condominiums, or retirement communities, the health care industry, and a host of other actors respond to these preferences?

Yet much of what these chapters have to say follows directly from accepted realities. One is called on to consider new twists on familiar questions about how various institutions—from the government to the workplace to the international economy—will adjust to the coming demographic changes. Just as the United States had first to scramble to find enough diapers, then enough classrooms and enough jobs for the baby boom that followed World

War II, it now faces the prospect of having to find enough health care and retirement benefits for the oldsters into whom the baby boomers have morphed. The extensions in life expectancy projected in this volume may simply promise—or threaten—to make those tasks more challenging.

What Sets Ethics Apart?

From an individual viewpoint, the ethical issues posed by molecular medicine may seem to differ little from those that arise in ordinary medical practice. If one assumes that patients remain free to accept or reject particular treatments, molecular medicine resembles traditional medicine in that it prevents or cures disease, relieves pain, and forestalls death. But that, of course, is not the end of the story. Medical developments over the past fifty years have made clear that not every remedy for disease, much less every lengthened life, is an unalloyed good. The prospect that science may soon produce whole new categories of medical interventions brings forward questions that go beyond the effects of molecular medicine on the lives of those who can easily afford the new interventions. How will they affect overall health care spending? Should scarce life-saving resources be allocated any differently to those whose need for treatment follows an artificially lengthened life than to other patients? Who will pay for the greater costs of longer life and perhaps more health care?

Such questions, of course, are not novel, but interventions that greatly lengthen life span could make their resolution much more difficult. Furthermore, all major social transformations create uncertainties, which may make ethically acceptable outcomes hard to reach. Molecular medicine raises basic questions about the ends not only of medicine but also of human life itself. Muddling through to the answers may not suffice.

Above all, ethical questions differ from those examined in the other chapters because ethics concerns not what we will do but what we should do—that is, what is good, just, and right. For example, suppose that science slightly improves the health—or more problematically, the power, wealth, or pleasure—of only a few people. Should that be regarded as a net improvement? Would it make any difference how such changes arose? For example, suppose that access differed because some could afford medical care but others could not. Alternatively, suppose that new techniques helped people only with certain inherited genetic susceptibilities. Would society be better with greater average life span and more chronic illness but also greater freedom of choice about how to live and to die? Questions of this sort will not be resolved by the presentation of more, or even "better," facts. Indeed, even the prediction that a particular state of affairs is unlikely does not end the matter, because the question remains whether the new biological knowledge should or should not be used in ways calculated to achieve a particular outcome, however improbable that outcome might be.

The coming changes in biomedical capabilities raise profound questions for individuals as well as for society. Over the past thirty years, most ethical commentary on medicine and the life sciences has focused on what people *have* the right to do, not what it would *be* right to do. Bioethicists have explored the ethical underpinnings of various rights—to reproduce, to die, to make informed choices among medical alternatives—but they have treated the exercise of such rights largely as matters of personal preference and individual morality. Even when they are asking, What is the good society? bioethicists seldom ask, What is the good life? Yet the biomedical developments that herald major increases in life expectancy make the latter question inescapable. Thus, although they are not the focus of this chapter, the implications of these technologies for individuals, not just what is meant by a *good* life but what is meant by a *human* life, cannot be ignored in the coming years.

An Ethical Approach

I begin by presenting a framework for ethical analysis and sketching some possible scenarios with differing consequences. Then I look at some of the intergroup and interpersonal issues raised by biomedical developments that could lead to major expansions in the life expectancy of the population or particular groups. At stake here are questions of equity both between age groups or generations and within age groups, especially regarding access to life-extending interventions. If means for life extension are developed and widely adopted, would the resulting transformation of society pose difficult or intractable ethical problems or issues? I then turn to the effects such developments could produce for individuals and how they could change what constitutes a good life. This section examines objections that have been raised regarding the whole longevity project—that is, the desirability of making longer life an objective of science—and its effect on human well-being, especially allegations that such an objective violates limits that are not only biologically but also ethically normative. One thread that unites these two parts is the conclusion that, in both realms, ethical evaluation turns not just on the social rules but also on individual actions and attitudes.

As an early foray into an emerging field, this chapter may succeed more in identifying issues than in resolving them. I do not withhold conclusions when I believe I have the means to reach them, but on many points answers are likely to emerge only from dialogue, as more comes to be known about how the new biomedical capabilities will be developed and employed.

The way social issues are addressed in the United States is more likely to highlight individual than social choices. In most other industrialized nations relevant issues are matters for common concern because services are provided collectively. In the United States, many of the questions about income support and health care that would be raised by a major increase in longevity are framed individually, rather than collectively, because a larger share of retirement income and health care is financed privately than in other developed nations. In this frame, the use of life-extending technologies will depend on individual choices—Do I want to spend the money? Have I selected a health plan that covers such interventions?—rather than on collective decisions designed to allocate resources fairly. So, although I assume that thinking about the issues as matters for rational analysis and principled resolution is worthwhile, they may not be posed in that fashion. Social policy in this arena may result not from collective determinations about resource allocation but from the collective effect of individual decisions that reflect varying degrees of knowledge about, and concern for, the consequences for the whole society.

A Method of Ethical Analysis

Many factors go into deciding whether efforts that tend toward, or even aim at, increasing longevity ought to be pursued. What can ethical analysis add to the picture? Ethics is concerned with the process of reasoning about the rightness of actions, the goodness of results, and (sometimes) the acceptability of a person's motive or intention or the nature of a person's character. One method that is frequently helpful in evaluating new biological developments is to begin by examining the purposes for which action is taken, then to scrutinize the means used, and finally to weigh the results achieved, both intended and unintended. If an act is intended to achieve an immoral or otherwise impermissible result, there is no need to evaluate its means. Likewise, when results would be achieved by forbidden means, one usually need not parse the consequences.[1] If the aims and means are acceptable, however, then ethical judgment depends on evaluating the consequences by weighing

1. The qualifier *usually* is intended to denote that, in some circumstances, philosophers argue for the acceptability of using immoral means to achieve imperative ends that cannot otherwise be reached; these situations are, however, unusual and embody classical ethical dilemmas (such as whether to torture a prisoner to get him to reveal the location of a ticking, hidden bomb).

the good and bad produced, and the benefits and the burdens in achieving it, in as rich and full a sense as the available evidence permits and as the importance of the decision at hand justifies.

This aims-means-results process is helpful, albeit not definitive. It can be employed whatever one's philosophical orientation. An evaluation of aims is most closely associated with teleological ethics. But it is also an appropriate analytical starting point for deontologists—those who derive duties from basic ethical principles, such as those often cited in discussions of bioethics: respect for persons, beneficence, and justice.[2] After all, even deontologists do not think that adhering to one's duties to another person validates seeking a forbidden end, although it may justify conduct that produces harmful side effects. Consequentialists—such as utilitarians—are usually thought to be concerned with weighing the costs and benefits of an outcome.[3] Nonetheless, even they typically accept a place for side constraints, which take the form of either extrinsic moral principles and rules (for example, Thou shalt not murder) or utility-based rules (for example, Keep your promises).[4]

To illustrate the use of this three-step method, consider human reproductive cloning. One of the most commonly cited aims is to increase reproductive choices for all couples or to offer those who lack gametes a chance to have a genetically related child—indeed, one that is virtually a genetic twin of its progenitor. Those who emphasize this goal see it as consistent with ones widely accepted in society. Conversely, those who see cloning as intended to enable one generation to determine the genetic makeup of the next find this

2. See National Commission for the Protection of Human Subjects of Biomedical and Behavioral Research (1978); Beauchamp and Childress (2001).

3. The basic principle of utilitarianism is that actions are right to the degree that they tend to promote the greatest good for the greatest number. J. S. Mill defines the good (utility) in terms of well-being, which rests on maximizing happiness and minimizing its opposite, based on measurements of pleasure, both intellectual and sensual. John S. Mill, "Utilitarianism," originally published in three installments in *Fraser's Magazine,* 1861. In Kenneth J. Arrow's elegant revision, utility is measured in terms of the degree to which people's preferences are satisfied. See Arrow (1951). The advantage of preference satisfaction over happiness is that it allows people to determine for themselves what has intrinsic value.

4. So-called rule utilitarians develop certain practice rules adherence to which is held to maximize utility as a general matter. This not only avoids the need to engage in complicated and time-consuming calculations in each case but also permits the articulation of rules that reflect other moral judgments that are a common (and usual) part of moral actions in everyday life (such as, Do not steal). This responds to a major critique of utilitarianism, namely, that the absence of such rules suggests that, whenever utility would be maximized, a step can be taken regardless of its harmful effects for some people. The adoption of rule utilitarianism, rather than act utilitarianism, nevertheless leaves open the question of whether it is possible to hold to a rule when, in a particular case, departing from the rule would produce the greatest good for the greatest number. In other words, can the utility principle be maintained—as it must to justify the rule—if utility is violated by adhering to the rule?

goal to be radical and unacceptable for medicine and indeed for society. The means used likewise divide analysts. Many find the means unexceptionable, provided that those whose eggs, nuclear DNA, and gestational abilities would be combined to create a cloned child are informed and voluntary participants. Those who regard embryos as full human beings see the means used to perfect human reproductive cloning as unacceptable because they would involve extensive experimentation in which hundreds or perhaps thousands of embryos would be created and then destroyed, either for study purposes or simply because of the inefficiency of the technology, as revealed through experiments in other mammals.

It is in evaluating the consequences that the divisions in analysis become most marked. (Evaluations of novel interventions always involve an element of conjecture.) Will the few individuals who happen to be genetic copies of someone else be seen by themselves and others no differently from other people created through sexual reproduction? Or will cloning result in children who are regarded as objects with characteristics chosen to please their parents' egos, dreams, or frustrated hopes, causing generations and relationships to become hopelessly muddled?

Such markedly different conclusions about the ethics of human cloning are hardly surprising, because people start with such divergent premises about embryos and reproductive rights. Yet even a radical procedure such as cloning, which excites heated debate, illustrates that careful analysis clarifies the source of disagreement and what information is relevant. When the topic is one that can be approached with more agreement on the premises and relevant moral principles, a more definitive ethical judgment can be expected.

Debates about the ethics of increased longevity will also be fueled by underlying differences. I believe that the dominant philosophical mode will be consequentialist, rather than the Kantian deontology that has characterized bioethics over the past quarter century, for several reasons. First, the principlist approach to bioethics is much better suited as an ethical system for individual physicians and researchers and the institutions of which they are a part than it is for resolving issues that involve either the rights and obligations of the members of a society or the appropriate allocation of collective resources. Indeed, the third principle in the usual bioethics trilogy (justice) is the least fully addressed. The reason is that its implications for individual professionals are either unclear or at odds with the generally accepted duties of physicians, especially the Hippocratic obligation to give primacy to the well-being of their patients over other interests. The second reason I expect that consequentialism will dominate analysis is that it is the prevailing mode of public policy analysis in liberal democracies.

The focus on consequences as the basis for judging the rightness or wrongness of increasing human life span reflects more than just the prevalence of utilitarian thinking, however. It is also because the aim and means of increased longevity do not provide clear points of controversy (though I come back to them later). It is not even clear that one can point to any policy, programs, or actions that are intended simply to increase longevity. Likewise, most—though not all—individual means used by biomedical scientists, physicians, and patients that might extend lives are morally unobjectionable. Even the critics of extending human life span recognize that such extension arises from the cumulative effects of medical choices that aim at legitimate ends and employ accepted means. Indeed, Leon Kass, probably the severest critic, seems to echo Justice Louis Brandeis's famous dictum about being most on guard against those who act from seeming benevolence when he worries that our ready acceptance of individually attractive medical developments blinds us to the ends to which the biomedical enterprise is leading us.[5]

I come back to Kass's concerns later, when I consider whether the effects of life-extending technologies on people provide ethical grounds for forgoing these technologies. But in dealing first with the intergenerational and interpersonal effects of greater longevity, I do not mean to suggest that a focus on consequences leaves us with no alternatives to utilitarianism, with its acknowledged faults.[6] The major competing approach comes from theories of justice. John Stuart Mill himself accepted a consequentialist version

---

5. Louis Brandeis's words were: "Experience should teach us to be most on our guard to protect liberty when the government's purposes are beneficent. . . . The greatest dangers to liberty lurk in insidious encroachment by men of zeal, well meaning but without understanding." *Olmstead* v. *United States*, 277 U.S. 438, 479 (1928) (Brandeis, J. dissenting). Kass sees danger because the changes that would lengthen life span are individually unobjectionable and even attractive; hence he fears we may be seduced by these tempting fruits of biotechnology, which have made us "many times over the beneficiaries of its cures for diseases, prolongation of life, and amelioration of suffering, psychic as well as somatic," while failing to recognize "that the powers made possible by biomedical science can be used for nontherapeutic or ignoble purposes, serving ends that range from the frivolous and disquieting to the offensive and pernicious." Kass (2003), p. 9.

6. Critics of using utilitarianism to ground policy decisions challenge its premise that it is possible to determine who will be affected by every action and to quantify the effects in each case, given that certain effects are difficult to measure; that it is difficult (impossible?) to express all effects in common terms (at least without distorting or misrepresenting what is essential about some of these effects); and that it is not uncommon for well-intended actions to have unforeseen bad consequences (as well as the converse), which would mean that one could not be certain of a policy's (utilitarian) rightness until its consequences had played out. Several responses have been mounted to these criticisms. First, the method does not have to be strictly applied to every action but only to important and seriously disputed actions; and second, when the question is not whether something should be done but which among several alternatives is preferred, it may not be necessary to reduce everything to a common metric but only to measure their effects on a comparative scale.

of justice based on utilitarian principles: Justice consists in adhering to laws and norms, which themselves are justified if they tend to maximize social utility. Today the dominant alternative account of the origins and effects of justice derives from John Rawls's influential book *A Theory of Justice*.[7] Rawls argues that one should ascertain justice through procedural fairness, by which he means that the social contract should be the one that a person would see as just from behind the "veil of ignorance"—that is, without awareness of the personal consequences of the choice. Two principles emerge from this method. The first is the principle of greatest equal liberty. According to this principle, each person is to have an equal right to the most extensive total system of equal basic liberties compatible with a similar system of liberty for all. The second principle imposes two requirements on the way that social and economic inequalities are to be arranged: that they give greatest benefit to the least advantaged (the difference principle) and that they attach to offices and positions open to all under conditions of fair and equal opportunity (the principle of fair equality of opportunity).[8]

On these principles, biomedical developments that could lengthen life would be judged ethically according to how the consequences of such developments are projected, both interpersonally and intergenerationally. It is often said that good ethics begins with good facts. Unfortunately, when it comes to the effects of molecular medicine on life expectancy, we have possibilities and projections but no certainties. We can, however, hypothesize several ways in which biomedical developments might increase life expectancy and affect human life. Hypothetical situations, which differ by the way they combine such features as the point in life when an intervention is used, the

7. Rawls (1971). In the tradition of Hobbes, Locke, and Rousseau, Rawls offers a distinctive social contract argument for justice derived from principles "that free and rational persons concerned to further their own interests would accept in an initial position of equality" (p. 11). Rawls propounds his principles (which he calls "justice as fairness") by arguing that they are the ones people would choose if they were situated behind a "veil of ignorance," which deprives them of information that would otherwise lead them to favor principles advantageous to their particular circumstances. Without such bias, Rawls argues that people will choose principles for social cooperation that are fair to all autonomous persons, with an interest in being free to choose and to revise their own ends and to pursue them effectively.

8. One of the criticisms of Rawls's theory that has particular relevance for an analysis of the ethics of increased longevity is that the difference principle has an implausibly strong assumption about how risk averse people would be in the original position. Is it likely that people would care only about minimizing losses and not about the greater gains available under a less egalitarian rule, particularly if the rule includes a floor of social and economic security below which no one would fall? Since the differences in life expectancy that could result from intervening with new biomedical techniques could generate social and economic inequalities, whether such differences were considered just or not could depend on the stringency of the difference principle.

pace at which senescence occurs, and the prevalence of disability during later years, provide a number of "models" to facilitate both the societal and personal analyses that follow.

Evaluating the Consequences of Prolonging Life

A century of advances in public health and medicine, from water purification and vaccines to artificial kidneys and mechanical ventilators, makes apparent that longer life has been a blessing for most people but a curse for some. Developments in medical care and in general living standards have radically reduced severe illness and death in early life. They have made old age not just longer but also more comfortable for many people. They have recast what it means to be old. For most parts of our society, old age begins later and is less burdensome than was true just one or two generations ago. Still, experience teaches that context is all: Something as simple as an antibiotic to cure pneumonia has vastly different meaning for a schoolchild than for an Alzheimer's patient. The importance of context emerges whenever a person considers whether to use life-extending techniques. What information do I have and how reliable is that information regarding the consequences of using particular techniques in my circumstances? What stopping rules will be available if the results are personally unsatisfactory? Context is likewise very important in thinking about life extension in population terms.

The ways that molecular medicine may increase average life expectancy can be analyzed through the various patterns of life they might produce and as manifestations of particular variables. Many of the contributors to this volume project relatively minor changes in average longevity, based on slow improvements in—and adoption of—techniques that retard aging. If actual developments follow these patterns, the ethical issues raised may be rather trivial. During the last century, average life expectancy increased by 40–50 percent without provoking ethical debate or even after-the-fact ethical handwringing. To be sure, "heroic" efforts with very sick dying patients and outcomes such as the growing population of elderly women in long-term care facilities have raised ethical concerns. Still, if life expectancy simply continues to edge upward, the ethical implications may never even come up for public debate. Instead, we will probably simply experience a series of ad hoc adjustments, such as a modest ratcheting up of the retirement age, which would be necessitated by practical problems and justified in narrow terms.

Although historic changes in life expectancy and in the proportion of the population classified as old have thus far provoked little angst, the past may

Figure 6-1. *Number of Deaths by Age at Death (holding total population constant)*

Hypothetical number of people (thousands)

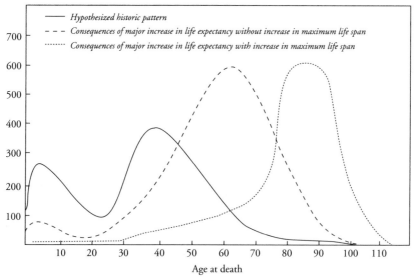

not foretell the future. Past advances simply extended to most people the survival rates and longevity previously achieved by a fortunate few (represented in figure 6-1 by the difference between the hypothesized historic pattern and the pattern that results from increased life expectancy without increase in life span). Possible future biomedical developments could produce a different pattern, in which a substantial increase in average life expectancy is accompanied by a significant number whose life spans exceed one hundred years, an age surpassed by only a tiny fraction (roughly 1 in 10,000) of the population in the past. Moreover, unlike earlier improvements in average life expectancy, which resulted largely from public health measures (sanitation, vaccination), future increases may come from efforts that are frankly described as part of a longevity project.

Just as the patterns set forth in figure 6-1 are merely heuristic, the hypothetical future states set forth below are intended as an aid to analysis, not as a forecast. If the contours of a supposed longevity project were clear, creating hypothetical futures would be unnecessary. In fact, the biomedical techniques that may boost average, and perhaps maximum, life expectancy are still emerging and remain diverse. Distinct futures may emerge, doubtless including some that are different from those I consider below.

Different means of intervening at different points over the course of people's lives could produce radically different life courses. Whether morbidity, disability, and diminished functionality accompany longer life spans is obviously of central importance, both because they are major determinants of the quality of life and because they affect how much people contribute to society or take from society in medical or social support. Dying could follow a drawn-out process of accumulating morbidities (such as compromised pulmonary, circulatory, and neurological functioning), a short, terminal period (with untreatable cancer, for example), or a sudden collapse.[9] Variables related to the timing of interventions will also influence how medical interventions affect a life course. Interventions could range from techniques that must be used before birth to those that could wait until a disease or disability occurs. Finally, some interventions could be so inexpensive and simple that they would be universally available (comparable to a blood transfusion), while others might have to be custom-made for each patient, rendering them expensive and perhaps so difficult or risky that only a few specialists could undertake them.

Combining these factors in various ways produces a wide range of patterns. Any evaluation of the ethics of using particular interventions will depend on how each intervention contributes to these patterns and how the patterns themselves are viewed. Playing out all the combinations would be tedious. I offer four life curves, that is, patterns of a life course in terms of functional level and general health for the average, unisex individual from birth to death. After describing these outcomes, I examine some additional variables relevant to reaching an ethical evaluation of different means of life extension, principally in terms of their consequences.[10]

Four Life Curves

Despite recent increases in average life expectancy in much of the world, "*healthy* life expectancy—that is, the period of life that is free from disease—

9. " 'We'd like to do away with much of the health care system,' says Charles Cantor, the chief scientific officer of Sequenom, the gene-discovery company that read my DNA. 'We'd like to keep people healthy until they suddenly go up in a puff of smoke. I don't think we'll quite get there, but we can get much better disease prevention.' " Nicholas D. Kristof, "Staying Alive, Staying Human," *New York Times,* February 11, 2003, op-ed.

10. Some of these variables (such as a lingering or a swift death) relate directly to differences in outcomes. Others could be characterized as differences in means. Yet such differences are not the sort that weigh heavily in the second step of the analytic framework. They are relevant for the different consequences they produce, not because one means is inherently more ethical than another. Thus I combine some of the variations into models while treating others as variables in addition to models, because it is useful to compare patterns of lengthened lives. There is no reason to regard the particular factors that produce these patterns (or models) as falling into a different ethical category from those I discuss separately.

Figure 6-2. *Three Variations on the Present Aging Curve*

Health status, average, unisex person (percent)

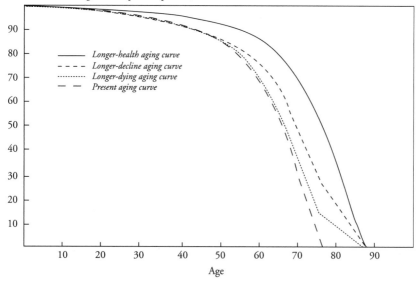

has remained the same," according to Ruud ter Meulen.[11] For the average person in a developed country today who lives to average life expectancy, the early years of life are marked by good health and high functioning (near 100 on the vertical axis; see figure 6-2).[12] Health declines little through the fifties. Then the curve heads down more sharply as disease conditions (including many, such as diabetes, pulmonary and cardiac insufficiency, and muscle weakness, resulting from poor environments and life-styles) limit functioning. Finally, there is a period of debilitation and chronic ill health (falling below 20 on the vertical axis of figure 6-2).

11. ter Meulen (1995).
12. The curve is smooth because it is an average and includes those who experience traumas or other illness, those who die prematurely, and those who survive well beyond the average. An alternative representation, which would show the deviation around this mean, might give a better sense of experience within a population, but it would also make the figure much more complex and interfere with its heuristic purpose, which is to convey graphically the alternative experiences of being healthy or ill over the course of a lifetime for people under different hypothetical models generated by various life-lengthening technologies. Another way of representing the information would be to chart, along the vertical axis, the percentage of the population in good health. Such a figure could make clear the burden of disease on the population and hence the relative consequences in terms of health care for the society as a whole. But the figure would lose an important quality by not being the life experience of a hypothetical average person under a particular set of biomedical and social assumptions.

The question, then, is whether extensions in life expectancy will raise or lower the time spent in illness and debility. In other words, would longevity be wasted on the old? Biomedical developments could affect the current pattern in several ways.[13] The first is more aggressive use of currently available therapies. Intervening aggressively toward the end of life would extend life expectancy by adding to the period of debility and ill health. This longer-dying model is not attractive. In fact, many people fear it already. To the extent that it is now a reality, it has caused many people to yearn for increased control over the circumstances of their deaths. The debate about how much control to place with individuals—from living wills to active euthanasia—is one of the most contentious in contemporary bio-ethics. While this scenario would not be sought as an objective, it could emerge as the unintended result of separate interventions, each of which, viewed individually, seemed to be an appropriate response to medical conditions and even dramatically improved patients' conditions. If these reparative interventions were so costly or risky that their use was usually limited to patients already suffering fairly severe consequences of disease, the result could be an extension of life expectancy exclusively through lengthening the dying process.

A much more attractive form of increased longevity is an extension of the relatively healthy years of middle age, after which decline and death would occur much as it does today. In this longer-health model, the curve would simply move to the right by an amount roughly equal to the extension in average life expectancy.

A third alternative, halfway between these two, would involve the same extension of life expectancy but through interventions that occur throughout life. By assumption, the healthy middle-age years would not increase as much as in the longer-health model, but the process of decline would be slowed. I believe that this longer-decline model is the most likely of the three, because it could result from various medical interventions for a range of chronic and acute conditions. Such interventions would prevent collapse and death but would not restore complete health.

Animal studies suggest a fourth alternative. These studies show that specific genes control the rate at which organisms age by affecting the speed at which cells break down glucose and in the process produce oxidant damage that in turn produces aging. In roundworms, combined mutations in several genes can produce up to sixfold extensions of life span, while also conferring

13. I am indebted to Margaret Battin for framing the first three alternatives, in comments on a draft of this chapter; and to Andreas Reis for assistance in graphing them.

Figure 6-3. *Three Variations of the Slower-Clock Life Curve*

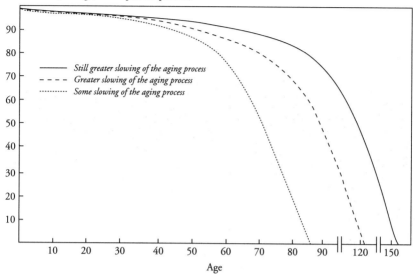

Health status, average, unisex person (percent)

protection against degenerative conditions. This slower-clock model would extend all life stages.[14] Clock slowing could extend various stages of life proportionally, with the same proportion of morbidity and resulting disability as now occurs, merely played out over more years. Alternatively, it could greatly extend youth and middle age, during which people could engage in productive activities, or an extended senescence, during which they would be dependent. If clock slowing were modest, the results might differ little from the three variations shown in figure 6-2, and the present curve would simply shift by an even percentage throughout its length (see figure 6-3). Given the dramatic changes in roundworms, clock slowing, if successfully applied from an early stage in development, could increase life span more than would the three models based on improvements in the capacity to repair various organs or to overcome specific diseases and disability. Were molecular manipulation to produce major changes in life expectancy, then the curves would move dramatically to the right.

14. If the evolutionary biologists are correct, the result would also be lower fecundity, but human reproduction already occurs at rates far below historic norms because improved life expectancy provides an incentive to limit reproduction artificially, which in turn leads to greater investment in each child, higher levels of development, and further increases in longevity.

Figure 6-4. *Two Variations of the One-Hoss Shay Model of Longer Health*

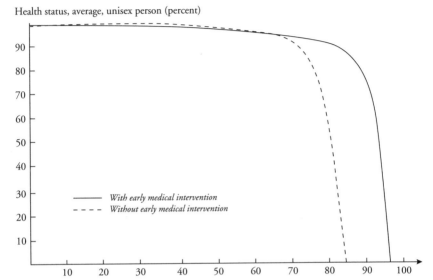

Health status, average, unisex person (percent)

Characteristic Variables

Besides the overall differences summed up in these four life curves, other variations could affect the desirability of particular interventions and the ethical acceptability of rules that allowed, aided, or prevented access to them. Suppose that the longer-health model results from techniques that work well for a number of years and then either cease being effective or are discontinued, whereupon death occurs promptly and without great pain or burden (see figure 6-4). Such an outcome would parallel the experience of the roughly 20 percent of the participants in the New England Centenarian Study who remain virtually illness free until nearly the moment of their death.[15] They resemble "the wonderful one-hoss shay" in Oliver Wendell Holmes's famous poem, which ran one hundred years and a day and then fell apart in a single day.[16] This model would also reflect the "compression of morbidity" pre-

15. Evert and others (2003). This group (32 percent of the male centenarians and 15 percent of the female centenarians) constitute the "escapers," while roughly two-fifths (44 percent of male subjects and 42 percent of female) are "delayers," in whom onset of age-associated illness did not occur until at least the age of eighty years, and the remainder (24 percent of males and 43 percent of females) are "survivors," who have a diagnosis of such illness before age eighty.
16. Holmes (1858).

dicted by James Fries, with the important difference that he views the human life span as fixed.[17] This state of affairs seems highly desirable as a means of conserving resources for health care and supporting people burdened by disabilities. Unfortunately, data give no indication that compression of morbidity is actually occurring.

Were such a technique to be developed, it would likely be widely adopted if it were at all affordable. Not only does it promise important social benefits, it would also grant people the sort of aging-and-dying scenario that many, perhaps most, people take as the ideal—a vigorous old age without lingering decline or a drawn-out dying process. One could imagine an intervention—say, a hormone pill that has to be taken regularly. The medicine eventually loses efficacy, and discontinuation produces rapid decline and death. In that situation, people could take the pill as long as it did good. The decline in effectiveness might be clinically noticeable to the patient or predicted presymptomatically through routine monitoring by a physician. At that point—or earlier, if the person wishes—the pill could be discontinued. Such passive euthanasia—or, as it is now usually termed, allowing to die—would permit people to direct the time and manner of their death. It would not require assistance from physicians or others, which remains controversial and, in the United States, has been formally legalized only in Oregon. The manner of death would be comparable to that of the 10–15 percent of patients on chronic hemodialysis who each year discontinue treatment, a decision that results promptly in a fairly gentle death.

The debate over federal funding of research using human embryonic stem cells highlights the hopes of some biologists that they are on the brink of creating "regenerative medicine" that "would draw on the rapidly expanding knowledge about . . . stem cells, and on genome-derived signals that influence cell behavior" as means to repair or replace damaged cells or organs.[18] Given how these repairs would occur, an appropriate name would be the auto shop model.[19] This name recognizes that cars ordinarily are not repaired until they malfunction, at which point the faulty part is frequently replaced. Regenerative medicine would thus extend beyond present-day organ transplantation both in the range of diseases treated and in the nature of the treatment (newly created cells and organs, rather than "used" ones).

17. Fries (1983).

18. Wade (2001), p. 119. These hopes include both the use of "excess" embryos from in-vitro fertilization clinics and cells created through somatic cell nuclear transfer (cloning).

19. See Okarma (2000), who envisions a therapeutic paradigm analogous to having a car come back from the repair shop with new parts.

Figure 6-5. *Two Variations of Longer-Decline Life Curve*

Health status average, unisex person (percent)

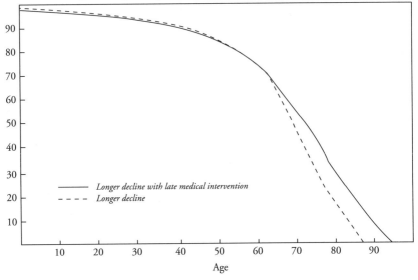

Because organ failure usually occurs late in life, this form of treatment would be reparative. It would do little to change earlier life experience through the normally healthy periods of youth and middle age. If successful, however, it could extend those periods and might indefinitely delay death, resulting in a variation on the longer-decline model (figure 6-5). If these interventions forestall imminent death but do as little as some current treatments—such as the artificial, implantable heart—the result might better be characterized as a version of the longer-dying model (figure 6-6). The major effect of such piecemeal replacement of organs, vital and otherwise, would be to change perceptions of aging. So many parts of a person might be replacements that it would be hard to know whether the person as a whole had aged or not—rather like antique cars the components of which have nearly all been replaced. At what point does the resulting car stop being an antique? Would it matter if the parts were new or salvaged from other vintage automobiles as, by analogy, the parts used in regenerative medicine would be?

Some Initial Conclusions about Consequences

These life curves give some specificity to the possible consequences of medical advances, but they provide no basis for balancing costs and benefits or

Figure 6-6. *Two Variations of the Longer-Dying Life Curve*

Health status average, unisex person (percent)

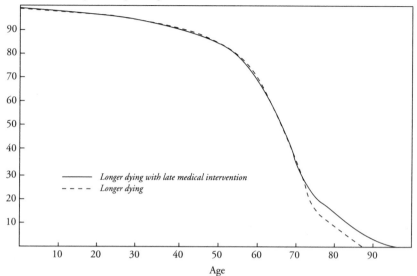

judging the distributional fairness of measures to produce those advances. To make wise choices about whether to spend money to develop and apply particular medical techniques that lengthen life, one needs to know the costs—both to develop and to employ the new techniques—and the outcomes. Outcomes include not only morbidity and mortality but also the effects on peoples' lives. For example, does increased life expectancy translate into an older and healthier work force or just a larger population of healthy or sick retirees?

Such information would be difficult and time consuming to develop. But the heart of the problem lies elsewhere—the decision is unlikely to be posed in such a fashion. U.S. health care policies often emerge from disconnected rather than systematic decisionmaking. Unless a formal longevity project—akin perhaps to the human genome project—were to be launched by the federal government, the occasion to think through the costs and benefits is unlikely to occur. Instead, individual researchers and, later on, individual physicians will offer individual patients various interventions. These will probably not be presented as a means of participating in a societal transformation or even of radically lengthening their own lives. Rather, these choices will be presented as a way to overcome some aspect of the aging process—such as a weak heart, a failing memory, an imminent cancer—that either affects patients' lives or that they fear may do so. Yet added together, individuals' choices may well transform the distribution of our population even when the individuals involved have had no occasion to weigh the consequences collectively.

Applying a utilitarian calculus in judging the ethics of various forms of life extension presents another problem. On utilitarian principles, longer health is clearly superior to longer decline, which in turn is superior to longer dying (see figure 6-2). This ordering holds because the burdens of illness are progressively greater as one moves from longer health to longer dying. Each indicates different levels of functioning, different qualities of existence for the average person. But life expectancy is the same in all three. A strong tradition sometimes called vitalism would hold the three life curves as equally valuable because every day of life is intrinsically as worthwhile as every other and infinitely better than the alternative (nonlife). This view has roots both in religious beliefs and in physicians' habits of mind. Some of the most heated ethical debates in recent years have occurred over evaluations of life-extending medical interventions between those who take a value-of-life approach and those who take a quality-of-life approach. The latter group would probably judge longer health superior to longer dying in terms of quality-adjusted life years. They would, in any event, judge the tail end of longer dying as undesirable. But such a conclusion would be anathema for the value-of-life group.

Evaluating the Means for Prolonging Life

Ethical evaluation of life-extending molecular medicine may center on the possible consequences, but means also need to be considered. Some debate may occur on whether the means are forbidden or illicit—for example, whether any steps to actively end life are permissible. But more attention will probably be devoted to the comparative desirability of various means and to their distributional effects. Controversy is likely over the relative desirability of interventions that produce reversible or temporary changes versus those that are permanent; interventions that are complex—and perhaps more burdensome—versus those that are simple—and therefore less burdensome; those that are expensive versus those that are not; and finally, interventions that are more easily subject to regulation, such as drugs and biologic agents that are licensed and sold, versus those that are hard to control, such as procedures that are created and applied by individual physicians (or even by nonprofessionals).

From a practical as well as an ethical standpoint, differences of these sorts may turn out to be very important. Take, for example, the ease with which life-extending interventions can be applied. If a treatment involves the transfer of an altered gene to most or all cells in the body, it may well be quite complicated. As a result it may not be widely available at an early date, either because physicians would be reluctant to use it often until its effects are carefully studied or because it would be regarded as a radical life alteration rather than just a medical intervention.

Level of Adoption of Intervention

A life-extending intervention that was used only on a few might greatly expand the maximum life span in those cases but have little effect on average life expectancy. How widely an intervention is used would determine the shape of the ethical discussion of two of the major issues: intergenerational equity (wider adoption produces a larger increase in the old-old population) and interpersonal equity (use by only a small percentage of the population raises questions of fair access). The more people who can afford a treatment, the more acceptable it is likely to be. Such an intervention is likely to raise few issues of interpersonal equity but many intergenerational ethical concerns.

How widely a powerful new technique is adopted shapes not only equity of access but also responsibility for the results. Suppose that an intervention, credited with extending life, is adopted by a few and that recipients are either willing experimental subjects or can pay for an intervention of proven efficacy. Might these circumstances not make any extension of life seem like something they had earned and any resulting advantage, financial or otherwise, seem more justified? An intervention that has to affect all organs to be successful—a gene transfer, for example—would raise additional complications. Such an intervention would probably require that it be applied prenatally through in-vitro fertilization and preimplantation genetic alteration. This mode of treatment would probably put limits on the frequency and speed of adoption. Use in the prenatal period, or even in childhood, would also necessarily delay for many years any rigorous evaluation of the extent to which the technique in question was actually safe and effective in extending human life.

Of course, once benefits from using an intervention become apparent, the desire for access may be driven by the sense that failure to use the technology may put one or one's children at a disadvantage (You'd be a fool not to do it!). The extent of the felt imperative to use an available innovation is, of course, influenced by the perceived benefits and risks as well as by cost. Ironically, arguments from equity may be self-reinforcing because they can affect demand by strengthening the impression that the intervention is desirable. As more people "want" the intervention, barriers to ready availability seem more inequitable.

Experimental Interventions

Whether an intervention has been proven effective or remains experimental raises two sets of issues. The first concerns predictability. The principal stated reason that health insurance plans deny coverage for experimental treatments is that they are too novel to be factored into actuarial calculations. Many promising new methods turn out not to be effective. Insurers do not feel obliged to pay for ineffectual interventions. Indeed, they may believe— often rightly—that they are thereby sparing their subscribers potentially harmful interventions. By the time that an intervention has become accepted therapeutically, insurers will ordinarily have had time to make the necessary actuarial projections and will face competitive and perhaps regulatory pressure to cover the new interventions. Insurers generally retain some discretion regarding interventions that are not central to a decent life or are of marginal medical value. They may classify such interventions—cosmetic surgery, for example—as a matter of life-style.

The second set of issues relates to the ethics of human experimentation. These issues have been a subject of public and professional scrutiny and of regulatory action for many decades. Any discussion of whether a technique to increase longevity is desirable must attend to the process by which it is developed and the risks that remain after formal research ends. As to the first, all novel medical interventions raise ethical issues. A large body of practical and theoretical literature addresses the ethics of research with human subjects. Many well-established—if not always flawlessly executed—processes and structures have evolved for overseeing such research and minimizing harm.[20]

The second concern relates to the risks inherent in medical interventions even after they have passed from experiment to clinical use. While all actions carry risk, danger commonly correlates with novelty. Some of the alterna-

20. In the view of some—for example, Kass (2003)—life extension is not a legitimate end of medicine. In that case, the usual justification for involving people in research and exposing them to risk would be absent, since neither relief of suffering, cure for disease, nor production of any scientific knowledge of value would be in prospect. Therefore those charged with protecting human research subjects and barring the gates of science against quackery should refuse to permit the research to proceed.

tives being proposed as means to achieve longer life seem especially novel and hence potentially risky because they aim at overcoming natural limits in biological functioning. For example, studies are under way to manipulate the production of the enzyme telomerase, which will preserve the length of telomeres and enable cells to go on dividing. But such manipulation requires caution because evolution seems to favor cell death to prevent mutations from being endlessly repeated. Indeed, cancer cells already experience the action of telomerase. Thus William Schwartz appends a warning to his hopeful predictions of a brighter, and longer-lived, future: "Techniques for stimulating telomerase activity may therefore maintain the integrity of telomere caps, prolong the life of cells, and extend the life of the organism, so long as uncontrolled, cancerous cell growth can be avoided."[21]

The risks in altering biology may not be immediately apparent. Therefore, even more than is usually the case, people using new life-extending techniques should be regarded as participants in a long-range study of the technique's effect and not simply as consumers of an approved intervention. Furthermore, a full account of the ethics of life extension must include justification for running the risks inherent in developing the means to extend life.

Ethics in an Aging Society

If life were greatly extended, would the resulting transformation of society pose difficult or intractable ethical problems or issues? I address four such concerns. First, would the resulting increase in the proportion of the population that is old (variously defined) distort the distribution of available resources? Second, would younger generations be unfairly burdened if longer life increased the number and life spans of dependent people? Third, would access to the technologies needed for extending life spans be equitable? Fourth, would such technology exert too much control over the dying process, thereby denying people a natural death?

Fair (and Wise) Distribution of Resources

Concerns about resource misallocation involve control over wealth and income as well as equity in health care expenditures. Increased longevity may have undesirable or unfortunate effects on the distribution of wealth (and the power that attaches to it), although these effects would be mitigated by

21. Schwartz (1998, p. 152).

premortem transfers to the extent that people believe that holding onto their wealth as they age is unwise for personal or economic reasons. In contrast, income support and payment for health care are usually accomplished through collective programs, both public (Medicare, for example) and private (employee fringe benefits, for example). Of these, health care costs have drawn particular attention, because the older the population the greater the cost of care to treat the sorts of acute and chronic health problems and disabilities that require medical, nursing, and related resources. These conditions increase with age, especially with the number of the old-old (today, those above age eighty).

The concerns about wasteful spending on the elderly emerged about thirty years ago. The source of these worries was less the growing elderly population than the increase in general health care costs. National health care expenditures nearly doubled as a percentage of gross domestic product, from 5.3 percent to 10.5 percent, between 1960 and 1982.[22] After some slowdown during the late 1990s, rapid cost increases resumed, because the forces pushing up expenditures—the development and adoption of new technologies that lead to more intensive treatment—show no sign of abating.

Although population aging contributes little to such inflation, considerable attention has been devoted to the large medical expenditures that elderly patients incur in their final few months of life. Large expenditures on those near death have led some people to question whether these resources could be more productively and fairly used for other patients. A study by James Lubitz and Ronald Prihoda shows that the 5.9 percent of Medicare beneficiaries who died in 1978 accounted for 27.9 percent of Medicare expenditures.[23] Moreover, Victor Fuchs points out that the high medical expenses of such patients are the principal reason that the medical expenditures of the elderly rise with age (though this calculation leaves out nursing home spending not covered by Medicare, which is also greater the older the population).[24] Others question the efficacy of such care as well as its cost.[25] Certainly, if patients derive no benefit from treatment or reject the care—directly or through an agent—treatment would be inappropriate, and spending money on it would be wrong.

If these conditions are not satisfied, the ethical picture is more complex.[26] Justice would not be served by allocating health care resources equally,

22. Scitovsky and Capron (1986).
23. Lubitz and Prihoda (1984).
24. Fuchs (1984).
25. Ginzberg (1984).
26. Scitovsky and Capron (1986).

because that policy would waste care on the healthy and provide too little care to the very sick. Nor would allocation by need be defensible; that rule would almost certainly result in excessive health care spending, because *need* can be confused with *want*. If equitable access to health care is what *just allocation* means, then everyone should have access to adequate care without imposing undue burdens on anyone in obtaining that care.[27] To give *adequate care* operational meaning, society must agree on what resources are available for this purpose. One means of determining the level and type of services that would constitute adequacy is the level and type of services purchased by people with good access to care, though such a consensus must take into account that much of the allocation of health care dollars occurs outside the market setting and that, in any case, even when health care is purchased by patients, the market for health care does not operate like normal markets. In this context, *need* is a comparative rather than absolute measure, and *adequate care* encompasses the ability of interventions to relieve pain and reverse lethal or crippling conditions. Whatever the formula, the greater need of the elderly for medical care provides a strong justification for allocating funds for their care.

Even with these qualifications, a utilitarian case can be made against devoting as much health care to the elderly as now occurs because current spending patterns fail to maximize the net benefit from the use of the resources. Jerry Avorn argues, however, that concerns about justice counter certain forms of utilitarian analysis in which any beneficial effect in a young person is valued more highly than the same effect in an elderly person, because the former will presumably enjoy the benefit for a longer period.[28] There is an even more serious barrier to using utilitarian analysis to justify the denial of treatment for dying patients. It is easy to look back and measure how much care was given at what dates to decedents, but it is impossible to predict which of a group of sick patients will die, say, six to twelve months in the future or, indeed, who will die by the succeeding day. Of those patients on whom most was spent, for whom the case of wasteful spending would seem to be most persuasive, more actually survived treatment than died.[29] Retrospective studies confuse patients who die with dying patients.

How many of those who died, one wonders, were recognized as being terminal patients, and how long before death was their status clear? Conversely, how many of the survivors were regarded as hopelessly ill by their physicians

27. President's Commission for the Study of Ethical Problems in Medicine and Biomedical and Behavioral Research (1983).

28. Avorn (1984).

29. Lubitz and Prihoda (1984).

but surprised them by recovering? One has to be cautious, therefore, not to equate the high medical costs at the end of life with the high costs of terminal care.[30]

While data do not show that health care resources are being wasted on old, dying patients, the study by Lubitz and Prihoda does foster concern that health care spending for the elderly is both unjustified and too high.[31] This concern, in turn, has stimulated philosophical inquiry on whether social spending, particularly for health care services, is unfair in generational terms and, in particular, whether limits should be placed on the use of all (or public) resources to this end.

Intergenerational Equity

On the face of it, the provision of extensive health services to the elderly does not serve the good that some theorists have argued health care is meant to advance—the opportunity to achieve all of one's other life goals.[32] On this rationale, resources would always be preferentially applied to the care of younger people, because they have more years to pursue their goals and, conversely, have had fewer opportunities already to do so. For such reasons, Daniel Callahan argues that limits should be set on what treatments are provided to patients after a certain age, at least through publicly supported programs.[33] After a person has lived out a natural life span, which Callahan suggests occurs by the late seventies or early eighties, medical care should no longer be oriented to resisting death but to the relief of suffering.

Norman Daniels reaches a somewhat different conclusion about care that supports but does not cure and that, hence, does little to advance the goal of opportunity.[34] He frames the question of justice between generations—in the sense of the competition for resources between children, working-age adults, and old retirees—as a problem to be examined in longitudinal terms. The question is not, he insists, one of the fairness of a particular allocation of funds (Medicare, Social Security) to the people who happen to be old today—that is, the members of a particular birth cohort. Rather, fairness

---

30. Scitovsky and Capron (1986, p. 70).

31. Lubitz and Prihoda (1984).

32. Daniels (1985, p. 104), defines the "fair equality of opportunity" that is promoted by meeting health care needs as helping to "guarantee individuals a fair chance to enjoy the normal opportunity range for their society."

33. Callahan (1987). It is apparent that, beyond the waste involved, Callahan regards many situations in which life-prolonging treatment is used as vain attempts to cling to life.

34. Daniels (1988).

should be measured by a "life-span approach," which aims for prudent allocation of resources among various stages of the life cycle of each person. Daniels thus asks whether public and private policies ensure that adequate resources are shifted from life stages in which they are not needed to life stages in which they are needed. Policies that do so through incentives to save and taxes to redistribute income encourage prudent behavior.

Daniels's concerns about the savings rate and the level of transfer payments are not central to an ethical evaluation of the issues raised by medical technologies that extend life. But one of his concerns—stability over time— is central. Shifting income from today's workers to today's retirees can be just only if today's workers have a fair chance of becoming tomorrow's retirees and if the benefits they will receive will be comparable to those provided for today's retirees. When there is reason to doubt that this will be the case, an injustice may arise.

In recent years, the concern over unfairness has centered on the impending retirement of the baby boomers. The security-over-time facet of Daniels's prudential life-span account dictates that an adequate reserve should be accumulated in the Social Security and Medicare systems to ensure that this large cohort receives retirement and health benefits comparable to that now provided, without imposing undue burdens on the then-working-age population. Failure to do so would be unjust either to the old in that generation (because benefits would have to be cut back) or to workers paying into the system (because their contributions would have to rise). While analysts— and politicians—disagree about the extent to which these conditions are being met, as well as about the appropriate and necessary steps to meet them, it is hard to escape the sense that failure to do so would be unfair.

If longevity were to increase gradually, gradual adjustments could deal with these problems. Modest reductions in Social Security benefits or increases in the rate of contributions, similar to those that would suffice to restore financial balance to Social Security as the baby boomers retire, could be made. Conversely, were increases in longevity to be rapid or discontinuous, large changes might be necessary. The resulting problem can be looked at from two vantage points.

The first is that of this newly long-lived group of elderly persons. For example, what would be a just way of treating their Social Security benefits? One approach might be to hold constant the expected present value of total lifetime benefits. Such a policy would require a later age of eligibility, lower annual payments, or some combination of the two. The difficulty with this view is that it treats Social Security like a savings account into which each worker has put a certain amount of money. In this version, it is appropriate for each worker to get back after retirement roughly what he or she has contributed, plus interest. Yet this is not the premise—much less the actual operating method—of the Social Security system. Instead, it is funded by current contributions, set to cover benefits for current retirees and partial, but much less than actuarially complete, reserves. Furthermore, changing Social Security because of a dramatic increase in longevity would also be unfair to the extent that access to the means for life extension are unequally distributed. That people who die young receive little or nothing from Social Security while other people collect benefits for decades is hardly the most lamentable aspect of the early deaths of the former group; in any case, any unfairness comes not from singling them out but from an inherent feature of insurance. In contrast, cutting back annual benefits because retirees are expected to live much longer would amount to attempting to achieve intergenerational equity by creating an interpersonal inequity to those who have not been able to have their lives lengthened by the new medical technology.

The second vantage point for deciding whether it would be right to reduce benefits paid to retirees or to increase current workers' Social Security taxes in order maintain benefits is from the viewpoint of the overall distribution of burdens and benefits in society. Would an increase in the proportion of resources allocated to the elderly—for example, by increasing taxes to pay the Social Security costs of the longer-lived retirees—be consistent with John Rawls's difference principle? If the least advantaged in society are not retirees, with their newly lengthened lives, but rather other groups, such as children of the working poor, then raising taxes to maintain benefits for the elderly would not meet this principle.

Once the population distribution stabilizes, there seems nothing inherently unjust if a society with many old members devotes more resources to supporting and providing health care to this group than does a population with fewer elderly. But for such an arrangement to be just, it requires institutions to allocate the burden fairly and to translate the problem of intergenerational justice to one of prudent planning for an expected life span. I believe that an essential precondition for such justice is that, to the extent feasible, those with increased life expectancies work—and contribute to the Social Security system—for a proportionately longer period of time. This precondition would obviously be much easier to meet if the pattern of longer lives is one of longer health (see figure 6-2) or, even better, its one-hoss-shay variant, longer health with early intervention (figure 6-4), than if patterns of longer dying and longer decline hold true (figure 6-2). If institutions have failed to act with sufficient prudence in light of the needs of the elderly population, then the justice of taking more resources from others in society could become a legitimate issue, especially regarding medical coverage.[35] Spending for medical care, in particular, may become almost infinitely expandable, while not achieving results that are worthwhile to patients.

The Burdens on the Younger Generation

I have thus far addressed concerns about fairness of the distribution of resources among groups in society. Another related issue deserves attention—namely, the ways the burdens of caring for the elderly are borne. A great deal of care of the elderly—as well as of other impaired members of society—falls on families and, within families, on women.[36] Whether this problem would be worse if longevity increases depends largely on what the resulting life curves look like. Lives burdened by protracted decline and dying would impose additional burdens on families—in particular, on wives, daughters, and daughters-in-law. The longer-health scenarios would delay, but not increase, the amount of dependence. The clock-slowing scenario (see figure 6-3 and also the longer-health curve in figure 6-2) might actually reduce the burden of care. Perhaps the most difficult situation is that of caregivers who are responsible for both their children and their parents at roughly the same time. This double burden is intensified for women who work outside the home. This situation not only increases the demands on their time but often leads them to postpone reproduction. The result has been a "sandwich generation" of people (especially women), now in their late thirties to early fifties, with both young children and old parents. If dependency is delayed more than reproduction as lives grow longer, and particularly if the duration of old-age dependence diminishes, the likelihood that prime-age adults—disproportionately women—have to care simultaneously for children and parents would be reduced.

What conclusions can be drawn about intergenerational equity? Assuming that a longevity increase does not occur abruptly, no inherent unfairness arises from a larger proportion of society being elderly. The issue would be whether social institutions promote prudent allocation of lifetime spending across all life stages, not whether those who happen to be young at any particular moment owe a particular level of support to those who are old. On Rawlsian principles one would qualify this conclusion: Shifting support from workers and their families to retirees would not be defensible if the

35. The obligation to engage in longer working lives might, to be either reasonable or fair, be said to generate a social obligation to provide means for people to "renew" themselves through opportunities for midlife education and shifting to a second or third career.
36. World Health Organization (2002).

former as a group are markedly worse off than the latter in terms of being able to fulfill their life opportunities. This constraint should receive serious attention, as the relevant social institutions are not neutral machines but facets of a political process in which the elderly may well exercise disproportionate power because of their numbers, accumulated wealth, and high voter turnout. If they exercise their power selfishly—not in line with Daniels's prudent life-span account but in service of the interests of those who happen at that moment to be old—then intergenerational concerns should not be brushed aside. Moreover, in such circumstances, medical developments that lengthen life and increase the number of elderly would themselves seem unjustifiable because they would only increase the inequities.

Equitable Access to the Technologies of Longer Life

If intergenerational problems do not loom large, what of interpersonal inequities? The question arises with respect to all medical innovations as they move from experiment to accepted practice. At what point do they become standard treatment that a competent physician should offer and that an adequate payment system would cover for all patients for whom the intervention would be beneficial? That there is no clear answer to this question, given the fractured nature of the American health care "system," is hardly surprising. No transparent formula exists for deciding when a new intervention should be guaranteed and when it may remain just an option for those who can afford to pay for it on their own. In many cases, private insurers wait for Medicare to act. Sometimes private health plans act before federal decision-makers. Some new treatments, such as in-vitro fertilization and other technology to assist reproduction, remain in limbo for years, with some insurers providing coverage and others refusing to do so, at least until forced by regulation or legislation.

To the extent that life-extending technologies are also of value in treating acutely ill patients, such technologies will likely be made readily available by physicians and reimbursed by public and private medical coverage. The harder cases involve the most interesting technologies, namely those that would be used for people who are healthy, not sick, and that would aim not at a single, defined disorder but at slowing or stopping normal aging. In this respect, technologies that aim at lengthening human life—rather than at curing a particular disease, with greater longevity being merely a side effect—resemble many forms of assisted reproduction, which insurers have been slow to include in health care coverage. Both are novel. Neither is a service that everyone wants or needs. Both are likely to be expensive. And both aim to correct something that can be regarded as a part of a normal life pattern, not a disorder for which medical care is mandated.

Would it be an instance of interpersonal injustice if a life-extending intervention were expensive, effective, and safe but available only to those who can pay for it with their own resources (that is, not covered by public or private health insurance)? Or would the incomplete availability of such an intervention be comparable to that of cosmetic surgery to erase the signs of aging? To answer this question, we must remember what is special about health care—that is, what makes its equitable availability a matter of social obligation in a just society. Access must be equitable (not equal) because needs and preferences differ. And it is not enough that a person need a particular treatment, in the sense that the treatment is a safe and effective response to a patient's condition, because both need and condition are malleable concepts that depend on the wishes and whims of patients and the ingenuity and values of physicians.

The daunting task is to move from what Daniel Callahan calls "expansive and open-ended generalities about health and individual need" to decisions about what medical interventions for what conditions must be included in any fair system.[37] Norman Daniels and Callahan argue that access to a treatment must be ensured when it is necessary—or at least appropriate in cost-effectiveness terms—to restore normal functioning for someone in like circumstances and thereby to enable that person to have a fair opportunity to enjoy and engage in his or her life pursuits.[38] Such principles were developed both to support an ethical claim to at least a basic, adequate level of care (Daniels) and to provide a rationale for limiting care in circumstances in which it does not meet the defined objective (Callahan). It is not surprising, however, that biomedical developments that could transform a central feature of normal function—namely, aging and death within an average life span of seventy to ninety years—confound these principles. Callahan notes that, in deciding what ought to count as normal, people should resist the implications of the modernizing view of old age, which would push back its frontier and subject it to no fixed standards of normal. Otherwise, that ideology combined with technological progress "could make Daniels's idea of a normal opportunity range for the elderly as an age group and my concept of a life-

37. Callahan (1990, p. 44).
38. Daniels (1985, pp. 26 ff). Drawing on Rawls's first principle, Daniels argues that, just as fair equality of opportunity can be impeded by features of the social system (such as the social class into which one is born or discriminatory practices in the labor market), it is also blocked when "diseases and disabilities" cause departures from "normal species functioning" that prevent an individual from pursuing the range of life plans that would otherwise be open to someone with his or her talents and skills.

span opportunity range for individuals intractable and useless as a standard for fair allocation among the generations."[39]

This problem is presented in an even more intractable form regarding interpersonal equity. If *normal* is used in a statistical sense, as Daniels suggests, then once life-extending technology has come into general use; failure to make it available to everyone, even those who cannot afford it, would be unfair. To avoid this problem, Callahan thinks that *normal* "should instead be given a normative meaning; that is, what counts as morally and socially adequate and generally acceptable."[40] Yet the standard of a natural life span, which is based on passing through certain important biographical stages that together make up a whole life, is itself subject to expansion even within the rationale Callahan provides. There is no reason to say that a person who was born in 1875 and lived to the point of average life expectancy did not live a natural life span in the biographical sense employed by Callahan. If a hundred years hence average life expectancy were 150 years for adults, there is every reason to think that appropriate adjustments would have been made in people's thinking about what constitutes each of the life stages, with a concomitant lengthening of the natural life span.

Once life-extending methods are widely adopted, being unable to obtain them would seem to be unfair discrimination. In Daniels's terms, as normal causes of death in old age become avoidable through routine medical intervention, these conditions would change status. They would become unacceptable interference with equality of opportunity, because the contours of normal species functioning would now be altered to encompass many more years. Indeed, the problem is not only that the norm of what is natural changes but also that longer life is already seen as having value, since old age permits activities that were incomplete to be finished and new interests to be cultivated. Appeals to a natural life span or normal opportunities simply fall apart as life expectancy expands. The tolerability of death in Callahan's terms is always relative to cultural expectations. Thus whether the health care system generates interpersonal justice regarding access to new life-extending technologies will depend upon the fairness of the processes used to detect when norms and expectations have shifted sufficiently to make barriers to equitable care unacceptable.

Intervention and Dying

Before moving from the societal level to examine the effects of greater longevity on individuals, we should note an ethical concern that straddles these two

39. Callahan (1987, pp. 136–37).
40. Callahan (1987, pp. 136–37).

realms—the potential connection between life-extending interventions and euthanasia. At first blush, the two seem to be opposites. Life-extending technologies aim to prolong life. Euthanasia ends it. But the former may feed the latter.

Current support for tolerating and even legalizing physician-assisted suicide and euthanasia reflects a popular idea that people should be able to control the circumstances of their deaths. It also grows out of distress that people feel when they contemplate others' protracted decline and dying, loss of dignity, and even loss of the ability to control decisions about their medical care. Life-extending interventions support people's sense of control and may also allow them to survive to a point at which they become aware of the accumulated limitations.

Proponents of allowing euthanasia point to patients sustained by medical interventions—such as kidney dialysis, artificial respirators, vasopressors, and antibiotics—who choose to die by declining further treatment. They argue that if such passive euthanasia—or as is usually said today, "allowing to die"—is permitted, then active euthanasia and assisted suicide should be permitted too. It is by now generally recognized that there is no moral, or legal, difference between stopping a particular intervention and not starting it in the first place. One reason for rejecting this difference is practical. Were it permissible to decline to initiate life-prolonging treatments but not to stop them once begun, physicians would be loath to offer—and patients and their families would be loath to accept—potentially life-prolonging therapy. Since "Don't Start" and "Stop" are treated as basically equivalent, many trials of therapy are begun on the slim, but still worthy, chance that they might succeed. All parties know that if the treatments fail they can be halted. Yet many of the most powerful methods that may be found to extend life—particularly those that involve genetic manipulation—cannot be halted because they are incorporated into the body. Thus patients offered such treatments may be loath to accept them unless they can be assured that should the result prove unacceptable they will be able to get free of their situation. Since passive cessation of treatment would not have the effect it has for the patient on a respirator, the only way to provide the relevant assurance would be to allow active termination of life, either through assisted suicide or euthanasia.

A Prolonged Life

The substantial increases in longevity that occurred gradually over the last century have not excited public or professional criticism because they were regarded as the fortunate secondary effects of efforts to prevent or cure specific diseases and to relieve suffering. Biomedical entrepreneurs go beyond the principle of adding life to our years rather than years to our life. That changes if biomedical entrepreneurs embark on a "quest to reverse time's toll."[41] But even as this ambition is asserted, critics are questioning whether increasing life expectancy is an appropriate goal of medicine. In this view, scientists' visions of a much longer life span represent not fitting hopes for humankind but rather a snare for the vain or the unwary. Several reasons are advanced for concluding that greater longevity ought not be regarded as an unqualified good. One is that the search for immortality is a pagan quest driven by the "essentially amoral and mindless dynamic of the technological imperative joined to an ignoble fear of death."[42] Others argue that life extension is an inappropriate goal for medicine and that a lengthening of life violates the natural order and the ethical dictates that derive therefrom.

These grounds for rejecting increased longevity share a sense that the current life span is acceptable and that efforts to lengthen it are wrong because they are, in effect, part of a larger project of seeking perfection and, specifically, immortality. Needless to say, many in biomedicine who work to find means of curing lethal diseases would not recognize their work in this description. Even some scientists working explicitly to slow the aging process would deny it. Yet simple denial does not refute the critics. The very innocence of the scientists—their claim not to be aiming for immortality but merely for overcoming lethal conditions—would, if believed, open them to the criticism that they are acting amorally and mindlessly, with their eyes only on technological advance. Further, the goals for extending the life span know no bounds. One researcher who studies aging in nematodes has already speculated about a human life span of 350 years.[43] If longevity is altered by X years now, why not by $X + Y$ years tomorrow, and so forth? There is no limit inherent in the process of lengthening life, so the end point would be virtual immortality.

Intolerable Consequences: Distracting the Soul

At the root of some objections is the worry that medicine, by trying to lengthen human beings' time on this earth, is enticing them with a false

41. Holden (2002).

42. Richard J. Neuhaus, at a University of Pennsylvania conference on the consequences of scientific control over life span, quoted in Nicholas Wade, "Arguments over Life and the Need for Death," *New York Times*, March 7, 2000, p. F4.

43. Tom Johnson, quoted in Holden (2002, p. 1033).

idol and keeping them from engaging in other essential tasks. Critics like Leon Kass not only reject the enterprise but are also convinced it is a perversion of the true goals of medicine. For these critics, the search for immortality—or at least for a very long youth—is at war with our heritage of aging, decay, and death. Seen thus, efforts to extend life span are but pathetic attempts to rewrite our history: Made in God's image, then, as punishment for eating from the tree of knowledge, cast out of the Garden lest we eat from the tree of life and become immortal, we long to overturn our God-given lot.

The critics' objection to efforts to prolong life span seems in part like the counsel one would express to a friend (or a psychiatric patient!) who is fixated on some unobtainable goal and fails to attend to important responsibilities. "It is not simply that our mortality as a whole makes it difficult for us to hold on to the pleasures of life," writes Callahan. "The very limited nature of those pleasures even at their very best—frustratingly bittersweet and evanescent— leads us to long for more."[44] But gaining more years will not satisfy that longing. According to Kass, "Once we acknowledge and accept our finitude, we can concern ourselves with living well, and care first and most for the *well-being* of our souls, and not so much for their mere existence. . . . To covet a prolonged life span for ourselves is both a sign and a cause of our failure to open ourselves to . . . any higher . . . purpose."[45]

However telling this almost pastoral concern may be when directed toward a particular person's vain grasping for "a little more," it is less clear that it provides a valid objection to the enterprise of life extension as a matter either of logic or of psychology. As to the former, were the objection valid, would it not follow that acts to shorten life (or at the very least to forgo interventions that would lengthen life) would be desirable because they would accelerate the virtues that flow from our mortality? As to the latter, if people routinely lived to be 100 or 120 rather than 70 or 80, why could they not still come in due course—just a little later—to the important work of a full human life, the taking up of the role and responsibilities of being an elder for one's family and community, which Callahan worries will be lost in the search for "prolongevity," or the aspiration for "some condition, some state, some goal toward which our earthly activities are directed" but that "cannot be attained during earthly life," as Kass puts it?[46]

44. Callahan (1987, p. 75).
45. Kass (1985, pp. 314, 316; emphasis in original).
46. Kass (1985, p. 312). Callahan (1987, p. 74) defines "prolongevity" as the alleged medical goal of "an indefinite extension of life."

Dangerous Means: Biological Objections

Even if a lengthening of life could be consistent with an acceptance of finitude rather than an expression of a longing for immortality, is it somehow
at odds with our biological destiny? Two concerns have been raised. The first
involves the simple danger of a longer life. Because evolution favors reproductive fitness, "there was no need to develop robust quality-control mechanisms allowing you to live beyond reproduction."[47] Thus rather than being
consistent with the usual goals of medicine, efforts to extend life could actually increase illness and suffering, because the longer people live the more
likely they will get sick. Yet this concern merely restates the goal of life extension: to find those means for a longer life that some members of our species
already possess and then to share those means with the rest of us. There are,
after all, some people who live very long lives and remain alert, vigorous, and
engaged right up to the end. Studies of centenarians strongly suggest that
genes—and not just "good living"—play some role in living long and
healthy lives.[48] Perhaps evolution did reward the genes these people happen
to possess. Perhaps also their long-lived forebears were available to supply
their children, grandchildren, and great-grandchildren the support and
guidance that comes with age and experience. For such benefits to accrue,
people of such lineage needed not merely to live long but to do so relatively
free of the burdens of degenerative diseases that would have made them a
drain on their progeny and thereby reduced the likelihood that their genes
would make it into future generations. If longevity is achieved by giving
everyone the benefit of such genes, perhaps the fear that living longer
inevitably means living worse might not be fulfilled.

Nonetheless, reply the critics, even when the lives of the old are not burdensome for them, they are inherently a burden on the rest of humanity.
The cycle of birth, maturation, procreation, and death has a wisdom, "the
eternally renewed promise," in the words of Hans Jonas, "of the freshness,
immediacy, and eagerness of youth."[49] He may well be right that "the greater
accumulation of prolonged experience" is no substitute for "the unique priv-
ilege of seeing the world for the first time and with new eyes . . . the wonder
which, according to Plato, is the beginning of philosophy." Yet beyond hop-
ing that such wonder is not the sole province of youth, I cannot see why
these two aspects of life—experience and discovery—are at war. If the question presented by the scientific enterprise were whether to adopt measures

47. George Martin of the University of Washington, quoted in Holden (2002, p. 1032).
48. Perls and Terry (2003).
49. Jonas (1984, p. 19).

that truly, rather than metaphorically, achieve immortality, then Jonas's concern would be more telling: In a world populated by people who live forever, there will be not only little room for new experience but also little space for new people. But in a world of (relative) plenty, can there not be a place both for long-lived, albeit not immortal, seniors and also new and eager juniors? It thus seems doubtful that, within reasonable limits, efforts to add years to human life would be so inconsistent with the species' natural functioning that they would amount to inadmissible means on either utilitarian or deontological grounds.

Illegitimate Ends: The Pursuit of Perfection

In the view of Leon Kass, the most prominent critic of the search for means to lengthen life, we should probably never have gotten to the questions of means and consequences because the goal itself is illegitimate.[50] Kass believes that the end of medicine is simply health, not the prolongation of life or even the prevention of death. He will have none of the modern view of health as a value or as a state of social and spiritual well-being. Rather, the goal of medicine is the "well-working of the organism as a whole."[51] The common view is that medicine has three aims: to treat illness (and more recently to preserve health), to relieve suffering, and to prevent death. To square his position with that view, Kass argues that aging and mortality are natural and inescapable parts of being human. Yet if Daniel Callahan's "natural life span" and Norman Daniels's "normal species functioning" do not work as devices to resolve questions of interpersonal equity in a world of greatly prolonged lives, then basing the good on that which is "natural" presents an even more severe problem when the changes one opposes could alter what is experienced as a natural life.

Thus a first and easy objection to critiques based on current experience is that they amount to nothing more than objections to change as such. Kass dismisses the suggestion that his position rests on rejecting all of medicine as unnatural. Yet if medical artifice produces a future world populated by millions of people who live as long as Jeanne Calment, the French woman who was 122 when she died in 1997, might not the residents of that world regard their longevity as being as natural as we regard ours? Still, rejection of the longevity project cannot be dismissed as a mere failure of imagination. To say that we might come to accept a different view of what it means to be

50. Kass (1985, p. 169).
51. Kass (1985, p. 174).

human is no comfort if the warm bath in which we think we are sitting is actually a cannibal's soup pot.

The question, then, is, Where is the science of life extension taking us? Fears voiced about our posthuman future are not fed alone by the work on longevity but arise also from the many ways in which scientists seem to be seizing control over human life.[52] As critics like Kass acknowledge, the intentions are typically beneficent: to restore function or to remedy innate human deficits and so forth. But the critics perceive a problem, nonetheless, and that is the ambition to achieve a *"full* escape from the grip of our own nature" in the drive to render people "better than well."[53] The problem is not simply one of hubris, of not having the wisdom to choose wisely, though that is part of the problem. In Kass's view, the problem is the very desire to escape what is inescapably human and to seek instead to be endowed with superhuman strength, beauty, and intelligence.

If research on life extension amounts to a quest for "ageless bodies," then Kass's concerns bear—and I suspect will receive—further attention.[54] A world in which hundred-year-olds are indistinguishable from thirty-year-olds is one that hardly needs the latter—and is one in which the transfer of knowledge and authority between generations would not happen without a struggle. It would also be, as Kass argues, a world with none of the preparation for, or acceptance of, death that is engendered by the natural process of decline. But if the result of the new technologies of life prolongation is not so much everyone living in full vigor until the day they die but rather lives encumbered by added years of decline and dying, Kass may have gotten the problem exactly backward.

52. The term *posthuman future* comes from Fukuyama (2002) and has been picked up by critics from the left as well as the right. See, for example, McKibben (2003).

53. The first quotation is from Kass (2003, p. 10; emphasis in original). The second quotation is from the title of Elliott (2003).

54. Kass (2003) characterizes developments that would lengthen life as part of a search for human "perfection," along with the use of cloning and genetic engineering to produce children. While I share many of his concerns about the reproductive technologies, I am not convinced that life-lengthening interventions belong in the same category. Techniques that produce longer life spans (not truly "ageless bodies," much less true immortality) do not aim to perfect human beings; unlike cloning, the differences they produce are quantitative rather than qualitative.

COMMENT
Margaret P. Battin

The prospect of extra-long life spawns a bloom of ethical issues, among them how to achieve intergenerational equity; how to balance health care entitlements with rising costs for the elderly; how to divide years of life between work and retirement; how to assign the responsibilities of young family members for care of the old; and how to answer philosophical questions about the meaning of life, the "naturalness" of the human life span, and the wisdom of "tampering" with nature. The chapters in this volume, especially Alex Capron's, touch on all these issues and in doing so share a common assumption: If extra-long life becomes possible, people will actually live it. Of all the authors in this volume, Capron comes closest to identifying this assumption explicitly.

This assumption is central not only to the ethical issues that Capron examines but also (and of particular importance in this volume) to economic and social policy forecasts. Yet this assumption is valid only under unlikely scenarios of how the human life span might come to be extra long; it is clearly faulty under other scenarios, and it is weak under the most plausible scenarios, the very ones we should be using in such forecasts.

Three Scenarios of Extra-Long Life

At least three scenarios of extra-long life can be imagined for future generations proximate to our own. In the most optimistic of these scenarios, the *longer-health scenario*, people will normally live substantially longer and will be in relatively good health until just before their death. The duration of healthy adult years increases, but the period of debility before death will not increase and may shorten. In the most pessimistic scenario, the *longer-dying scenario*, most or all of the extension of the human life span will consist in physical disintegration and severe debility. What is now the unfortunate plight of some would become normal for most: a protracted preterminal and terminal period. Intermediate between these two scenarios is the *longer-decline scenario*, in which an increase in longevity will involve an extended descent from good health to death, during which physical and mental deterioration is spread out over a sustained period of time.

Capron addresses the ethical issue that confronts our own generation: whether to pursue medical techniques that would foreseeably lengthen the human life span. Are such efforts wise? That is, would benefits exceed costs, and would the outcome be distributively just? The answers hinge on the central assumption above, and it is thus imperative that we explore this assumption in the light of well-founded projections about the future.

Means of Extending the Human Life Span

Capron and the other authors in this volume explore the many ways by which the human life span might be expanded. Improved disease prevention; life-style regulation; dietary matching of individual needs with available foodstuffs; understanding of human physiology and the way it is affected by exercise, stress, and caloric intake; and better management of depression and mental illness might all contribute to longer life. So might improved supportive care, including better management of cardiac dysfunction, respiratory support techniques, management of electrolyte imbalances, and repair of nervous system function. Specific advances in disease prevention and treatment can be anticipated, and some are already on their way, including improved regulation of sugar metabolism and the prevention of diabetes, better control of blood pressure, vaccines for cancer, more precise targeting of therapeutic drug regimens, and improved imaging in diagnostics and treatment.

The point so easily ignored is this: Not all ways of extending the life span point toward the same outcome scenario. Some—improved disease prevention, better diet, and better understanding of exercise, stress, and mental illness—herald the scenario of longer health. On the other hand, if longer life is realized through medical techniques that are invasive or that use drugs with serious side effects, longer dying may be the outcome. The implications of some potential technologies are unclear: Stem-cell-farmed replacement organs, for example, could lead either to longer health (if the function of multiple interactive organ systems is improved by the replacement of one or more parts) or to longer dying (if repeated surgeries required to replace various failing organs contribute to an overall decline in health).

Advances in genetics offer additional routes to extended life spans but may also point to different outcomes. Genetic diagnosis—beginning with carrier screening before conception, continuing with prenatal diagnosis and early childhood examination, and extending to early-adult diagnosis—will make it possible to identify and avoid genetic traits that lead to early death. For some conditions this promise has been realized. The incidence of Tay-Sachs disease, a condition that causes death in early childhood, has already been reduced among Ashkenazi Jews to below the rate for the general population. Genes have also been identified for cystic fibrosis, breast cancer, and early-onset Alzheimer's disease. Deselection of such disease genes, although it would reduce mortality among the young and thus lengthen life expectancy of populations as a whole, does not affect end-of-life scenarios for those who reach adulthood. Other genetic interventions, however, might be used to favor genes predisposing for longevity; or for reduced susceptibility to environmental toxins; or for avoiding life-threatening social behaviors; or for preventing aging-related telomere shortening.

The human life span is also sensitive to external factors (climate, air, soil, background radiation, and infectious disease). Many changes in these factors could decrease human longevity, but others could operate to extend it: for example, warming trends that made available a range of new foodstuffs or atmospheric changes that counteracted human-caused pollutants. Unlike at least initial developments in medicine or genetic technology, changes in these factors, if they occur, are likely to operate on a very large scale, and yet it is difficult to say whether they would herald longer health or longer dying.

What Will Future Generations Know?

People of proximate coming generations are likely to be reasonably conversant with their world, to have adequate information about their own health and health prospects, and to understand why their life expectancy has increased. They will also know what past human existence was like. Our successors will be at least as knowledgeable as we are about, for example, the processes of human psychology, the reasoning powers of the human mind, and characteristic human errors in reasoning, like the tendency to argue from anecdotal cases rather than base-rate information, to overemphasize recent evidence, and to use seemingly irrational discount rates. They will know how optimism embellishes perception of the future and how fear can infect their choices. In short, they will be in general moderately self-aware, reasonably rational creatures capable of making choices—sometimes good ones, sometimes not so good—about their lives.

Let us also imagine our successors as culturally literate, familiar with writings in history, literature, sociology, and theology that bear on issues about length of life. For example, they will have read Cicero's *On Old Age*. They will know the views of both Seneca, who supports suicide as the responsible act of the wise man, and Thomas Aquinas, who denounces suicide as the worst of sins. They will have read Jonathan Swift's account in *Gulliver's Travels* of the Struldbruggs, who were lucky enough to be immortal—or so Gulliver thought, until it turned out that immortality meant perpetual, unceasing decay. People in future generations—at least some of them—will also be philosophically sophisticated: For instance, they will know Bernard Williams's account of the Makropulos case and his reflections on "the tedium of immortality"; they will know Daniel Callahan's writings on the overuse of health care at the end of life; and they will understand Norman Daniels's Rawlsian reconstructions of justice in health care. They will have seen plays, films, and other works of past generations such as *Whose Life Is It, Anyway?* and *Soylent Green.* And they will have read plenty of trashy novels about treachery and stealth and evil physicians who make a mockery of death and dying. Of course, they will also have read accounts of triumph over illness, disability, aging, and the like. They will know the hopeful literature and the grimly realistic as well.

In short, they will know what we know and more. Thus, because we know at least part of what they know, we have some basis for predicting how they might behave when facing the prospect of extra-long life.

Questioning the Central Assumption

To restate the central assumption: If extra-long life becomes possible, people will actually live it. But it is possible that future generations will not, after all, live the "extra-long" part of their potentially extra-long lives. To see why, it is instructive to compare the different scenarios of possible extra-long life.

Suppose that longer life usually yields longer health. Under this scenario, neither the wisdom (in Capron's cost-benefit terms) nor the justice (in distributive terms) of extra-long life will be at issue. Added life will be a clear benefit. People not only will live longer but will also be able to work longer. They will thus not impose increased burdens on the young, either directly or through publicly supported pensions or health care programs. Although there will be many old people, most of them will be old only in number of years, not in health status. To be sure, the population structure will change, as family structure becomes more vertical, but this change will not mean added burdens for the younger generations.

If longer health is the scenario of the future, people can be predicted to choose to live extra-long lives, and no party or institution will try to keep them from doing so since there will be virtually no negative social impact. This scenario provides an answer to Capron's moral question, Should we pursue the techniques that will lengthen life? If those techniques promise longer health, the answer seems to be a resounding yes.

Suppose, however, that longer life usually takes the form of longer dying, that most people will face a protracted period of preterminal and terminal decline—say, an extra twenty or thirty years in a hospital wing or a nursing home or the back bedroom of an overburdened, resentful family member's house, reduced in physical and intellectual capacity, limited in activities of daily living, perhaps unable for extended periods to engage in social interaction or to recognize family members or to experience life's pleasures. The early and middle years of life might be much the same as they are for us now, but life would conclude with a far more extended period of senescence and medical dependency. The cost-benefit balance will be negative; issues of justice will be exacerbated as the many, many very old strain societal resources and consume ever greater shares of the health care pie. If this longer-dying scenario is the picture of the future, the answer to Capron's moral question about whether techniques for extending life expectancy should be developed seems to be a clear-cut no.

But suppose techniques for extending the human life span are developed anyway or that increases in longevity result from exogenous processes. What can we predict about whether these potentially extra-long lives will actually be lived? While it might seem that such a question can be answered only with sheer speculation, we already know how the present generation behaves in more limited versions of such situations, and we can assume that proximate future generations will have some of the same self-perceptions and cultural backgrounds and, hence, be likely to act in much the same way.

This leads us to expect that future generations will use some of the same mechanisms for avoiding overly prolonged life that the present generation does—and for the same reasons: to avoid suffering, indignity, loss of control, and pain. For example, among the mechanisms now used to avoid overly prolonged life in situations of terminal illness are living wills and durable powers of attorney for health care—two types of advance directive, legally recognized in virtually all states, that allow people to reject in advance certain life-prolonging treatments or to designate a surrogate with legal powers to act on their behalf. With both directives competent patients can decide, before they become incompetent, that their lives are not to be prolonged even though it is technically possible to do so. These instructions may direct the physician to issue a "do not resuscitate" (DNR) order; they may stipulate that specific treatments such as dialysis or the use of a respirator are to be withheld or withdrawn; or they may be used to accept pain control but refuse antibiotics, or accept antibiotics but refuse surgery, and so on. While advance directives are at times used to request rather than reject treatment, they are used primarily to curtail rather than extend life.

Pain control measures, especially opiates, are also often used in a way believed to hasten death, though there is some controversy about the pharmacology. Escalating doses of morphine, for example, are used under the principle of double effect to control pain, despite the foreseen but unintended possibility that they will eventually suppress respiration and bring about death. In 1997 the U.S. Supreme Court explicitly acknowledged the legality of this use of pain medication.[1] Although data are not as readily available on decisions about dying in the United States that involve the alleviation of symptoms with possible life-shortening effect, about 20 percent of deaths in the Netherlands occur in this way.[2] In the United States and elsewhere, terminal sedation is also sometimes used for patients in intractable pain: The patient is sedated into unconsciousness and artificial nutrition and hydration are withheld, with the result that the patient dies.[3]

Patients sometimes seek direct means of ending life. During the first five years after the legalization of physician-assisted suicide in Oregon, 129 people used this means of hastening their deaths.[4] A physician may provide a competent, terminally ill patient who has requested it, under legal safeguards, with a prescription for a lethal drug. In the Netherlands, where physician-assisted suicide and voluntary active euthanasia have long been legally tolerated and are now legal, an estimated 2.4 percent of annual deaths are attributable to voluntary active euthanasia provided by the physician at the request of the patient; 0.2 percent are attributable to physician-assisted suicide.[5] In the United States, a national study shows that a substantial proportion of physicians report that they receive requests for physician-assisted suicide and euthanasia and that about 6 percent have complied with such requests at least once.[6] Another study estimates that one in five physicians has received at least one request for assistance in helping a terminally ill patient die and that, despite the fact that doing so has not been legalized in any state except Oregon, between 3 percent and 18 percent of these physicians acceded to these requests.[7]

---

1. *Vacco* v. *Quill*, 521 U.S. 793, 117 S.Ct. 2293 (1997); *Washington* v. *Glucksberg*, 521 U.S. 702, 117 S.Ct. 2258 (1997); decided jointly.

2. van der Wal and others (2003), table 1.

3. Bernat, Gert, and Mogielnicki (1993).

4. Hedberg, Hopkins, and Kohn (2003).

5. Onwuteaka-Philipsen and others (2003).

6. Meier and others (1998).

7. Meier and others (2003), p. 1537.

To anticipate how many people in the future will fail to live as long as they can, one must also anticipate how they will be treated by others—that is, how often other parties will choose shorter lives for them. Contemporary medicine routinely includes DNR orders, the withholding or withdrawing of life-support equipment, the use of opiates under the principle of double effect, and both legal and clandestine assisted suicide and euthanasia. In some cases the patient is aware of and requests or accepts these practices, but in other cases the patient is incompetent, confused, not informed, or otherwise unaware of them, and decisions are made on the patient's behalf by others: family members, physicians, or designated surrogates. Thus some of these practices are voluntary on the part of the patient, some are nonvoluntary, and many occupy a gray zone in between. Although many very ill and old people seem to want to hang on to life indefinitely, resisting death, nevertheless the majority of deaths occurring in institutions in this country (and the majority of deaths do occur in institutions) are "negotiated" in a way that involves a shorter life than would otherwise have been possible for that person. The medical and legal euphemism is that these patients are "allowed to die."

How frequent such decisions are is difficult to determine. In the United States, it has been estimated that some 70 percent of deaths in institutional settings involve some form of negotiated strategy.[8] The most recent comprehensive Dutch study, covering a six-year period ending in 2001, finds that of all deaths in the Netherlands, about 20.2 percent involved the withholding or withdrawing of life-sustaining treatment; in another 20.1 percent, pain and symptoms were alleviated with doses of opioids that may have shortened life. The ending of life without a current explicit request, a violation of Dutch law, occurred in about 0.7 percent of all deaths (though in virtually all cases with the prior request of the patient or when the patient was no longer capable of communication). Altogether, some 43.7 percent of all deaths—a figure approaching half—appear to have involved decisions that probably or certainly allowed or caused death to occur sooner in order to avoid a dying process regarded as worse.[9] Roughly similar pictures are believed to be true of other advanced industrial democracies in Europe, Australia, and elsewhere.[10] A study of six European countries released in 2003 reveals that the frequency of end-of-life decisions (including decisions about withholding

8. Stell (1998), citing the amicus curiae brief filed by the American Hospital Association in *Cruzan* v. *Director, Missouri Department of Health*, 497 U.S. 261 (1990).

9. van der Wal and others (2003); Onwuteaka-Philipsen and others (2003).

10. Deliens and others (2000); Kuhse and others (1997); van der Heide and others (2003).

or withdrawing care, alleviation of pain and suffering in a way that might foreseeably hasten death, euthanasia, physician-assisted suicide, and direct termination of life without an explicit current request) ranged from a low of 23 percent in Italy to a high of 51 percent in Switzerland.[11] The ending of life without the patient's explicit request happened more frequently than voluntary, active euthanasia in five of the six countries studied (Belgium, Denmark, Italy, Sweden, and Switzerland; all except the Netherlands) and was the only form of doctor-assisted death recorded in Sweden.

Thus even now lives are often less long than they could be. To be sure, they are not very much less long. In the Netherlands, the best-studied site of these end-of-life practices, relatively little life is forgone; in about 50 percent of cases of euthanasia, physician-assisted suicide, and life shortening without explicit request, life is shortened by an estimated twenty-four hours or less; in another 30 percent, life is shortened by less than a week, and only about 9 percent involve shortening life by more than a month.[12] A generously estimated average by which life is curtailed by direct termination of life, practices that account for about 3 percent of total deaths, is 3.3 weeks.[13]

Clearly, abbreviations of this modest sort have little impact on overall longevity; an extra-long life that is shorter on average by 3.3 weeks is still extra long. However, the amount of possible life not actually lived by future generations might be much greater. Not only does the estimated sacrifice of 3.3 weeks by today's Netherlanders not include deaths that occur earlier as a result of "allowing to die," but today's Dutch, like inhabitants of advanced nations generally, face a comparatively short preterminal and terminal phase. Proximate future generations for whom extra-long life becomes possible could face the scenario of longer dying, a protracted period no better in quality of life than that which some contemporary people now seek to avoid. Although measures to curtail or terminate life may now be used sparingly in advanced nations, they are already in place and are used, with professional and public knowledge and acceptance, to spare people deaths that could be much worse than the deliberately chosen death.

Although some such measures doubtless are rooted in self-interest or greed, second-party decisions to allow a patient to die or to assist in causing death are typically not malevolent. Rather, they are seen as benevolent choices made by concerned family members, physicians, or others to spare the patient a much worse death. It is rapidly becoming a culturally accepted view that

---

11. van der Heide and others (2003), p. 3.
12. Onwuteaka-Philipsen and others (2003).
13. Emanuel and Battin (1998).

when all that remains is a painful process of dying, it may not be in the patient's interests to continue living; the patient may refuse to continue to live; or if not able to make that choice, others may do so on his or her behalf.

Thus if medical, genetic, and environmental science produces a longer-dying scenario, we should expect both that people will find the likely end periods of their lives not worth living and voluntarily elect not to continue them, and also that others will make such choices on their behalf. Under the longer-dying scenario, the amount of life forgone will likely be greater than it is now. We should also anticipate that medical, legal, and social attitudes and policies will conform to the view that longer dying is not acceptable. To anticipate that individual behavior and social institutions will evolve in this fashion is not to put forth a slippery slope argument, which predicts whole-sale nonvoluntary deaths; rather it is to argue that the very considerations that underwrite currently accepted practices—that it is a good thing to spare people bad deaths—will find application in the future if generally bad deaths strung out over extended periods of time—that is, longer dying—is what they face.

The present provides a basis for predictions about the future. Few people now enjoy longer health—that is, a long life span with good health until right before death. Instead, the vast majority of people in the United States, and indeed in the developed world in general, die of degenerative diseases (especially heart disease, cancer, and stroke), which often exhibit long terminal declines.[14] However, few people now suffer the much longer terminal decline that will characterize the longer-dying scenario of the future. Good ends today are not always as good as they could be if longer health were genuinely the case—that is what contemporary medical science tries to achieve; and bad ends today are shorter and easier than what longer dying might impose. Yet we already often forgo these even shorter end stages. Would not the members of proximate future generations behave in much the same way? If longer health were the norm, it would be enthusiastically lived; if longer dying were the norm, it would likely not be lived at all.

These predictions also provide some basis for speculating about the impact of future scenarios of extra-long life on the economic and social policy issues the chapters in this volume explore. If longer health is the scenario, people will live extra-long lives but constitute no extra burden. If longer dying is the scenario, their very extensive care, Social Security, and health care costs could constitute a real burden, but people are unlikely to be willing to live such lives. Thus the impact of longer health and longer dying on

14. Field and Cassel (1997), chap. 2.

social institutions and programs might be similar. Exactly how much future generations may choose to curtail life if they face longer dying is unclear, but we cannot rule out the possibility that they would shorten life enough to call current economic forecasts into question, especially those that see the social costs of extra-long life as an immense, unsupportable burden about to spiral out of control. The assumption at the heart of such forecasts—that if extra-long life becomes possible people will actually live it—is persuasive only under one scenario, that of longer health. It is unpersuasive under the alternative that predicts these huge burdens, longer dying.

Longer Decline, the Plausible Scenario

I have so far explored two stark alternative future scenarios in order to highlight the ubiquitous problematic assumption that runs throughout discussions of extra-long life: the scenario of longer health, attractive in all ways and a burden to none; and the scenario of longer dying, attractive in no way and a burden to all. The more probable outcome, however, of mixed advances in medical science, genetics, environmental science, and other new fields we cannot yet anticipate—variously exacerbating and offsetting each other's advantages and disadvantages—is the longer-decline scenario. This intermediate scenario is the most plausible but, paradoxically, yields the least secure predictions. If longer decline materializes, we cannot reliably predict whether future generations will elect to live out whatever extra-long life becomes possible for them. Nor will it be an easy choice for them or for their caretakers, medical managers, or policymakers. Unlike longer health and longer dying, longer decline really does bode an "uncertain demographic future."

References

Arrow, Kenneth J. 1950. *Social Choice and Individual Values.* Yale University Press.

Avorn, Jerry. 1984. "Benefit and Cost Analysis in Geriatric Care: Turning Age Discrimination into Health Policy." *New England Journal of Medicine* 310 (20): 1294–301.

Beauchamp, Tom L., and James F. Childress. 2001. *Principles of Biomedical Ethics,* 5th ed. Oxford University Press.

Bernat, James L., Bernard Gert, and R. Peter Mogielnicki. 1993. "Patient Refusal of Hydration and Nutrition: An Alternative to Physician-Assisted Suicide or Voluntary Active Euthanasia." *Archives of Internal Medicine* 153: 2723–28.

Callahan, Daniel. 1987. *Setting Limits: Medical Goals in an Aging Society.* Simon and Schuster.

———. 1990. *What Kind of Life? The Limits of Medical Progress.* Simon and Schuster.

Daniels, Norman. 1985. *Just Health Care.* Cambridge University Press.

———. 1988. *Am I My Parents' Keeper? An Essay on Justice between the Young and the Old.* Oxford University Press.

Deliens, Luc, and others. 2000. "End-of-Life Decisions in Medical Practice in Flanders, Belgium: A Nationwide Survey." *Lancet* 356 (9244): 1806–11.

Elliott, Carl. 2003. *Better than Well: When Modern Medicine Meets the American Dream.* W.W. Norton.

Emanuel, Ezekiel J., and Margaret P. Battin. 1998. "What Are the Potential Cost Savings from Legalizing Physician-Assisted Suicide?" *New England Journal of Medicine* 339 (3): 167–72.

Evert, Jessica, Elizabeth Lawler, Hazel Bogan, and Thomas Perls. 2003. "Morbidity Profiles of Centenarians: Survivors, Delayers, and Escapers." *Journals of Gerontology Series A: Biological Sciences and Medical Sciences* 58: M232–37.

Field, Marilyn J., and Christine K. Cassel, eds. 1997. *Approaching Death: Improving Care at the End of Life.* Washington: National Academy Press.

Fries, James F. 1983. "The Compression of Morbidity." *Milbank Memorial Fund Quarterly* 61 (Summer): 397–419.

Fuchs, Victor. 1984. "Though Much Is Taken: Reflections on Aging, Health, and Medical Care." *Milbank Memorial Fund Quarterly* 62 (Spring): 143–66.

Fukuyama, Francis. 2002. *Our Posthuman Future: Consequences of the Biotechnology Revolution.* Farrar, Straus, and Giroux.

Ginzberg, Eli. 1984. "The Elderly Are at Risk." *Inquiry* 21 (4): 301–02.

Hedberg, Katrina, David Hopkins, and Melvin Kohn. 2003. "Five Years of Legal Physician-Assisted Suicide in Oregon." *New England Journal of Medicine* 348 (10): 961–64.

Holden, Constance. 2002. "The Quest to Reverse Time's Toll." *Science* 295 (5557): 1032–33.

Holmes, Oliver Wendell. 1858. "The Deacon's Masterpiece; Or, The Wonderful One-Hoss Shay: A Logical Story." In *Autocrat of the Breakfast-Table.*

Jonas, Hans. 1984. *The Imperative of Responsibility.* University of Chicago Press.

Kass, Leon R. 1985. *Toward a More Natural Science: Biology and Human Affairs.* Free Press.

———. 2003. "Ageless Bodies, Happy Souls." *New Atlantis* 1 (Spring): 9–28.

Kuhse, Helga, and others. 1997. "End-of-Life Decisions in Australian Medical Practice." *Medical Journal of Australia* 166: 91–96.

Lubitz, James, and Ronald Prihoda. 1984. "The Use and Costs of Medicare Services in the Last Two Years of Life." *Health Care Financing Review* 5 (3): 117–31.

McKibben, Bill. 2003. *Enough: Staying Human in an Engineered Age.* Times Books.

Meier, Diane, and others. 1998. "A National Survey of Physician-Assisted Suicide and Euthanasia in the United States." *New England Journal of Medicine* 338 (17): 1193–201.
———. 2003. "Characteristics of Patients Requesting and Receiving Physician-Assisted Death." *Archives of Internal Medicine* 163: 1537–42.
National Commission for the Protection of Human Subjects of Biomedical and Behavioral Research. 1979. *The Belmont Report: Ethical Principles and Guidelines for the Protection of Human Subjects of Research.* Government Printing Office.
Okarma, Thomas B. 2000. "Prospects for Cellular Therapies in the Treatment of Chronic Disease." *Journal of Commercial Biotechnology* 6 (Spring): 300–07.
Onwuteaka-Philipsen, Bregje D., and others. 2003. "Euthanasia and Other End-of-Life Decisions in the Netherlands in 1990, 1995, and 2001." *Lancet* 362 (9381): 395–99.
Perls, Thomas, and Dellara Terry. 2003. "Genetics of Exceptional Longevity." *Experimental Gerontology* 38: 725–30.
President's Commission for the Study of Ethical Problems in Medicine and Biomedical and Behavioral Research. 1983. *Securing Access to Health Care.* Government Printing Office.
Rawls, John A. 1971. *A Theory of Justice.* Harvard University Press.
Schwartz, William B. 1998. *Life without Disease: The Pursuit of Medical Utopia.* University of California Press.
Scitovsky, Anne, and Alexander M. Capron. 1986. "Medical Care at the End of Life: The Interaction of Economics and Ethics." *Annual Review of Public Health* 7: 59–75.
Stell, Lance. 1998. "Physician Assisted Suicide: To Decriminalize or to Legalize, That Is the Question." In *Physician Assisted Suicide: Expanding the Debate,* edited by Margaret P. Battin, Rosamond Rhodes, and Anita Silvers. Routledge.
ter Meulen, Ruud H. J. 1995. "Solidarity with the Elderly and the Allocation of Resources." In *A World Growing Old: The Coming Health Care Challenges,* edited by Daniel Callahan, Ruud H. J. ter Meulen, and Eva Topinková, 73–74. Georgetown University Press.
van der Heide, Agnes, and others. 2003. "End-of-Life Decision-Making in Six European Countries: Descriptive Study." On behalf of the EURELD Consortium. *Lancet* 362 (9381): 345–50.
van der Wal, Gerrit, and others. 2003. *Medische besluitvorming aan het einde van het leven.* Utrecht, Netherlands: Uitgeverij De Tijdstroom. Summary in English in Onwuteaka-Philipsen and others (2003).
Wade, Nicholas. 2001. *Life Script: How the Human Genome Discoveries Will Transform Medicine and Enhance Your Health.* Simon and Schuster.
World Health Organization. 2002. *Ethical Choices in Long-Term Care: What Does Justice Require?* Geneva.

BARRY P. BOSWORTH
BENJAMIN KEYS

7 Increased Life Expectancy: A Global Perspective

THE ECONOMIC EFFECTS of population change are currently matters of considerable global concern. Most nations are in the midst of substantial demographic transitions induced by sharply lower fertility and mortality rates. However, there is a great diversity across countries and regions. And because economic effects differ at various stages of the process, demographic change has had widely varying economic and social consequences.

Most industrial countries have experienced low fertility rates for several decades and have achieved relatively high life expectancy. Consequently, they are most concerned with what they see as the economic burden of providing for a rapidly aging, economically nonproductive elderly population. There is a general perception that the graying of the population will slow economic growth through reduced increase in the working-age population and lower rates of saving and capital formation.

The developing world is at an earlier stage in the demographic transition, where they anticipate substantial near-term benefits. The working-age population is still growing rapidly because of past high fertility. At the same time, child dependency rates are falling because birth rates have declined. This combination provides the opportunity to raise rates of saving and capital accumulation. Lower mortality rates among the young and the middle-aged also imply increased returns from investments in education and other forms of human capital.

247

These differences between the demographic situation of the rich industrial societies and that of the developing world have important implications for economic interactions between the two regions. Some analysts think that consumption of a large retired population will drive down saving in the rich industrial economies and create a global capital shortage just when investment needs are surging in the developing world.[1] If saving declines faster than investment in the aging industrial societies, they will become more dependent on the rest of the world, requiring resources to be transferred from poor countries to support the consumption of the rich. Others see a quite different future and foresee that a slowly growing or even declining working-age population will reduce investment within the industrial economies, creating a glut of saving and economic stagnation.[2]

Humanity is now faced with the prospect of major innovations in the field of biology that could lead to substantial further reductions in mortality and morbidity. How will these reductions affect the demographic transition currently under way? Will they simply extend and accelerate existing trends? Or will they change the process in some more significant way? In particular, how would such changes affect the economic relationship between the developed and developing portions of the world economy?

We examine three aspects of the relationship between increased life expectancy and global economic performance. We start by using population projections from the United Nations to examine past and projected changes in the world's demographic structure and to highlight its cross-country diversity. These projections provide the basis for examining the demographic implications of increased longevity. We next summarize the current state of the research on the macroeconomic effects of demographic change, focusing on how increased life expectancy, anticipated and unanticipated, affects saving and investment in the industrial countries (and thus their trade balance with the rest of the world). Finally, we use the panel data on saving and investment of eighty-eight countries, representing 95 percent of the world's gross domestic product (GDP) and 85 percent of the total population, to examine how demographic changes influence national rates of saving and investment. We use those results to evaluate the potential for international capital flows to moderate the economic effects of population aging in the industrial countries.

We conclude that the effects of a major increase in longevity would be borne largely by the high-income regions, for which further increases in rates of aged dependency would make existing retirement practices untenable. The

1. OECD (1996).
2. Cutler and others (1990).

direct effects on developing countries will be modest because they will not have a large proportion of their populations in the older age brackets (those most affected by greater life expectancy). However, the developing world would be disadvantaged by a greater global scarcity of capital, as aging leads to substantial reductions in saving. We find evidence that national rates of saving and investment are both negatively affected by increases in dependency rates. The current account deficit, which exactly equals the excess of investment over saving plus any public sector budget deficit, would become extreme for many high-income countries. These economic trends would force even larger adjustments of national retirement policies than would be required if past trends continue.

We consider neither possible changes in labor force participation by the older population (the subject analyzed by Gary Burtless, this volume) nor the implications of greater cross-border migration. In addition, the proportion of the population of the high-income regions that survives beyond the normal retirement ages of sixty to sixty-five is already high, given current medical technology, and it is likely that increased life spans will, as in the past, add to the length of retirement. Labor force participation rates are determined largely by the incentives embodied in existing retirement programs. In the absence of policy change, retirement ages are unlikely to rise in line with increased longevity.

United Nations projections do incorporate assumed future rates of migration. We do not address the potential for changes in migration in response to increased longevity. Most of the international consequences of population aging can be addressed through the mobility of capital and technology rather than of labor. With recent reductions in the cost of transportation and communication and the removal of trade barriers, for example, Japan can move its factories to China as an alternative to large-scale immigration.[3]

Demographic Trends

The growth and structure of the world's population has changed dramatically over the past 150 years. Those changes were driven first by a major decline in human mortality, as nutrition and sanitation improved and health technology advanced. Then, after a lag, fertility rates fell sharply. A revolutionary increase in longevity began near the end of the nineteenth century,

3. The movement of factories does not deal directly with employment in industries that produce nontradables; but labor is free to move among sectors. Thus we can expect aging to be accompanied by a shrinking of the tradables sector and a shift of employment to nontradables.

Table 7-1. *Life Expectancy at Birth, by Development Level, 1950–2050*[a]

Years

Region or country	1950	2000	2050	Change 1950–2000	Change 2000–50	2000 population in millions
World	46.5	66.0	76.0	19.5	10.0	6,057
High-income regions	66.2	75.6	82.1	9.4	6.5	1,191
Middle-income regions	41.8	66.8	76.6	24.9	9.8	4,207
Low-income regions	35.5	51.4	69.7	15.9	18.2	658
G-7 countries						
United States	68.9	77.5	82.6	8.6	5.1	283
United Kingdom	69.2	78.2	83.0	9.0	4.8	59
France	66.5	79.0	84.0	12.5	4.9	59
Germany	67.5	78.2	83.4	10.7	5.2	82
Italy	66.0	78.7	82.5	12.7	3.8	58
Canada	69.1	79.0	82.8	9.9	3.8	31
Japan	63.9	81.5	88.0	17.5	6.5	127
Russian Federation	64.6	66.0	76.9	1.4	10.9	145
China	40.8	71.2	79.0	30.4	7.8	1,275
India	38.7	64.2	75.4	25.6	11.1	1,009
Brazil	50.9	68.3	76.9	17.4	8.6	170

Source: United Nations (2001).

a. High-income countries, as defined by the United Nations, are all regions of Europe plus the United States, Canada, Australia, New Zealand, and Japan, with a population of 1.2 billion in 2000. Middle-income countries had a population of 4.2 billion in 2000 and include China and India. Low-income countries are the forty-eight least-developed countries, as defined by the United Nations, and had a population of 650 million in 2000.

as life expectancy in Western Europe and North America began to rise above a historical average of about forty years. Comprehensive global data are available after 1950, by which time much of the improvement was already evident in the high-income regions (see table 7-1).[4] However, life expectancy

4. Population data are drawn from United Nations (2001). High-income countries are the UN's most-developed nation grouping, which includes all European countries, the United States, Canada, Australia, New Zealand, and Japan. The low-income group comprises the forty-eight countries the UN classifies as least developed. The middle-income group is the less-developed group minus the forty-eight least-developed countries; it includes, among others, China and India.

remained at about forty years or less elsewhere. Since 1950 life expectancy has risen spectacularly in a group of countries now classified by the United Nations as middle income. By 2000 life expectancy in China increased by thirty years and in India by twenty-six years. The result has been a substantial convergence in life expectancy across countries.

Life Expectancy and Fertility

Improvements in life expectancy in the industrial countries are projected by the United Nations to slow by about one-third compared to the 1950–2000 experience (table 7-1). These assumptions are slightly more optimistic (longer lives) than those of the Social Security Administration for the United States, but they do not incorporate any discontinuous improvements in longevity. The rate of improvement in the middle-income countries slows more substantially as they approach the frontier of experience, but there continues to be room for substantial gains among the least-developed nations.

The increase in longevity initially caused a surge in population growth but was followed by equally large declines in fertility—from an average of about five births per woman to around three (table 7-2). In high-income countries that process is largely complete; in many the fertility rate has fallen below simple replacement (just over two births per woman). The decline in fertility in middle-income countries has been particularly rapid since 1965, largely because of the one-child policy adopted by China. At the world rate of 2.8 births per woman, there is still room for significant reduction. The UN projects the world fertility rate to decline steadily until it reaches the replacement rate by 2050. The fertility transition is still in its very early stages for the least-developed regions, where fertility rates are projected to fall rapidly over the next half century.

Dependency Rates

While lower fertility and mortality rates imply that the average age of the population will rise in all countries, the differences in the timing of the changes across countries translate into substantial diversity in rates of both child and aged dependency (table 7-3). For high-income countries the aged dependency rate (the number of persons over age sixty-five divided by persons ages fifteen to sixty-four) is expected to double by 2050 to near 50 percent. Although the increase will be even more dramatic in less-developed countries, the aged dependency rate in those nations will not reach levels currently experienced in the high-income countries until 2050. Furthermore,

Table 7-2. *Fertility, by Development Level, 1950–2050*[a]

Children per woman

Region or country	1950	2000	2050	Change 1950–2000	2000–50
World	5.0	2.8	2.1	−2.2	−0.7
High-income regions	2.8	1.6	1.9	−1.3	0.4
Middle-income regions	6.1	2.8	2.1	−3.3	−0.7
Low-income regions	6.6	5.5	2.5	−1.1	−3.0
G-7 countries					
United States	3.4	2.0	2.1	−1.4	0.1
United Kingdom	2.2	1.7	1.9	−0.5	0.2
France	2.7	1.7	1.9	−1.0	0.2
Germany	2.2	1.3	1.6	−0.8	0.3
Italy	2.3	1.2	1.6	−1.1	0.4
Canada	3.7	1.6	1.9	−2.1	0.3
Japan	2.7	1.4	1.8	−1.3	0.3
Russian Federation	2.8	1.2	1.8	−1.6	0.5
China	6.2	1.8	1.9	−4.4	0.1
India	6.0	3.3	2.1	−2.7	−1.2
Brazil	6.2	2.3	2.1	−3.9	−0.2

Source: United Nations (2001).

a. *Fertility* is defined by the United Nations as the average number of children a hypothetical cohort of women would have at the end of their reproductive period if they were subject during their whole lives to the fertility rates of a given period and if they were not subject to mortality.

because of continuing declines in the birth rate, the overall dependency rate—children plus the aged—will be substantially lower in the less-developed countries in 2050 than it is today. For the world as a whole current projections indicate that the aged dependency rates will rise but that the total dependency rate will not change.

Even within the G-7 countries (the United States, the United Kingdom, France, Germany, Italy, Canada, and Japan), the degree of aging and the sources of change are quite diverse. By 2050 dependency rates will range from highs of 71 percent in Japan and 68 percent in Italy to lows of 35 percent in the United States and 41 percent in Canada. In Japan and Italy, a large decline in the working-age population accounts for half of the rise. In the United States and Canada, in contrast, the work force is projected to continue to grow. In Great Britain and France, it will remain roughly unchanged.

Table 7-3. *Dependency, by Development Level, 1950–2050* [a]

Percent

Region or country	Aged dependency			Child dependency			Total dependency		
	1950	2000	2050	1950	2000	2050	1950	2000	2050
World	8.6	10.9	24.7	56.7	47.5	33.1	65.2	58.4	57.7
High-income regions	12.2	21.2	46.5	42.2	27.1	26.9	54.4	48.3	73.4
Middle-income regions	6.8	8.5	22.6	63.1	49.2	24.3	69.9	57.8	46.9
Low-income regions	5.9	5.8	9.8	73.8	80.2	45.2	79.7	86.0	54.9
G-7 countries									
United States	12.8	18.6	34.9	41.7	32.9	30.7	54.5	51.5	65.6
United Kingdom	16.0	24.1	47.3	33.4	29.1	26.0	49.4	53.2	73.3
France	17.3	24.5	46.7	34.5	28.7	27.9	51.7	53.2	74.6
Germany	14.5	24.1	54.7	34.6	22.8	21.9	49.0	46.9	76.5
Italy	12.6	26.7	68.1	40.2	21.1	21.8	52.8	47.8	89.8
Canada	12.2	18.5	40.9	47.4	28.0	27.5	59.6	46.5	68.4
Japan	8.3	25.2	71.3	59.5	21.6	24.5	67.8	46.8	95.8
Russian Federation	9.5	18.0	47.1	44.5	25.8	23.0	54.1	43.8	70.1
China	7.2	10.0	37.2	54.1	36.4	26.7	61.3	46.4	63.9
India	5.8	8.1	22.9	67.4	54.4	33.8	73.2	62.5	56.7
Brazil	5.4	7.8	28.7	74.9	43.6	32.0	80.3	51.4	60.7

Source: United Nations (2001).

a. Aged dependency rates are the percentage of population over age sixty-five divided by the working-age population (ages fifteen through sixty-four). Child dependency rates are the percentage of population under age fifteen divided by the working-age population.

These changes translate into slowing future rates of population growth in all major regions of the world. However, the deceleration proceeds from dramatically different current rates of growth. As shown in figure 7-1, high-income regions are expected to experience absolute population decline only after 2025, and the rate of contraction is small. More important, the growth in the working-age population (figure 7-2) turns negative within the next decade, and the rate of decline is quite substantial, averaging a minus 0.5 percent annually after 2020. Meanwhile, the population and the labor force will both continue to expand in middle-income countries, though at much

Figure 7-1. *Actual and Projected Population Growth Rates, by Development Level, 1950–2050*

Percent

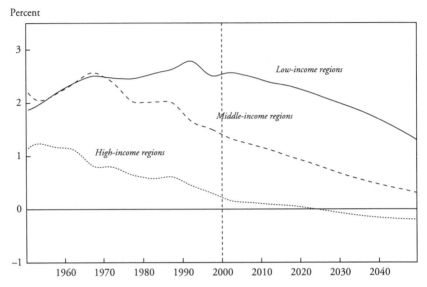

reduced rates. Finally, even with continued decline in birth rates, population and labor force growth in low-income regions will remain high.

Mortality Rates

How would the above outlook be affected by a sharp reduction in mortality rates, such as that which might result from a biomedical breakthrough? First, in high-income countries it would have relatively minor effects on the population below age sixty-five because the survival rate to age sixty is already 85 percent. However, survival rates fall off rapidly thereafter—only 50 percent are expected to reach age eighty. Thus the effects of a radical decrease in mortality rates would be concentrated among the very old. For middle-income countries the age profile of survival rates is largely parallel and quite close to that for more developed regions—about 75 percent survive to age sixty. Thus the effects would be similar to those in the more developed countries. The much lower life expectancies in low-income regions are strongly influenced by high infant mortality—an average of 17 percent of newborns in low-income regions do not survive to age five, compared to 1 percent in

Figure 7-2. *Actual and Projected Working-Age Population Growth Rates, by Development Level, 1950–2050*

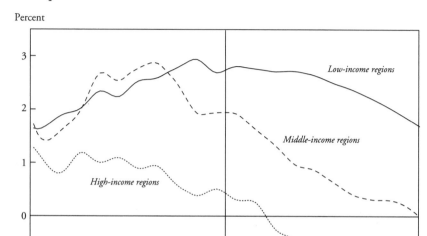

Percent

Source: See figure 7-1.

high-income countries. The survival rate to age sixty in these countries is only 50 percent. For many years to come, improvement in life expectancy in low-income regions will be affected far less by future discoveries than by their ability to apply currently available medical technologies and nutritional practices to reduce the mortality rate of younger persons.

To a large extent the applicability of any technological breakthrough in poor nations will depend on its cost. Expensive individual treatments will be used only in the richest societies and, depending on methods of payment, may be used only by their richest members. Low-cost improvements, on the other hand, similar to the low-cost measures of sanitation and public health that have found wide applicability in countries such as China, could have significant implications in the broad category of middle-income countries. For advances that are costly to develop but cheap to produce, there is a third possibility—that developers try to use laws governing intellectual property rights to restrict their use as a means of extracting monopoly rents. As with drugs for the treatment of AIDS, the issue is likely to be highly divisive. How rapidly such therapies spread is likely to depend more on politics than medical science.

Scenarios

In developing a hypothetical scenario, we treat the assumed improvements of Henry Aaron and Ben Harris (this volume) as an outward shift of the current survival rates among the elderly. As shown by their scenario for the United States (figure 7-3), the changes in the population under age fifty would be small. Thus we model the biomedical advances as raising future survival rates of those who are alive at age forty-five to age forty-nine. We compute implicit survival rates in 2050 for this cohort in the UN projections for all regions. We then scale those rates up by the proportionate U.S. difference between the Aaron-Harris projections and a baseline case. The U.S. survival rates projected by the Social Security Administration (SSA), which were used as a baseline for comparison by Aaron and Harris, differ significantly from those of the United Nations (figure 7-4).

The UN survival rates are higher than the SSA's and similar to those of the U.S. Census Bureau. As a result we constructed two alternative projections of the biomedical breakthrough, which show the implications for potential changes in dependency rates (table 7-4). In 2050 the aged dependency rate of high-income countries would be increased from 46 to 54 percent of the working-age population if the adjustment were based on UN

Figure 7-3. *U.S. Population, by Age, Two Projections, 2050*

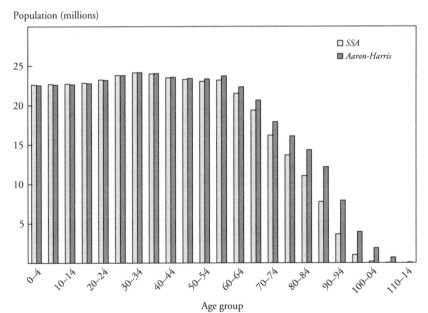

Population (millions)

Figure 7-4. *Implicit U.S. Survival Rates from Age Fifty,*
Three Projections, 2050

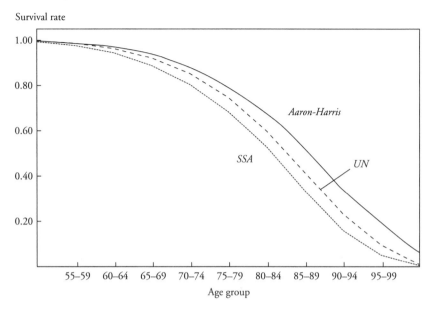

Survival rate

projections for the United States (AH 1). It would rise to a more dramatic 64 percent if we use the difference between Aaron-Harris and SSA (AH 2). Changes are only about a third as large for middle-income countries and are very small for the least-developed countries because relatively few of their populations will be in the age categories affected by expanded longevity. This scenario differs in one important aspect from the general pattern of increases in the aged dependency rate in the UN baseline because no offsetting drop in child dependency rates would occur.

Japan's population structure would be greatly altered by a biomedical breakthrough. The Japanese aged dependency rate is already high (71 percent) and could reach a staggering 117 percent of the working-age population. Japan combines a low birth rate with high life expectancy. As a result, a very large proportion of its population is in the age brackets that would be quickly affected by a major change in longevity. China also would experience a larger rise in the dependency rate than the typical middle-income country. The effect in the United States, however, would be slightly less than the average of the other high-income countries.

Comprehensive global data on the proportion of the population of various ages that is working do not exist. However, changes as large as those shown in table 7-4 for the aged dependency rates in high-income countries could be

Table 7-4. *Dependency in 2050, by Development Level, Three Projections*[a]

Percent

Region or country	Aged dependency			Child dependency			Total dependency		
	UN	A-H 1	A-H 2	UN	A-H 1	A-H 2	UN	A-H 1	A-H 2
World	24.7	27.3	30.7	33.1	33.0	32.9	57.7	60.3	63.6
High-income regions	46.5	54.1	64.1	26.9	26.9	26.8	73.4	81.0	90.8
Middle-income regions	25.3	27.7	30.8	30.6	30.5	30.4	55.9	58.2	61.2
Low-income regions	9.8	10.4	11.3	45.2	45.1	45.0	54.9	55.5	56.3
United States	34.9	40.5	47.9	30.7	30.7	30.6	65.6	71.2	78.4
Japan	71.3	91.2	117.1	24.5	24.5	24.4	95.8	115.7	141.4
China	37.2	41.2	46.4	26.7	26.7	26.6	63.9	67.9	73.0

Source: United Nations (2001); Henry Aaron and Benjamin Harris, this volume.

a. Aged dependency rates are the percentage of population over age sixty-five divided by the working-age population (ages fifteen through sixty-four). Child dependency rates are the percentage of population under age fifteen divided by the working age population. A-H 1 is the adjustment for Aaron-Harris, relative to the UN projections; A-H 2 is the adjustment for Aaron-Harris relative to the SSA projections.

offset if the definition of the working-age population is extended by about
two additional years, from sixty-five to sixty-seven for the Aaron-Harris projection 1 and about five years for the Aaron-Harris projection 2. In Japan,
the change would be much more dramatic: Retirement age would have to
be extended for an additional ten years to offset the effects of the assumed
increase in longevity on the aged-dependency ratio.

Overall, the primary effect of a major increase in longevity would be to
widen the emerging demographic disparities between the rich and old societies of the industrial world and the young and poor societies of the developing world. For the rich economies, greater longevity would exacerbate an
existing trend toward much higher rates of aged dependency. The effect
would be much smaller in developing countries. As explained more fully in
the following sections, the divergent trends may significantly expand capital
flows between rich and poor countries, as the former seek to finance a longer
retirement by investing in the latter.

Economic Effects

Declining fertility rates, low and possibly declining population growth, and
the attendant aging of the population give rise to fears of economic stagnation
in the advanced economies. Demographic change can affect the economy
through several channels. Economic growth will slow because the labor force
will grow slowly or shrink. Furthermore, labor productivity peaks between
ages forty and fifty and then drops (quite rapidly at later ages). Thus an aging
population may be an unproductive population.

Growth of the work force is but one contributor to rising output. In most
economies, increases in the stock of capital and general improvements in the
efficiency of production—multifactor productivity—are of equal or greater
importance. Thus the economic effects of demographic change depend sensitively on how it affects saving and capital formation. Will the rising consumption needs of the elderly drive down national rates of saving? And if so,
how will reduced saving compare with the lower investment needs of a stag-
nant work force?

Saving

According to the standard life-cycle hypothesis, saving follows a hump-shaped
curve, starting at low or negative rates among young adults then rising as people accumulate wealth and, finally, becoming negative as retirees use up their

accumulated assets. In the early stages of the transition, a decline in child dependency rates might cause consumption to be shifted from the child-rearing ages to later stages of life. Thus rates of saving should be systematically related to changes in the age structure of the population. In addition, aggregate income growth should influence saving. Increased growth raises the relative importance of young income-earning households relative to the elderly, who are retired and dissaving. Several studies suggest, for example, that highly favorable demographic developments—a decline in the child dependency rate, in particular—explain much of the extraordinary growth performance of the East Asian economies. These demographic events, which triggered a sharp rise in saving, supported rapid increases in investment.[5] That same process, operating in reverse, suggests that saving rates will fall throughout the high-income economies because of rising future rates of aged dependency.

Investment

The concerns about the effect of demographic changes on investment follow from the neoclassical model of economic growth, in which the growth of output is determined by three factors: growth in the labor force, labor-augmenting technical change, and increases in capital per worker. In the long term, capital stock must expand in line with output to avoid a progressive decline in the rate of return. Thus the sustainable rate of growth in output and capital stock is given by the combination of labor force growth and labor-augmenting technical change.[6] A slowing of growth in the labor force or in technological advance implies a reduced rate of capital accumulation and a lower rate of investment. An aging population, with a lower rate of growth of the work force, can devote a smaller proportion of its output to capital accumulation.

Linkages

Several studies explore the economic effects of population aging on national rates of saving and investment. A 1990 study by David Cutler and others examines the issue of population aging in a closed-economy model, where saving can be invested only domestically.[7] Reduced labor force growth results in

5. Bloom, Canning, and Malaney (1999); Higgins and Williamson (1997); and the studies they review.

6. Cutler and others (1990). Under the assumption of a fixed capital-output ratio, we can also assume that the share of investment in output is proportionate to output growth.

7. Cutler and others (1990).

lower investment and decreased profitability of saving. Under these assumptions, increases in saving cannot offset the economic costs of a rising aged dependency rate because it would lead to a perpetual fall in the rate of return. The optimal social response to population aging and lower rates of labor force growth under these conditions is to reduce saving and increase current consumption.

This dismal and somewhat paradoxical result follows from two assumptions. First, increased longevity is assumed to offer no utility beyond the opportunity to consume over a longer period of time: There is no trade-off between consumption and leisure. If the increased longevity simply means a longer retirement, the gain in longevity does not raise lifetime income. As longevity rises, average annual consumption falls. However, with a trade-off between consumption and leisure, individuals would respond to the increased consumption needs of a longer life in part by delaying retirement. The larger labor force would support a higher rate of capital accumulation, negating some of the decline in the rate of return. Second, this study assumes that society has already optimized its saving in equilibrating current and future benefits of consumption. Thus any effort to raise saving and investment in anticipation of increased retirement costs drives down the rate of return to capital, negating any gains. If one assumes that the consumption of the young is as good as the consumption of the old, there is also no social benefit of transfers from the young to the old.

The 1990 study differentiates between the effects of aging due to a decline in fertility and the effects of aging due to an increase in longevity. In the long run, both cause aged dependency rates to rise and average per capita consumption to fall. However, reduced fertility also implies lower labor force growth, which reduces the rate of saving required to sustain a given level of capital per worker. The goods not required for investment may be consumed, providing a partial offsetting gain in per capita consumption. In contrast, an increase in longevity during retirement years yields no net economic benefits to society. Any effort to meet the increased consumption needs of the elderly is fully offset by the consumption losses to the young.

A 2000 study by Douglas Elmendorf and Louise Sheiner analyzes how a small, open economy should respond to increased longevity.[8] An open economy can invest its own saving abroad as well as at home, thereby avoiding any induced decline in the rate of return. This study concludes that, although it would be desirable to increase current saving in anticipation of higher future dependency rates, the increase would be small. Judged solely in con-

8. Elmendorf and Sheiner (2000).

sumption possibilities, increases in longevity are not good news. However, the study relies on the assumption of no trade-off between consumption and leisure and also on the assumption that both the developed and developing worlds were in a prior equilibrium of optimal saving and capital.

A second 2000 study, by Orazio Attanasio and Giovanni Violante, examines a process closely related to the question we are exploring: the implications of demographic transition in older, high-income countries and a young developing region.[9] The authors assume that there is no public pension system or other way to share the costs of supporting retirees across generations. In the older region, labor force growth is slowing and the aged dependency rate is rising. In the young region, fertility and child dependency rates are falling and labor force growth is accelerating. Using an overlapping-generations model, the study shows that, without trade (closed economy), demographic change will induce large transitional changes in saving and wages. In the absence of trade between the regions, the older region raises saving in anticipation of the costs of consumption in retirement, but the response is limited because added saving drives down the return on capital. In the younger region, the rising proportion of the working-age population will boost per capita income, but the shortage of capital slows the realization of the gains.

When the study introduces trade between the two regions, the demographic disparities create substantial opportunities for joint gains from the expansion of cross-border resource flows. These benefits can be realized without labor mobility. Transfer of capital and technology is sufficient. In the younger region, capital mobility accelerates the gains by speeding capital accumulation. In the older region, capital mobility helps maintain the return to capital.[10] The Attanasio and Violante study emphasizes the benefits of factor mobility more than does the Elmendorf and Sheiner study because the former concentrates on the short-run period of transition to an equilibrium. It is also more realistic in incorporating large initial differences in capital per worker, and thus rates of return, between the rich and the poor regions.

From the perspective of the Attanasio and Violante study, the demographic transition is not all bad news. The diversity of timing around the globe suggests that trade can help alleviate the costs to older societies and accelerate economic growth in younger societies. Of course, factor mobility

---

9. Attanasio and Violante (2000); also see Bryant and Velculescu (2002).

10. Attanasio and Violante (2000) introduce open capital markets at a time of substantial difference in the rate of return to capital in the two regions, which magnifies the benefits of the capital transactions.

does not solve the fundamental economic problem that increased longevity requires that consumption be supported over a longer lifetime, but it does help sustain the return to saving. For some time, increased saving by the young and the near-old in anticipation of increased longevity in the high-income countries would increase saving more than the consumption of the old would decrease it. A portion of that saving would flow to young, developing economies, accelerating their economic growth.

Many analysts resist the notion that trade between old, rich countries and young, poor countries could lighten the economic burden of population aging and yield general benefits. They stress the political and financial market barriers to expanded investment in the emerging market economies.[11] They doubt that financial market improvements in the developing world can occur fast enough to support larger capital inflows. They also stress the risks to developing countries of reliance on such inflows.

In fact, international capital flows have been growing apace in recent decades. Much of that growth has taken the form of foreign direct investment, which has proved to be stable and generally beneficial. These flows are likely to continue increasing if returns to saving decline significantly in aging economies. In countries such as the United States the scope of capital markets spread steadily over the last century—from localities, to regions, to the nation. This process is likely to continue in the international sphere if there are gains to be realized.

Other studies stress the impact of the demographic changes on incentives to invest in human capital.[12] Reduced mortality for people of working age increases incentives to invest in education. These incentives are particularly important in countries during the early stages of the demographic transition.[13] In addition, investing in one's children can serve as an alternative to saving for one's own retirement. Several simulation studies show that the effects of reduced mortality on education decisions can be economically significant.[14] In addition, intergenerational transfers between the young and the old are still very important in most societies.[15] Thus investment by parents in the education of children has elements of both self-interest and altruism and serves as an alternative to retirement saving. More broadly, future

11. Holzmann (2000); Rodrik (1998).

12. Ehrlich and Lui (1991); Kalemli-Ozcan, Ryder, and Weil (2000).

13. To the extent that increased labor skills and physical capital are complements in the growth process, improvement in the educational level of the work force will also help maintain the return to capital.

14. Kalemli-Ozcan, Ryder, and Weil (2000) and citations therein.

15. Ehrlich and Lui (1991).

generations will enjoy significantly higher income because their parents invested in their education.

The view that increased longevity among the elderly is economically bad news is unduly pessimistic. That view presumes that longer lives increase the future consumption needs of the retired with no compensating income gains and that they drive down rates of return, at least in a closed economy. That framework ignores the significant opportunities for beneficial exchange between regions with differing patterns of demographic change. It also often ignores the possibility that healthier, longer-lived people may work longer.

Empirical Estimates

Even if population aging in industrial countries slows economic growth and lowers saving and investment, the practical question is, How much? The answer remains a matter of debate. The standard life-cycle model yields a straightforward prediction that national saving will fall in response to population aging. The neoclassical growth model equally clearly predicts that increased longevity will reduce investment.

A 1998 study by Matthew Higgins embodies both assumptions.[16] This study uses both national saving and investment functions of the proportion of the population in five-year age brackets, from ages zero to four, up to ages seventy and older.[17] The model is applied to saving and investment data for a sample of a hundred countries over varying periods, extending from 1950 to 1992. The results provide evidence of strong demographic effects on both saving and investment. In addition, the positive effects of population on investment peak at earlier ages than do the effects of population on saving. This study suggests that demographic shifts would alter the balance between saving and investment—and of its mirror image, the nation's net current account balance with the rest of the world. Investment demand tends to

---

16. Higgins (1998); also see Higgins and Williamson (1997). The role of demographic change in economic growth is stressed in many studies. As examples, see Coale and Hoover (1958); Mason (1988); Masson (1990); Lindh and Malmberg (1999). Special attention is devoted to Asia, where there have been dramatic changes in both demographic structure and rates of economic growth. Prominent examples are Fry and Mason (1982); Bloom and Williamson (1998); Bloom, Canning, and Malaney (1999).

17. Because of concerns about multicolinearity among the demographic variables, Higgins (1998) uses a third-order polynomial to capture the age profile and includes the rate of growth of output per worker to capture the income effects.

exceed domestic saving in young countries, especially those with rapidly
growing populations, while investment declines in older countries as growth
in the labor force begins to slow. Higgins's results indicate that saving and
investment for the economies of the Organization for Economic Cooperation and Development (OECD) will fall 5–7 percent of GDP on the average
over the next quarter century.

In contrast, analysis of survey data from individual households casts doubt
on the simple life-cycle model. Studies of several industrial countries show
that, contrary to the predictions of the model, the elderly do not deplete assets
but continue to save. Furthermore, the influence of life-cycle effects on saving is small.[18] Instead, different birth cohorts of workers appear to have systematic differences in rates of saving, which suggest a complex relationship
between age and saving. Despite a large empirical literature, the relationship
between demographic change and saving continues to be an issue of substantial dispute.

To explore this issue further, we developed a panel data set covering
eighty-eight countries with annual information on the age structure of the
population, GDP, saving, and investment over the period 1960–99. The
sample accounts for about 95 percent of world GDP in the 1990s and about
85 percent of the world's population. The information on saving, an extension of data put together by the World Bank, is at the national level with no
division between the public and private sector.[19] We focus on the national
saving rate for three reasons: public saving and private saving are partial substitutes; inflation distorts the measurement of public versus private saving
because nominal interest rates include an element of principle repayment;
and many countries do not produce separate estimates of public and private
saving.[20]

The empirical model that we estimate is that of Higgins, which has many
antecedents in the demography literature. Rates of saving (S/Y) and rates of
investment (I/Y) are both related to real income growth and the age distribution of the population:

$$S/Y = a_0 + b_1 \, DGDP + \Sigma \, c_i \, POP_i \text{ and}$$

$$I/Y = a_1 + b_2 \, DGDP + \Sigma \, d_i \, POP_i,$$

18. Poterba (1994); Deaton and Paxson (1997).
19. Available at www.worldbank.org/research/projects/savings/data.htm [3/21/03].
20. The data on saving should be better than that available to Higgins (1998), and we are able
to extend the analysis through the 1990s.

where *DGDP* is the rate of growth of real GDP and POP_i represents the shares of the population in various age brackets.[21] Like Higgins, we used a third-order polynomial in age to capture the demographic effects.[22] We also converted all data to five-year averages. Thus we have a maximum of eight observations per country spanning four decades. With the panel data set, we can examine the patterns of change both over time and across countries.

The Time Dimension

The time-series estimates of the equations are based on a fixed-effects estimation, where the intercepts, although unique for each country, have common slope coefficients. Thus the age profile is assumed to be the same across all countries. Changes in the aggregate saving rates reflect several underlying processes. First, the aging of the population would impart a life-cycle pattern on aggregate saving. Second, there may be systematic differences among birth cohorts. For example, the generations that lived through the Great Depression may be more attuned to saving than younger cohorts. Third, some saving determinants affect all cohorts but may be changing over time. Statistically it is not possible to distinguish among all three effects—age, cohort, and trend—since any one effect can be represented as a linear combination of the other two. We specifically include the age effects and test for cohort and trend effects by including a trend variable.

Figure 7-5 illustrates the results of a model that includes all eighty-eight countries. These results are similar to those of Higgins's. They indicate that demographic structure influences both saving and investment.[23] The derived coefficients of the age distribution seem consistent with expectations. Although the implications for the current account can be approximated by the difference between the estimated effects of saving and investment, one can also directly estimate the effect of demography on the current account. It is noteworthy that the peak of the age profile for investment precedes that for saving, with the result that the current account is in deficit for young

21. While the relationship between saving and the age distribution of the population has an obvious theoretical rationale, it is not so clear for investment. What should matter for investment is the rate of growth in the work force, which is reflected in the growth of GDP. We have some concern that the correlation with investment may actually be operating through the effects of demography on saving in a world of limited capital mobility.

22. This was used initially by Fair and Dominguez (1991).

23. An *F* statistic for the combined contribution of the three coefficients of the polynomial implies significance at the 0.01 level.

Figure 7-5. *Time-Dimension Regression, Country Fixed Effects, Eighty-Eight Countries, Five-Year Averages*[a]

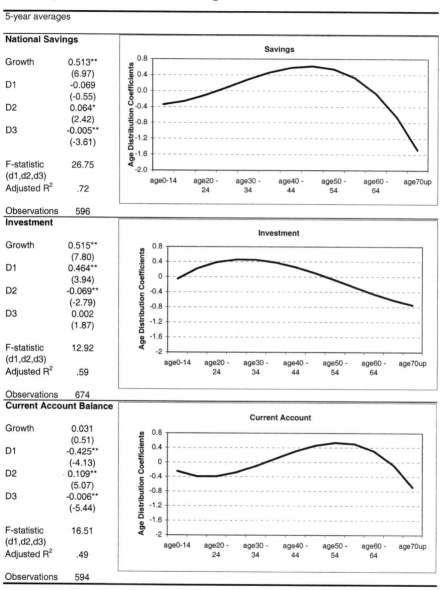

5-year averages

National Savings

Growth	0.513**
	(6.97)
D1	-0.069
	(-0.55)
D2	0.064*
	(2.42)
D3	-0.005**
	(-3.61)
F-statistic (d1,d2,d3)	26.75
Adjusted R^2	.72
Observations	596

Investment

Growth	0.515**
	(7.80)
D1	0.464**
	(3.94)
D2	-0.069**
	(-2.79)
D3	0.002
	(1.87)
F-statistic (d1,d2,d3)	12.92
Adjusted R^2	.59
Observations	674

Current Account Balance

Growth	0.031
	(0.51)
D1	-0.425**
	(-4.13)
D2	0.109**
	(5.07)
D3	-0.006**
	(-5.44)
F-statistic (d1,d2,d3)	16.51
Adjusted R^2	.49
Observations	594

a. Growth measured as annual real growth in GDP; t statistics in parentheses.

* 5% significance; ** 1% significance.

populations before turning positive at later ages. The coefficient on the trend term is statistically insignificant and is deleted from the final results.[24]

The economic significance of the demographic effects can be illustrated by using the coefficients to project rates of saving in the three income regions. Figure 7-6 illustrates the results of this exercise, using coefficients from table 7-4. The specific saving and investment rates are not particularly meaningful, as they are simply calibrated to the arithmetic averages of the sample. It is the *changes* in saving and investment that are most revealing. First, although demographics contributed very little to changes in saving and investment in the 1950–2000 period in the high-income economies, they are projected to lead to very large declines in the future. Rates of saving are projected to decline by 15–20 percent of GDP by 2050. The fall in investment is comparable. The current account balance is projected first to move into a small surplus and then to decline.

Second, saving and investment rates also move together in the middle-income countries, but saving rises far more than investment. As a result, the current account moves into substantial surplus. Rates of saving are also projected to rise in the low-income regions. Thus net trade balances shift substantially among the three regions. Increased surpluses in the middle- and low-income countries offset the shift toward current account deficits in the high-income economies. Overall these empirical results are supportive of the expanded cross-border capital flows outlined in the model of the Attanasio-Violante study.

How would these results be altered by an accelerated rate of improvement in longevity? We can calculate the effects of the increased longevity indicated by the Aaron and Harris projections of table 7-4 for 2050 using the same age coefficients used to construct figure 7-6. The implied saving, investment, and current account balances for 2050 are shown for the three income groups in table 7-5. An increase in the proportion of the population that is elderly implies even larger declines in saving and investment than previously indicated. Under Aaron-Harris projection 2, which has the largest changes in demographic structure, the national saving rate would be lowered by an additional 11 percentage points for the high-income countries to a negative 8 percent of national income.[25] For the middle-income and low-income groups, the drops would be smaller—4 percentage points and 2 percentage

24. The inclusion of income growth in the current period raises some concerns about possible estimation biases arising from the use of endogenous variables as regressors. However, the use of instrumental variable estimation, such as lagged income change or the simple exclusion of the income term, has no discernible effect on the age profile, which is the focus of our interest.

25. Again, the emphasis should be on the changes, as the levels are only approximations.

Figure 7-6. *National Saving, Current Account, and Investment,*
by Development Level, 1950–2050

National saving rate

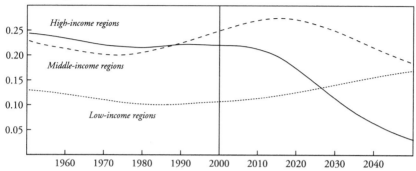

Current account balance

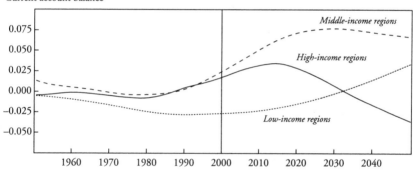

Investment rate

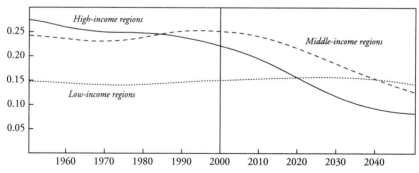

Table 7-5. *National Saving, Investment, and Current Account Balance, by Development Level, Four Projections*[a]

Percent

Region or country	Saving rate				Investment rate				Current account balance			
	UN 2000	UN 2050	A-H 1 2050	A-H 2 2050	UN 2000	UN 2050	A-H 1 2050	A-H 2 2050	UN 2000	UN 2050	A-H 1 2050	A-H 2 2050
Time dimension results												
High-income regions	22	3	-2	-8	22	8	6	2	0	-5	-8	-11
Middle-income regions	25	18	16	14	25	13	12	10	0	6	5	4
Low-income regions	10	17	16	16	15	14	14	13	-5	3	3	2
United States	18	5	1	-5	21	12	9	7	-3	-7	-9	-11
Japan	30	-1	-11	-21	28	10	5	0	2	-11	-16	-21
China	39	20	17	13	37	18	16	14	2	2	1	-1
Cross-national dimension results												
High-income regions	22	9	6	3	22	20	20	21	0	-11	-14	-18
Middle-income regions	25	20	19	17	25	23	23	23	0	-3	-5	-6
Low-income regions	10	16	16	15	15	19	19	19	-5	-3	-3	-3
United States	18	9	7	4	21	20	20	20	-3	-10	-13	-16
Japan	30	10	3	-3	28	26	26	26	2	-17	-23	-30
China	39	25	23	21	37	33	33	33	2	-8	-10	-12

Source: United Nations (2001), tables 5 and 7.

a. Projections are calibrated to rates of saving and investment of the late 1990s. The high-income countries are calibrated by an average of the OECD nations. The middle-income countries are calibrated by an average of the Latin American and East Asian countries in the sample. The low-income countries are calibrated by an average of the African nations in the sample. A-H 1 is the adjustment for Aaron-Harris relative to the UN projections; A-H 2 is the adjustment for Aaron-Harris relative to the SSA projections.

points, respectively. The declines in investment would be only half as large as those for saving. The results are even more striking for individual countries. The U.S. national saving rate would fall by about 9 percentage points, and that of Japan would become highly negative.

These results imply an impossibility—that the current account would deteriorate in all three regions. Because world trade flows must balance, some additional adjustments are inescapable. Our model does not provide a framework for predicting the form of those adjustments—sharply increased saving by the young in anticipation of longer retirement, a change in pension policy to restrict consumption by the elderly, a sharp increase in interest rates to curtail investment and encourage saving, or delays in retirement, for example.

The Cross-National Dimension

The population characteristics of countries differ more at a point in time than over time. In particular, the prospective variation among countries in the age structure of the population is larger than the change that was observed from 1960 to 2000. To reduce the influence of short-run fluctuations, we created ten-year averages of the data. Thus we can look at changes in the relationships across decades as well as across the sample of eighty-eight countries. The regression results, based on all of the countries and four decades of data, are shown in figure 7-7.

We augmented the original model by adding per capita income to the list of explanatory variables. Because countries with high income tend to have relatively old populations, it is important to include per capita income to avoid attributing the higher saving rates found in rich countries to demographic characteristics.[26] Once again, a significant effect of demographic change on national rates of saving is indicated, but the results are more damped than those based on the time series.[27] Not surprisingly, life expectancy is highly significant in the saving equation. This result suggests that rates of saving are systematically higher in societies with high life expectancy. In contrast to the time-series results, however, demography does not seem to affect investment. The positive association between life expectancy and investment is also puzzling. Overall, the cross-national analysis suggests that aging has a larger neg-

26. Income is GDP per capita, and it is measured in common international prices using the 1985 benchmark of the Penn World Table. We also included income-squared to allow a nonlinear relationship between income and saving.

27. The demographic variables are jointly significant at the 0.01 level for saving and the 0.05 level for investment.

Figure 7-7. *Cross-Country Regressions, Eighty-Eight Countries, Ten-Year Averages*[a]

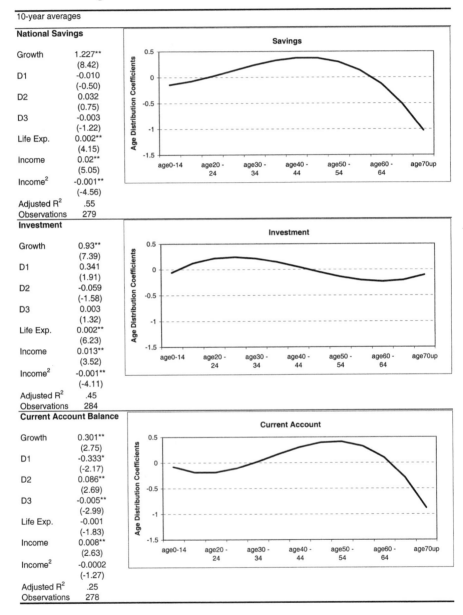

*5% significance; **1% significance.

a. Growth measured as annual real growth in GDP. Income is measured as GDP per capita. *T* statistics in parentheses.

ative impact on national saving than on investment, pushing aging societies toward substantial trade deficits.

The cross-national analysis implies considerably smaller changes in saving rates in response both to normal aging embodied in the UN projections and to increased longevity (table 7-5). Under the UN demographic projections, the rate of saving in 2050 for the high-income countries is 6 percentage points higher than it is in the time-series analysis. In general, the estimates of the decline in saving between 2000 and 2050 are one-third to one-half smaller under the cross-section analysis than under the time-series analysis. The projected fall in the rate of investment is also much attenuated. The revisions to the outlook for the middle- and low-income countries are smaller. Cross-section regressions indicate that the rate of saving in the middle-income countries would fall 5 percentage points between 2000 and 2050 and that the investment share would barely change. The resulting implications for the current account suggest reduced opportunities for net capital flows among regions. If demographic changes have little effect on investment but reduce saving, the current account balance would tend to deteriorate everywhere, an anomalous result that suggests heightened global competition for capital.

Similarly, the changes in rates of saving and investment resulting from improvements in longevity are smaller under cross-section than under time-series analysis. The cross-section regressions indicate that reductions in national saving are only about two-thirds as large as under the time-series analysis, and there is no reduction in investment. On the other hand, the implied changes in current account balances are larger than those of the time series. Hence accelerated aging would push the global economy toward greater capital shortage as lower rates of saving in the rich countries are not offset by equivalent reductions in investment or increases in saving in the rest of the world.

Caveats

For several reasons one should view these strong apparent demographic influences on both saving and investment with caution. First (and most important), when one disaggregates the regional data into subregional groups the coefficients change considerably. Most of the support for a relationship between demographic change and saving is found in the regressions for the developing countries, particularly those of East Asia and Latin America. The coefficients for both the aged dependency and child dependency rates are statistically insignificant for the high-income OECD countries. Yet the greatest degree of projected change in life expectancy is in the OECD countries.

Thus we do not have any direct evidence of strong demographic effects for the countries that matter the most.

Second, saving and investment may not be sufficiently independent at the national level to support estimates of independent relationships from the time-series data. While global trade has been expanding faster than global GDP, the transfer of goods and services across national borders still faces considerable frictions. Thus saving and investment are forced to move together. As a result, the forces that affect saving are likely to exercise similar effects directly on investment to a greater extent than would occur if goods moved without significant obstruction from national borders.[28]

Third, although we are particularly interested in the influence on saving and investment of changes in longevity, we found no statistically significant effects over the 1960–2000 period in the time-series analysis. Thus we could not differentiate between changes in the aged-dependency rate caused by reduced birth rates and those caused by greater longevity. Longevity was highly significant in the cross-national regressions, however.

Conclusion

Whether or not a medical revolution based on molecular biology occurs, the world economy is going to have to adjust to a dramatic increase in longevity and an aging population. Quite apart from any research breakthrough, the high-income countries will face a major challenge to provide for the consumption needs of the elderly. Large declines in rates of national saving and investment are likely, as is the need to borrow from or sell off assets to the rest of the world. The portents of demographic change for the developing world are more favorable, where dramatically reduced child dependency will more than offset increases in the number of the aged. While aging populations will tend to lower saving and investment everywhere, the changes will be much smaller in middle- and low-income countries.

We believe that increased longevity will pose formidable challenges only to the high-income countries. Even for them, these challenges are an intensification of trends with which they must cope in any case. Even if longevity rises only gradually, current practices with respect to retirement will become increasingly costly and difficult to sustain. The consumption costs of an aging

---

28. The high correlation between saving and domestic investment was noted by Feldstein and Horioka (1980), using data for the 1960s and 1970s; and although the correlation has declined over time, it remains very evident in the international data. For a contrasting argument, see Taylor (1994).

population will depress saving rates well below investment requirements by midcentury. The direct effects of increasing longevity would be relatively small in regions with relatively young populations and few elderly members.

Our simulations emphasize the importance of either increasing saving in anticipation of longer retirement or inducing people to delay retirement. Increased saving would offer substantial benefits in a world beset by capital shortage. Large variations in national saving are apparent but seem to depend to a large extent on cultural differences.[29] Research has not identified policies that reliably can increase saving. The history of U.S. policy may be read as a cautionary tale of failed efforts to promote saving through tax incentives. As a result, most of the discussion of responses to population aging has focused on efforts to encourage later retirement.

This chapter measures aging and the pressures of retirement in terms of the aged-dependency rate, or the ratio of the population over a normal retirement age of sixty-five to the working-age population. In fact, retirement ages differ widely. The participation rate among males at ages fifty-five to sixty-four in the OECD countries averages 62 percent but varies from about 45 percent in Finland, France, and the Netherlands to 84 percent in Japan and 74 percent in Sweden (column 1 of table 7-6).

Early retirement has been associated with high income and long life expectancy.[30] The tendency of high-income countries to adopt public income support and retirement programs that reduce the rewards of continued work by older workers contributes to this pattern. Several studies find a strong correlation between retirement ages and such national retirement policies as the standard retirement age, replacement rate, and incentives for delayed retirement under public pension systems, the duration and size of unemployment insurance benefits, and labor market conditions.[31] The results of one such study are summarized in columns 3 and 4 of table 7-6. This research suggests that nations could induce workers to delay retirement by appropriate changes in their pensions systems. But only part of the variation shown in table 7-6 can be explained by differences in those identifiable factors. Just as with saving, cultural or national practices seem to play a large role. For reasons that go beyond simple political barriers to change, it is likely to prove difficult to achieve major increases in retirement ages through the altering of public programs.

29. Poterba (1994) and the citations therein.
30. For a study that incorporates large differences in economic development see Clark, York, and Anker (1999).
31. Gruber and Wise (1997); Blöndal and Scarpetta (1999).

Table 7-6. *Labor Force Participation, Male Workers Ages Fifty-Five through Sixty-Four, OECD Countries, 1985–95*

Country	Participation rate	Difference from mean	Portion explained	Portion unexplained
Australia	60.9	–1.1	1.8	–2.9
Canada	64.4	2.4	1.6	0.8
Finland	46.5	–15.5	–3.5	–12.0
France	45.7	–16.3	–3.2	–13.1
West Germany	58.6	–3.4	1.6	–5.0
Ireland	67.7	5.7	0.3	5.4
Italy	50.7	–11.3	–7.3	–4.0
Japan	83.7	21.7	2.9	18.8
Netherlands	44.5	–17.5	–0.7	–16.8
Norway	74.3	12.3	8.7	3.6
Portugal	64.4	2.3	–1.8	4.1
Spain	61.5	–0.5	–9.4	8.9
Sweden	73.7	11.7	0.7	11.0
United Kingdom	66.6	4.6	4.9	–0.3
United States	67.0	5.0	5.1	–0.1
Average[a]	62.0			

Source: Blöndal and Scarpetta (1999).

In our analysis of the demographic trends incorporated in the UN projections, we find some reasons for optimism. The aging of the high-income countries would be complemented by increases in the working age populations in the poorer developing portions of the world. A growing need to expand saving in the rich countries in anticipation of retirement could be accommodated by a growing work force and a need for added capital in a younger developing world. On the other hand, a major increase in life expectancy, occasioned by a biomedical breakthrough, would increase the economic burden in all countries. From a global perspective, it is not evident that a major increase in life expectancy of the very old should be applauded.

COMMENT
Martin Baily

The question this volume addresses is, What would happen if the increase in life expectancy occurs at a faster rate than is currently the case? Such an improvement in life expectancy would result in a rapid increase in the number of retirees, assuming the retirement age stayed the same. But unlike the baby-boomer issue, the effect of increased life expectancy would not be temporary; there would be more retirees indefinitely.

I was a discussant of the paper by David Cutler and others at the Brookings Papers meeting in 1990 and found the results counterintuitive. Two demographic issues were discussed in the paper. The first was the impact of the baby-boom generation, which is a bulge passing through the demographic snake and causing a temporary surge in the number of retirees as boomers age. The paper concludes that the prospect of the baby-boom retirement bulge does not justify a higher saving rate today. The mathematical model was surely correct, but it is hard to ignore the intuition of the Bible story in which there are seven fat years and seven lean years, making it optimal to save during the fat years and use the savings to increase consumption in the lean years. Mathematically, the reason for the results of Cutler and others is that, as the baby-boom generation passes into retirement, the growth of the labor force declines. If there has been extra saving and capital accumulation, the marginal product of capital will be driven down. The intuition of saving more for the boomers' retirements is correct in a sense but is offset in an optimal growth model by the disincentive to save created by the decline in the return to capital.

As a discussant I challenged the authors to look at the possibility of saving and buying foreign assets, which could avoid the problem of the decline in the rate of return to capital. They responded to that in the final version of the paper, making a point also stressed in the chapter by Barry Bosworth and Benjamin Keys. Other OECD countries besides the United States have a worse demographic problem than we do, so in fact global equilibrium would be reached with Europe investing in the United States. This is of course what has happened, although the explanations of the capital flows are not usually given in demographic terms. The United States has run a large current account deficit and increased its net foreign indebtedness, while Europe has increased its holdings of U.S. assets. This means of course that as the United States services that indebtedness, it will help Europe's demographic problem at the expense of slightly worsening its own.

Two other objections to the model by Cutler and others are noted by Bosworth and Keys. First, the model assumes that the United States is currently choosing an optimal saving rate. If the country is not saving enough now, then it should increase its saving rate. Second, the model does not examine the trade-off between consumption and leisure.

It seems intuitive that if life expectancy increases the optimal amount of work would also increase. This could take the form of an increase in working life or an increase in hours worked per year; it would depend on people's wishes (utility functions). In many optimal growth models, individuals choose to spread their consumption out evenly over time. If people can expect to live a hundred years rather than seventy-five, it is likely that they will choose to accept some reduction of consumption per year and some increase in work life or work intensity, rather than making all the adjustment in the form of lower consumption per year. This would be a partial result, holding everything else constant. There may be changes in the other direction; for example, if leisure is a superior good, then people will choose longer retirements or fewer work hours as the economy becomes richer.

A more complex model would incorporate the effect of declining health with age. There is an obvious reason why education and work are concentrated in the early years of adult life, since that is when most of us are most productive. Other authors in this volume point to the possibility that an increase in life expectancy could involve just an extension of the period of dying. In this case, people's ability to work falls off just as quickly with longer life as it does with current life expectancies. According to Larry Katz, speaking at the Brookings panel meeting in the spring of 2002, the evidence suggests that this is not the case. People are remaining healthier at least through age sixty. This reinforces my view that, other things equal, the optimal response to increased life expectancy is for people to work more.

Another complication is that the decision to continue to participate in the labor force is often a family decision, not an individual decision. In the United States, male labor force participation has declined and early retirement has increased, but the overall labor force participation of the population has increased. The actual response of the U.S. labor force to longer life expectancies and other changes has not been to increase the length of work life per worker but instead to increase the intensity of work for families.

A few words about Bosworth and Keys's empirical results. I do not understand the structural model that led to the estimated equation. An equation with the investment rate (or even the saving rate) on the left side and the GDP growth rate on the right side calls to mind regressions in the literature with GDP growth on the left and investment on the right.

A second concern grows out of a study of the impact of demographics on saving that I participated in while at the McKinsey Global Institute. A thorny issue we had to deal with in that study was separating out age effects and cohort effects in their influence on saving rates. If people in a certain age bracket display a high saving rate on average, is this because of their age or because they grew up in the Great Depression and developed a frugal mindset? I am a user of this literature, not a contributor to it, but the experts in the area certainly lectured me about the importance of allowing for both age and cohort effects, and I wonder whether this issue has been dealt with adequately in the Bosworth and Keys estimates.

I go back now to the extent to which the international financial system, or the global flow of capital, permits a net benefit from shifting resources between countries with different demographic profiles. As Bosworth and Keys point out, developing countries—with large numbers of young people—have different demographic profiles from those of the United States. Bosworth and Keys say that these demographic differences should not have driven capital flows up until now, because the large cohort of young people is only just entering the work force. That is a good point. But even if capital flows would not have been expected, based on demographic differences, neoclassical economics suggests large capital flows should have occurred because of differences in capital endowments. The developing countries have relatively low capital-labor ratios and therefore should, with neoclassical assumptions, have relatively high rates of return to capital. This is Robert Lucas's famous paradox: Why is capital not flowing rapidly to India?

A few years ago I decided to believe the neoclassical model and put some of my retirement funds into an emerging market mutual fund. For every dollar I put into the account, there is now fifty cents. The fund managers may have made bad decisions, but I think most emerging market funds would show similar results. Fortunately it was not a lot of money, but it was enough for me to no longer guide my portfolio choices by academic models. Clearly, the returns to invested funds in emerging markets have not been high in recent years, even though capital-labor ratios are low. Understanding why this is the case is an essential precursor to an analysis of the potential for capital flows driven by demographic differences.

A series of industry case studies of Brazil, Russia, India, and Korea show that these countries' institutional arrangements and policies help explain why many have not achieved better rates of economic development and why the rates of return to capital investment may be lower than those in the United States. Institutional and policy failures account for the Lucas paradox. In India, specifically, laws restricted foreign ownership of Indian assets.

Although these laws are changing, there are still many barriers to the flow of capital and many reasons why the returns are low even on the capital already in place. The Lucas paradox can be understood by the policy and institutional environment and does not need a model with externalities or increasing returns. If these policy problems could be overcome, there is a huge potential for a large welfare gain to both developing countries and the United States. The biggest problems are not in financial markets, which are looking for high returns. Rather they are within the developing countries themselves.

Turning back to high-income countries, the figures in the Bosworth and Keys chapter make it clear that Europe has a different aging pattern from that of the United States. If this country has a baby-boom problem, they have a looming demographic disaster. At the same time, the European Union has a lower level of productivity than that of the United States and a much lower level of labor force participation. According to data from the Conference Board, the EU in 2001 had 67 percent of the GDP per capita of the United States, 87 percent of the GDP per hour of the United States, and 77 percent of the hours worked per capita of the United States. The lower labor input comes partly from shorter hours per employee and partly from fewer employees per capita.

What would happen in Europe if life expectancy were to increase rapidly? Presumably, if such a trend emerged in the United States it would also emerge in Europe, which has a health care system that in some respects is better than that of the United States: less advanced on the leading edge, perhaps, but more comprehensive. A rapid increase in life expectancy could render the European economic paradigm unworkable. That paradigm has been to maintain equality and to subsidize withdrawal from the labor force, while accepting the cost in terms of reduced labor force participation and early retirement.

As Gary Burtless mentions in his chapter of this volume, retirement age is partly dependent on incentives to retire. Europe provides strong incentives for early retirement, forces retirement in some cases, and provides free health insurance (the United States does have Medicare, but that is not provided until age sixty-five and is not complete coverage). Further, labor income is taxed heavily in some European countries. There is some question whether Europe can afford its retirement provisions even under current life expectancies. If these turn out to be sharply understated, the financial burden on the working population would become even higher and would test the limits of European willingness to pay taxes.

That does not mean Europe has to follow the example of the United States, which is pretty stingy in its provision for the elderly and the poor. There may be alternative ways of encouraging more labor force participation and longer working lives. Sweden has had some success in using active labor market policies, including being tough on those who choose not to work.

A final point on the United States: There is a question of whether Social Security and Medicare benefits will be cut as the baby boomers retire. That is always possible, but one factor going against it is that the propensity to vote rises with age (up to a certain point). There will be a significant increase in the number of people in retirement or near retirement, and there will be an even greater increase in the number of voters in that age bracket. Politicians proposing cuts in programs for the elderly might have a hard time at the polls.

References

Attanasio, Orazio P., and Giovanni L. Violante. 2000. "The Demographic Transition in Closed and Open Economy: A Tale of Two Regions." Working Paper 412. Inter-American Development Bank.

Blöndal, Sveinbjörn, and Stefano Scarpetta. 1998. "The Retirement Decision in OECD Countries." Working Paper 202. Paris: Organization for Economic Cooperation and Development.

Bloom, David E., David Canning, and Pia N. Malaney. 1999. "Demographic Change and Economic Growth in Asia." Working Paper 15. CID, Harvard University.

Bloom, David E., and Jeffrey G. Williamson. 1998. "Demographic Transitions and Economic Miracles in Emerging Asia." *World Bank Economic Review* 12: 419–55.

Bryant, Ralph, and Delia Velculescu. 2002. "Population Aging and Public Pension Systems: A First Look at the Cross-Border and Global Effects." Brookings Institution. Paper prepared for International Forum of the Collaboration Projects, Economic and Social Research Institute, Government of Japan, February, 2002.

Clark, Robert, Elizabeth Anne York, and Richard Anker. 1999. "Economic Development and Labor Force Participation of Older Persons." *Population Research and Policy Review* 18 (5): 411–33.

Coale, Ashley J., and Edgar H. Hoover. 1958. *Population Growth and Economic Development in Low-Income Countries.* Princeton University Press.

Cutler, David, James Poterba, Louise Sheiner, and Lawrence Summers. 1990. "An Aging Society: Opportunity or Challenge?" *BPEA, 1:* 1–73.

Deaton, Angus, and Christina Paxson. 1997. "The Effects of Economic and Population Growth on National Saving and Income Inequality." *Demography* 34 (1): 97–114.

Ehrlich, Isaac, and Francis T. Lui. 1991. "Intergenerational Trade, Longevity, and Economic Growth." *Journal of Political Economy* 99 (5): 1029–59.

Elmendorf, Douglas W. and Louise M. Sheiner. 2000. "Should America Save for Its Old Age? Fiscal Policy, Population Aging, and National Saving." *Journal of Economic Perspectives* 14 (3): 57–74.

Fair, Ray C., and Kathryn M. Dominguez. 1991. "Effects of Changing U.S. Age Distribution on Macroeconomic Equations." *American Economic Review* 81 (5): 1276–94.

Feldstein, Martin, and Charles Horioka. 1980. "Domestic Saving and International Capital Flows." *Economic Journal* 90 (358): 313–29.

Fry, Maxwell, and Andrew Mason. 1982. "The Variable Rate-of-Growth Effect in the Life-Cycle Saving Model: Children, Capital Inflows, Interest, and Growth in a New Specification of the Life-Cycle Model Applied to Seven Asian Developing Countries." *Economic Inquiry* 20: 426–42.

Gruber, Jonathan, and David Wise, eds. 1997. *Social Security Programs and Retirement around the World.* University of Chicago Press.

Higgins, Matthew. 1998. "Demography, National Savings, and International Capital Flows." *International Economic Review* 39 (2): 343–69.

Higgins, Matthew, and Jeffrey G. Williamson. 1997 "Age Structure Dynamics in Asia and Dependence of Foreign Capital." *Population and Development Review* 23: 261–93.

Holzmann, Robert. 2000. "Can Investments in Emerging Markets Help to Solve the Aging Problem?" World Bank. Paper prepared for conference "The Graying of the Industrial

World: Assessing the Economic, Political, and Strategic Implications of the Simultaneous Aging of the Major Industrial Nations," January 2000.

Kalemli-Ozcan, Sebnem, Harl E. Ryder, and David N. Weil. 2000. "Mortality Decline, Human Capital Investment, and Economic Growth." *Journal of Development Economics* 62: 1–23.

Lindh, Thomas, and Bo Malmberg. 1999. "Age Structure Effects and Growth in the OECD, 1950–1990." *Journal of Population Economics* 12 (3): 431–49.

Mason, Andrew. 1988 "Saving, Economic Growth, and Demographic Change." *Population and Development Review* 14 (1): 113–44.

Masson, Paul. 1990. "Long-Term Macroeconomic Effects of Aging Populations." *Finance and Development* 27: 6–9.

OECD (Organization for Economic Cooperation and Development). 1996. *Future Global Capital Shortages: Real Threat or Pure Fiction?* Paris.

Poterba, James. 1994. *International Comparisons of Household Saving.* University of Chicago Press.

Rodrik, Dani. 1998. "Who Needs Capital Account Convertibility?" In *Should the IMF Pursue Capital Account Convertibility?* edited by Stanley Fischer and others. Essays in International Finance 207. Princeton University Press.

Taylor, Alan M. 1994. "Domestic Saving and International Capital Flows Reconsidered." Working Paper 4892. Cambridge: National Bureau of Economic Research.

United Nations. 2001. *World Population Prospects, 2000.* New York: United Nations.

Contributors

HENRY J. AARON
Brookings Institution

MARTIN BAILY
Institute for International
  Economics

MARGARET P. BATTIN
University of Utah

BARRY P. BOSWORTH
Brookings Institution

GARY BURTLESS
Brookings Institution

ALEXANDER M. CAPRON
World Health Organization and
  University of Southern
  California

DORA L. COSTA
Massachusetts Institute of
  Technology

WILLIAM G. GALE
Brookings Institution

ALAN M. GARBER
Stanford University and Veterans
  Affairs Palo Alto Health Care
  System

DANA P. GOLDMAN
RAND Corporation

STEPHEN GOSS
Social Security Administration

BENJAMIN H. HARRIS
Brookings Institution

285

BENJAMIN KEYS
Brookings Institution

JOHN T. POTTS
Massachusetts General Hospital

WILLIAM B. SCHWARTZ
University of Southern California

JOHN B. SHOVEN
Stanford University

NICHOLAS WADE
New York Times

Index

targeted, 32. *See also* Antibiotics; Treatment methods

Pharmaceuticals—specific: Gleevec, 32, 57; herceptin, 117; statins, 38, 109, 110, 118; transretinoic acid, 32

Pima Indians. *See* Native Americans

Population issues: age distribution, 78–79, 80–82, 251, 271; demographic transitions, 247; longevity and, 251; models and methods for modeling, 91–92; population projections and implications, 99–102, 253. *See also* Baby boom generation; Global issues

Prevention, 118–20

Prihoda, Ronald, 220, 222

Proteins: in Alzheimer's disease, 47–48; amino acids and, 18; appetite and, 44; C-reactive proteins, 37; definition of, 19; genes and, 18, 33; immunotherapy and, 34; pathologic proteins, 3, 47; RNA and, 23; role of, 18, 24–25, 33; signaling, 33; thermogenesis, 44–45; in treatment, 24

Proteomics, 24

RAND Health Insurance Experiment, 114

Rawls, John, 205, 224

Regenerative medicine, 25–26, 53–54. *See also* Stem cells

Reproduction. *See* Fertility, fecundity, and reproduction

Research: biomedical research, 105–06, 210; clinical trials, 34–35, 48; genetic engineering, 34; longevity and evolution, 49–51, 52–58; projecting progress in, 28; treatment trials, 122

Retirement issues: age of, 275, 280; baby boomers, 277; costs, 13; delay of, 126, 131; economic issues, 275; educational factors, 163; family factors, 163–64; international issues, 153–59; life expectancy, mortality,

and longevity, 6–7, 68, 127, 128, 249, 261, 277; savings and, 275, 276; Social Security and, 196; theoretical issues, 132–35; United States, 143–53, 160–61; wages, income, and consumption, 137–41. *See also* Labor and labor market issues; Pensions and pension plans

Ribonucleic acid (RNA), 19, 23, 41–42

Ribosomes. *See* Cells

Risk analysis, 21–22

RNA. *See* Ribonucleic acid

Ruvkun, Gary, 56

Sardinia, 50

SARS. *See* Severe acute respiratory syndrome

Schwartz, William, 219

Science, 13–14

Seneca, 237

Senile dementia, 5. *See also* Neurodegenerative diseases

Severe acute respiratory syndrome (SARS), 16–17

Sheiner, Louise, 261, 262

Single-nucleotide polymorphisms (SNPs), 19, 21

Social Security: age of receiving benefits, 8, 162, 167, 168, 173–74; beneficiaries, 166; benefits, 151, 162, 163, 168–69, 172, 173–74, 281; costs and expenses, 8, 9, 170–74, 188; Medicare and, 176; mortality and longevity, 169–71, 173–74, 188, 194, 195–96, 223–24; normal retirement age (NRA), 150, 151, 152, 168b; Old-Age, Survivors, and Disability and Hospital Insurance (OASDHI), 89, 168, 169, 170–71, 173, 175; outlays and population aging, 142, 167, 223–24; primary insurance amount (PMI), 168b, 169, 173–74, 188; problems of, 167, 169, 171–74, 194, 223–24; reforms, 160–61; retirement issues,